Practical Management of the Elderly

SIR FERGUSON ANDERSON

OBE KStJ MD FRCP(Glas, Edin, Lond)
HonFRCP(Ireland, Canada) FACP
Emeritus David Cargill Professor of Geriatric Medicine
University of Glasgow

BRIAN WILLIAMS

MD FRCP(Glas)
Consultant Physician in Geriatric Medicine
Gartnavel General Hospital, Glasgow
Honorary Clinical Lecturer in Geriatric Medicine
University of Glasgow

FIFTH EDITION

BLACKWELL SCIENTIFIC PUBLICATIONS

OXFORD   LONDON   EDINBURGH

BOSTON   PALO ALTO   MELBOURNE

© 1967, 1971, 1976, 1983, 1989 by
Blackwell Scientific Publications
Editorial offices:
Osney Mead, Oxford OX2 OEL
  (*Orders*: Tel. 0865 240201)
8 John Street, London WC1N 2ES
23 Ainslie Place, Edinburgh EH3 6AJ
3 Cambridge Center, Suite 208
  Cambridge, Massachusetts 02142, USA
667 Lytton Avenue, Palo Alto
  California 94301, USA
107 Barry Street, Carlton
  Victoria 3053, Australia

First published 1967
Second Edition 1971
Third edition 1976
Japanese edition 1976
Fourth edition 1983
Fifth edition 1989

Set by Times Graphics, Singapore
Printed and bound in
Great Britain by
Billings & Sons Ltd, Worcester

DISTRIBUTORS
USA
  Year Book Medical Publishers
  200 North LaSalle Street,
  Chicago, Illinois 60601
  (*Orders*: Tel. 312 726-9733)

Canada
  The C.V. Mosby Company
  5240 Finch Avenue East
  Scarborough, Ontario
  (*Orders*: Tel. 416-298-1588)

Australia
  Blackwell Scientific Publications
  (Australia) Pty Ltd
  107 Barry Street
  Carlton, Victoria 3053
  (*Orders*: Tel. (03) 347 0300)

British Library
Cataloguing in Publication Data

Anderson, *Sir* Ferguson, *1914*–
  Practical management of the elderly.—
  5th ed.
  1. Old persons. Diseases
  I. Title II. Williams, B.O. (Brian
    Owen), *1947*–

618.97

ISBN 0-632-01941-7

Contents

Preface

This book is intended as a guide to the doctor, nurse, social worker, caring staff and students interested in their elderly patients. No attempt has been made to discuss in detail the symptoms and signs of disease; the main concern has been practical management.

The methodology of geriatric medicine is described with reference to the preventive as well as the curative aspects. The purpose behind this book is the hope that the interest of those caring for the elderly may be stimulated to face the difficulties which confront the older person.

Dr Brian Williams is a co-author of this text and I wish to thank him for all his help, initiative and drive. To Mrs Martha Williams both authors owe heartfelt gratitude for her most useful advice and for reading the script with meticulous care. The splendid guidance of Dr W. M. Doig and Dr R. S. Chapman is gratefully acknowledged.

1
Old Age

Elderly citizens play an important part in modern society, and it is our duty to try and keep such people fit. There is now an old person in every third house in any town, and it must be the prime aim of a physician to endeavour to keep older people healthy and happy in their own homes.

The outstanding thesis of modern geriatric medicine is that old people who are ill are unwell not because they are old but because there is some disease process present. Ageing itself is a very slow and symptomless affair, not clearly understood, and certainly varying from person to person. There is probably an increasing introspection with age and a greater awareness of the physical body and fear of the unknown future. It is worth recording that ageing is not a steady decline but there seems no doubt that it occurs, as it were, in steps, and the tread of the step is not level so that the old people may enjoy quite suddenly a phase of much better health than they have had in previous years.

It is essential to realize that 'normal' attributes change with age, so that iatrogenic disease is not produced by trying to modify an age-adjusted attribute to that of a young person. Doctor-induced illness of another variety is seen in the elderly who tend to believe implicitly and remember what they were told when young. No one really ever recovers from a dropped stomach or a displaced womb or a damaged heart valve. There is something almost macabre about the nonagenarian who has never really been well since some doctor told her about her distended and misplaced bowels.

An attempt has been made in this book to give advice to those who care for elderly people. It will be abundantly apparent that knowledge of this subject is still insufficient, and when in doubt it is wise to be guided by common sense. If some new theory or new drug seems to stretch to the utmost previous beliefs and opinions it should be regarded with extreme caution.

In the United Kingdom there are now two and one-half times as many people aged 85 and over as there were 30 years ago. The size of this group will continue to increase throughout the rest of the century. Those aged 85 and over spend an average of 12 days a year in hospital compared with just 1 day a year for nearly all those under 55. There has been a real and significant fall in mortality even among those aged 85 and over. In the USA the recent percentage falls in mortality in this age group exceeds those in all other age groups over 25.

People with chronic conditions including mental illness live longer now and an increase in the life expectancy of those with dementia has been reported. Thus more rather than fewer resources will be needed to cope with the growing numbers of very elderly people.

No attempt is made here to explain the processes of ageing, which are complex and not clearly understood. It must be accepted, however, that the concept of when a person is old has changed and no individual should be considered in this category until over 80 years of age. Nevertheless, due deference must be paid to the well-recognized fact that chronological age is of little value in the accurate assessment of a person's physical and mental health. It is important to recognize that age does not affect all organs and systems in the same way and that the biological age of various organs is not uniform throughout the body because involution may not start at the same time or progress at the same rate in all tissues. Paget named this differential ageing 'errors in the chronometry of life'. Ageing is, however, associated with decrements in the functional capacity of a number of organs and systems. Gradual reduction in reserve capacity, characteristic of growing old, is based on the progressive loss of functioning cells in specific organs. This is associated with senescent changes at cellular level involving genetic and biochemical mechanisms.

Most of the physiological characteristics important in regulating the internal environment are maintained, even in advanced age.

Studies of body water content distributed mainly in muscle and very little in fat and bone show a systematic fall in lean body mass with advancing age. The intracellular water decreases in the ageing human, and this is a reflection of the reduction of metabolizing cells in the elderly. In older people both systolic and diastolic levels of blood pressure increase; myocardial reserve is diminished and excess demands may induce cardiac failure more readily in the old than in the young. There is an increased peripheral resistance to blood flow. With ageing, renal function gradually deteriorates and as all functions of the kidney decrease at about the same rate it can be concluded that nephrons are lost in their entirety, and although the remaining units are adequate to maintain renal function under resting conditions, reserve capacities are subsequently reduced in the ageing individual. The passage of material generally decreases with age, e.g. the blood flow through organs diminishes as seen in decreased renal plasma flow; diffusing capacity of gases in human lungs is lessened by approximately 8% per decade. Vital capacity diminishes as people grow older; this has been partly explained by diminution in muscle strength, and it is possible that the excessive dyspnoea on exertion in old people is attributable to a reduction in the vital capacity of the lungs, brought about by increased rigidity of the thoracic cage.

Loss of bone tissue from the skeleton in both sexes leads to thinning of the cortex of the long bones and to a diminution of radiographic density in all bones. This process is accelerated at the menopause in females and by the time old age is reached they have lost more bone than men. With increasing age muscle power lessens and there is a significant decrease in the power of the grip of both hands of men and women. From middle age on the ability to change the focal length of the lens of the eye is impaired due to changes in the muscles of accommodation and to a loss of elasticity of the lens.

Around one-half of people 65 years and over have impaired hearing especially to high frequencies. Intellectual performance declines with age and psychometric tests may be affected by physical health.

There is also diminished information coming from impairment of vision, hearing loss and poorer sensory signals from the limbs. In spite of these changes the body adapts well to these losses which occur almost imperceptibly and at rest the individual even in extreme old age feels as well as a much younger person.

Age-related deficit is demonstrated when the individual is stressed. Body temperature, blood pH and blood glucose do not change with age under resting conditions. If the temperature is caused to increase by work or older people are given a sugar or alkaline load, alterations in temperature, sugar and pH are greater in the elderly and more time is required for the return to resting levels.

Incidence of auto-immune phenomena increases with advancing age. It is not clear that primary intrinsic ageing processes occur in cells of the immune system or that immunological failure is part of normal ageing. Sensation of pain, febrile response to inflammatory reaction and response to tissue injury may be decreased in ageing individuals.

All ageing individuals are progressively less likely to survive a given amount of tissue injury.

In summary the ageing individual shows loss of reserve capacity in individual organs and loss of elasticity in many tissues, e.g. skin, bone, arteries and lungs. The mind also reveals an inability to adjust rapidly to changing circumstances: an inelasticity of thought.

Surveys as in the USSR of the 80s and over have confirmed the preponderance of females with seven times as many women aged 100 and over as men. A feature noted in almost every survey is the difference of opinion between the doctors and the old people examined with regard to their state of health. Fewer old people consider themselves unfit and those who live a long time are still active and continue to take part in their housekeeping or work within their capacity (Chebotarev & Sachuk 1964). In the USA studies from a Jewish Old Age Home showed by a rigorous selection process that there is a supremely fit group of the elderly who after testing in the most comprehensive way were shown to be as fit as people much younger (Birren *et al*. 1963).

In a population aged 85 years and over in Finland examined in 1972 to 1978 and again in 1982 it was shown that the percentage of hospital in-patients had increased three-fold and the functional capacity of the subjects had deteriorated in ability to walk and mental function. Dementia or confusion, anaemia, femoral neck fracture and cataract were signifi-cantly increased (Haavisto *et al*. 1985).

Early on in the work of the Rutherglen Centre it was realized that within a population regarded as healthy by usual standards there existed a sub-group who were particularly healthy – the gerontocrats.

The Duke study (Busse 1966), which had as a primary objective the effect of ageing upon the nervous system showed that a sudden decline in intelligence and an alteration in the EEG suggested the onset of a process of deterioration and approaching death. When studied longitudinally the importance of physical health as a factor in depression became increas-ingly evident. Lastly, the longitudinal study provided little support for the disengagement theory. Relatively active elderly subjects were more likely to maintain morale than those who were inactive.

Some 600 people in Ontario aged 70 years and over were surveyed by Schwenger (1971) using public health nurses. Those in rural areas were less healthy but did not worry so much about their health and life expectancy of men past middle age might actually be decreasing in comparison with women where it was increasing regularly. The very old, the women of 80 years and over, were showing signs of forming what has been called a biological and psychological elite.

There does seem to exist in an old age a super class of people who rep-resent normal ageing almost untouched by disease. The complete evalu-ation of their metabolism may help in the understanding of this mysterious process. A fundamental problem in geriatric medicine, includ-ing psychiatry, is to determine how to extract ageing from other factors producing overt manifestations of disturbance.

Laboratory findings

Haemoglobin

The overall average value found in health at Rutherglen was 12.5 g for men and 12.0 g for women: the Sahli content used was calibrated so that

100% = 14 g haemoglobin in 100 cc of blood. Caird (1973) stated that the haemoglobin concentration does not change significantly with age. According to the World Health Organization (1972) the haemoglobin levels below which anaemia may be considered to be present are 13 g/dl for adult males and 12 g/dl for adult non-pregnant females and these criteria should be adopted for old people. The standard haematological indices (PCV, MCHC, MCV) are unaffected by age and so are the appearances of the blood film.

Erythrocyte sedimentation rate

Mean values rise steadily with age in healthy people and are higher in women than in men, and no convincing cause may be found in old people for values as high as 35–40 mm/h (Milne & Williamson 1972). The isolated finding of a raised ESR is an indication for repeating the test after a few weeks and only a persistent rise should be regarded as an indication for further investigation. However Griffiths *et al.* (1984) suggest that an ESR exceeding 19 mm in the first hour in elderly men and 22 mm in the first hour in elderly women warrants investigation. Among the conditions to be considered Exton-Smith & Overstall (1979) raised the possibility of polymyalgia rheumatica, giant-cell arteritis or myeloma. According to Kenny *et al.* (1985) serum C-reactive protein concentration is superior to the ESR as an objective, non-specific marker for disease activity in the elderly.

Biochemical tests

Caird (1973) found the mean values and range for serum sodium, potassium, chloride, bicarbonate, magnesium, bilirubin, inorganic phosphate, total protein, albumin and globulin were identical in older and younger people. For a second group of measurements the range of normal values is not the same in the elderly as in the young. Blood urea in people over 65 has a normal upper limit of about 60 mg/100 ml (10 mmol/l) and random blood glucose, 3.4–9.3 mmol/l. An upper limit of normal for serum creatinine is 1.9 mg/100 ml (169 μmol/l). Levels below 7.7 mg/100 ml (0.46 mmol/l) are normal for serum uric acid. The serum cholesterol concentration rises with age and after the menopause is higher in women than in men. There are probably considerable variations in normal levels in old age associated with nutritional differences but in urban Scotland over 40% of women and 8% of men over the age of 65 have a serum cholesterol level of over 300 mg/100 ml (7.8 mmol/l). These high values are not associated with coronary artery disease or with hypothyroidism. There is no evidence that lowering the serum cholesterol is of benefit to an elderly person. Range for serum calcium is for men 8.5–10.5 mg/100 ml (2.1–2.6 mmol/l) and for women 8.7–10.7 mg/100 ml (2.17–2.67 mmol/l). A serum alkaline phosphatase over 20 K–A units/100 ml is abnormal and an indication for a search for liver or bone disease, and a value of 15–20 K–A units is of uncertain significance. Normal values for the serum acid phosphatase are probably the same in the elderly as in middle age, and this also applies to the other commonly estimated serum enzymes such as aspartate transaminase, alanine transaminase or lactic dehydrogenase.

Information about the attributes of older people is gradually increasing and may in time lead to fundamental discoveries in other fields of medicine. People can be very fit in advanced old age and this knowledge is of vital importance in the health education and orientation of the doctor and the general public.

REFERENCES

Birren J.E., Butler R.N., Greenhouse S.W., Sokoloff L. & Garrow M.R. (1963) *Human Ageing*. US Department of Health, Education and Welfare, Public Health Services, Publication No. 986.

Busse E.W. (1966) The effect of ageing upon the central nervous system. Abstracts of papers presented at the *7th International Congress of Gerontology*. Vienna. p. 40.

Caird F.I. (1973) Problems of interpretation of laboratory findings in the old. *British Medical Journal* **4**, 348.

Chebotarev D.F. & Sachuk N.N. (1964) Sociomedical examination of longevous people in the USSR. *American Journal of Gerontology* **19**, 435.

Exton-Smith A.N. & Overstall P.W. (1979) *Geriatrics*. Lancaster, MTP.

Griffiths R.A., Good W.R., Watson N.P., O'Donnell H.F., Fell P.J. & Shakespeare J.M. (1984) Normal erythrocyte sedimentation rate in the elderly. *British Medical Journal* **289**, 724.

Haavisto M.V., Heikinheimo R.J., Mattila K.J. & Rajala S.A. (1985) Living conditions and health of a population aged 85 years or over: a five-year follow-up study. *Age and Ageing* **14**, 202.

Kenny R.A., Saunders A.P., Coll A., Harrington M.G., Caspi D., Hodkinson H.M. & Pepys M.B. (1985) A comparison of the erythrocyte sedimentation rate and serum C-reactive protein concentration in elderly patients. *Age and Ageing* **14**, 15.

Milne J.S. & Williamson J. (1972) Haemoglobin, haematocrit reading, leukocyte count and blood grouping in a random sample of older people. *Geriatrics* **27**, 118.

Schwenger L.W. (1971) Sociomedical care of the aged. *World Medical Journal* **3**, 42.

World Health Organization (1972) *Nutritional Anaemias*. WHO Technical Report Series No. 503. Geneva, WHO.

2
The Preventive Approach

In 1906 Korenchevsky became interested in preventive medicine as it applies to the elderly after a visit to an infirmary for old people in Moscow. He saw there so many pathological changes that he thought people could age in a more physiological way. It has become apparent that if more knowledge about the ageing process (gerontology) was available more active preventive measures might be found to assist in the slowing down at least of the age-related changes. Geriatric medicine (clinical gerontology) is concerned with the ageing individual who has developed pathological diseases in addition to the physiological changes of ageing. This subdivision is said to have been introduced by Galen as physiological or 'normal ageing' and pathological or 'sick ageing'.

Geriatric medicine has been defined as a branch of general medicine dealing with the health and with the clinical, social, preventive and remedial aspects of illness in the elderly. Rhee (1974) states that the relevance of geriatric medicine lies in that geriatric care should be preceded by an assessment of the physical, mental and social factors responsible for disabilities at higher ages, and feels that physicians practising geriatric medicine justify their speciality only if they diagnose correctly the risk situations which lead to or aggravate states of dependency.

An essential element in this work is the necessity for a team approach. The doctor must be aware of the different abilities and functions of the health care team. Nurses, social workers, occupational therapists, physiotherapists and colleagues in many different aspects of medicine have a particular part to play. One of the main objectives of geriatric medicine is the endeavour to maintain health and thus allow older people to remain in their own homes for as long as they are fit and desire to be there. The second is to make the maximal effort when the elderly individual is unwell to restore that person to the best level of fitness and to ensure continued surveillance. The practice of geriatric medicine is intimately concerned with continuity of care.

Health maintenance

Prevention of illness is an important part of the methodology of geriatric medicine and one of the tenets is that the self-reporting of illness is not always a satisfactory method of detecting disease at an early stage and that many older people have remediable complaints and if treated and supervised can be kept in the community. It is thus essential to teach all who work with the elderly in the early detection of disease.

Most people living in a so-called developed country can now anticipate a long life. Mehigan (1978) found that 35% of beds in a 500-bed teaching hospital were occupied by patients suffering from the effects of cigarette smoking and 25% more were used for the treatment of illnesses induced by the abuse of alcohol or drugs, accidents, obesity or faulty dietetic habits: the lifestyle diseases. If the new generation of older people are to enjoy continuing good health then the general public especially the young people must receive education in health maintenance; health education must be regarded as the best method of primary prevention.

Better health in old age is achieved by treating correctly conditions like hypertension in middle age. It is now recognized that smoking is a factor in the causation not only of lung and heart disease but also of stroke. Obesity especially for men is not conducive to long life; it does not appear to be so harmful to women.

Exercise is important at all stages in life and the exercise capacity of older people can be improved by training. Physical retraining programmes in late middle age may produce not only improvements in cardiovascular and muscular fitness but also may bring about histological changes like those of younger patterns in muscle biopsy. Practical guidance on the prescription of exercise and the expected response to it in elderly patients has been given (Shephard 1987). Ignorance of the basic facts of nutrition is prevalent in elderly women and possibly more so in elderly men and 16% of people 65 years and over needed dietetic advice (Andrews *et al.* 1971). The groups especially at risk were those with physical disability, the recently bereaved, old people socially isolated and those with depression. The danger of alcoholism in old age is considerable especially in the groups mentioned above.

The importance of foot care should be stressed; feet should be thoroughly dried after washing and a little talcum powder placed between the toes. Those with diabetes or peripheral vascular disease must take particular care and obese elderly people will require help with the cutting of their toe-nails. Readily available chiropody services are important for older people.

It is essential to try and reduce accidents in the elderly and this is a worthwhile exercise in the prevention of illness. These accidents usually occur in the elderly individual's own home, where over 80% of fatal accidents take place. In the attempt to prevent an accident it may be necessary to go over the whole days routine activity of the old person to discover the danger point and to be able to give advice on improving habits. Many of the elderly persist in hurrying and must be taught to do things more slowly and carefully; this is often very difficult. Many have no sense of smell and safety taps for any gas apparatus should be installed where necessary.

Women are more prone to accidents than men and falls are the most common cause with poisoning and burns and scalds taking second and third places. Falls are often associated with a decline in postural sense which may occur with increasing age. The elderly frequently cannot correct their balance once they have stumbled and this, associated with the osteoporosis of ageing, explains the high incidence of fracture. The fall may be accidental or associated with a drop attack or other concomitant disease. Accidental falls are commonly caused by lack of handrails on stairs, insufficient illumination, polished floors with loose rugs, electric flex too long and trailing across the floor or inappropriate footwear. Drop attacks (Sheldon 1960) without warning or loss of consciousness are accompanied by a flaccid state of leg and trunk muscles. The aetiology is obscure but may be due to cerebral ischaemia and thus almost any serious illness can cause a fall in the elderly. Myocardial infarction, anaemia, heart block, latent chest infection and neoplasm are some examples. On occasion the fall may be caused by therapy as, for example, a hypotensive agent being prescribed with excessive zeal. The patient with a history of falls presents a problem in diagnosis which demands investigation. Diagnosis is essential; not only must any injury be treated which has occurred as a result of the incident, but search must be made to find out why the patient fell. Scott (1976) confirmed that elderly individuals who had fallen had the results of the fall treated extremely well, but there was a virtual absence of medical examination directed towards finding the cause of the fall.

The more active life of many old people brings new types of accidents; elderly drivers must as well as wearing seat-belts use neck restraints. They should consult their own doctors about their driving ability and general practitioners must be on the alert for warning signs of visual defects or increasing mental frailty.

Poisoning due to household gas does occur and the incidence is higher in the winter months. Old people have a poor sense of smell and this may be largely responsible for household gas poisoning.

Burns and scalds are usually due to clothing catching fire or are caused by a fall into the fire.

The importance of this whole subject lies in preventive measures.

The first essential is good housing for the elderly with efficient illumination and carefully planned architectural design so that un-necessary steps and steep staircases are avoided. The door of the lavatory should not be directly opposite a staircase, and for the elderly handrails on both sides of the stairs are necessary while rails round the WC are required. There should be a sufficient number of electric plugs to avoid long trailing electric wire, fireguards on the fires and safety gas apparatus. Electric plugs should be at waist level to avoid unnecessary bending.

The patient's hearing and vision should be tested and, if defective, hearing aids and spectacles provided. Older people should be encouraged to wear proper shoes or boots and not house slippers.

If a patient complains of unsteadiness and falling every effort should be made to reach the correct diagnosis and where this is possible appropriate therapy given. If no reason for the falling can be discovered, then the patient should be told to avoid changing posture suddenly. If he is getting out of bed he should do it as it were by numbers – sitting up first, then putting the legs over the side of the bed, waiting in this position for a minute or two, then standing. Inquiry must be made, however, to make sure that no drugs are responsible for the giddiness.

It should also be emphasized that the patient should not turn his head rapidly or look up quickly and stretching up to high shelves should be avoided.

Health education should also draw attention to urinary incontinence and indicate that advice should be sought from the doctor if this occurs as many older people accept this as a part of the ageing process.

An essential part of health education is the need to provide motivation for the older person and the following measures were undertaken to try and enhance mental health and may be examined critically to see if they could be applied more widely.

Reassurance on physical health was found to be a reasonable method of allaying anxiety. Older people are much helped by kindly encourage-ment after they have received a complete and thorough physical examin-ation preceded by a careful history of their past illnesses and experience. This type of reassurance based on knowledge helps the elderly, many of whom have secret and unexpressed fears of disease. If plenty of time is given to them so that they may describe accurately their troubles and anxieties, this too is of great assistance. Advice can now be given to them on the method of living they should adopt bearing in mind their estimated physical ability. Such people can be recalled at intervals for some months for repeated encouragement and continued guidance. Reflective consideration by the individual in the evolution of present problems is beneficial.

Interpersonal hostility within a household is one of the causes of emotional disturbance; these difficulties between parent and daughter or son may be clearly revealed on questioning. A conference between the old person, their relatives and the doctor may be necessary to formulate a way in which the stress situation within the home might be alleviated or eradicated. A doctor with experience in such matters outwith the family circle will be able to see the total picture more clearly and can frequently redirect the household in a smoother way of life. This, as would be anticipated, can be a very time-consuming procedure but is often very worthwhile. Many husbands immediately following retirement enter an apathetic stage which may lead to difficulty in diagnosis. The possibility of physical disease must be excluded, the thought of a depressive illness should be considered and finally advice may need to be given that the husband requires stimulation by his wife to do more to look after himself properly and to help in the house. A wife may have to receive complete reassurance regarding her husband's physical and mental health before she will apply the necessary robust encouragement. Liaison with the padre or minister of the patient's religion may on frequent occasions be of value and a stimulation of the patient's interest in religious affairs will often be of great help. Unfortunately, many elderly people lose touch with their church as they grow older, in many instances because of physical disability. Every effort should be made to maintain contact with the appropriate religious organization. The caring member of a family in which there is an elderly invalid should receive regular relief in order to maintain social life and to have some freedom for personal pleasure. Voluntary agencies such as Crossroads in the UK provide care attendants on a regular basis free of charge.

Home visiting by either trained and skilled visitors such as health visitors, social workers, or, if such help cannot be obtained, by well-intentioned volunteers does improve the patient's mental health and prevent loneliness. The local authority or the local Age Concern (Old People's Welfare Committee) can arrange to keep the old person under surveillance. A change of dwelling by removing to protected or warden-supervised housing may be of value if friendship and company is required and if there is anxiety about living alone.

A wider spectrum of accommodation should be provided by local authorities so that the fit old person is not usually admitted to a residential home with all facilities provided. An intermediate type of accommodation between this and special housing for the elderly is useful – a room given to the older person where personal belongings and furniture could be brought and where there might be a younger old person to each six or seven older people who would supervise their welfare. In such accommodation the residents would do their own shopping, be responsible for all meals, with the exception of a mid-day lunch. This would encourage independence and yet provide supervision and companionship while preserving a place of one's own. It would also prevent the sapping of individuality which tends to accompany hotel-like existence. Such schemes have been successfully run by voluntary organizations, e.g. Abbeyfield Society.

This type of home has to be close to shops and preferably available to elderly people born and bred in the area so that they remain among friends and familiar surroundings.

More sheltered housing with an intercommunication system to a warden is urgently required. If such accommodation were more widely available many beds in residential homes and hospitals would be freed (p. 339).

Any change in social conditions, e.g. from one's own home to a sheltered house or from a sheltered house to a geriatric unit or nursing home should be an occasion for a comprehensive physical examination. Complete assessment of physical, mental and social health is essential before any such move.

The advice of a psychiatrist specially interested in the elderly can be of the greatest help and should be sought early rather than later. It is often very difficult to persuade older people and their relatives of the need for this step. The psychiatrist will often wish to admit an older person for complete assessment and also, on occasion, to give the relatives a rest. The constant care of a confused old person is very arduous and is indeed a task without respite. The modern geriatric unit can offer a diagnosis and quite frequently therapy and cure. In some areas specialized psychogeriatric units exist and they are most useful; on occasion admission to a mental hospital will be essential for specialized treatment. The home for the mentally frail is a most useful adjunct to the geriatric unit and the mental hospital (p. 349).

Older people need constant stimulation to undertake the development of interests and hobbies; with perseverance this aim can be achieved, and this will be of great benefit to the patient's mental health. Study can stimulate mental function and there are now a wide range of courses in many subjects available for older people.

Many older people are depressed and this is frequently undetected. A constant watch must be kept as treatment is commonly successful.

Clubs, either in the form of lunch clubs, afternoon clubs or all-day clubs, have a most important role to play in the maintenance of mental health. Many conveners of these clubs note when an old person does not attend and send a member of their visiting committee to the old person's home to find out what is happening. As bereavement is a common cause of severe and lasting depression, someone has to encourage the old person to come back again to meet their companions and friends. There may well be a period of withdrawal but if the club has a well-organized home visiting service it should be possible to bring the former member back to the community. Old people with a sound religious belief are greatly helped by this during the difficult time.

Retirement is for many a time of stress and some, a relatively few, achieve success and contentment through disengagement from their previous level of activity. In practice when disengagement takes place it is usually due to an adverse home environment or physical incapacity. In an industrial society in which men and women are educated to work it is necessary to regard the promotion of activity in old age as fundamental for the attainment of a healthful life.

Certain facilities are available with the aim to maintain physical and mental health:
Education for retirement.
Hobbies and crafts centres.
Re-employment bureaux.
Retired employees' associations.
All-day clubs.
Telephone reassurance schemes.
Friendly visiting.
Sheltered housing.
Homes for the physically or mentally frail.
Television and radio programmes.
Immunization.

Education for retirement

The Scottish Retirement Council founded in 1959 is a voluntary body which exists to:
1 Study the problems of the elderly worker and, in co-operation with employers and appropriate bodies, statutory and voluntary, to promote education for retirement by providing courses for this purpose.
2 Promote occupational activities for men and women in retirement, and to provide facilities for hobbies and handicrafts.
3 Provide information and advice services on the above matters by the publication of the results of the Council's research and the dissemination of literature published by the Council and other bodies on these subjects.

The courses meet in new technical colleges for higher education and each course consists of six full day sessions on, for example, consecutive Tuesdays; the employer thus releases the employee from work with pay 1 day a week for 6 weeks. The forenoon sessions are from 9.30 a.m. till 12.45 p.m. and the afternoon sessions from 1.50 p.m. till 5 p.m. No fees are charged for the course but a small one is made for lunch, morning coffee and afternoon tea. The older people mix with the young students and much is gained from this association.

Since October 1959, 18 410 people (13 227 men and 5183 women) have taken part in 984 courses. Unanimously they have expressed appreciation of the courses and have declared themselves as feeling better equipped to confront and plan for their retirement. They have strongly recommended the courses both to their employers and to those working beside them at the same stage in their careers. The courses are offered to all employees willing to attend the course.

In the light of the experiences of the Scottish Retirement Council it is suggested that greater benefit is likely to be derived by those who attend a course some 2 to 5 years before the date of their retirement.

Living in retirement courses have also been useful and these bring individuals out of their own homes to meet others and so form a new group of people who become interested in one another and often form the basis of a new day club.

A report (1981) on Retirement Education in Scotland described ways of attempting to strengthen the intellectual and physical well-being of retired people in Scotland by means of a flexible, systematic service of education for the retired.

Hobbies and crafts centres

There are five hobbies and crafts centres in Glasgow and two are situated in schools which were given by the Corporation of Glasgow when new schools were built; the others are in local community centres. At these centres the men have facilities for woodwork, work in metal and basket work. They can make furnishings for their own homes, toys for the grandchildren or presents for their friends. They receive no payment for this work but every year a sale of work is held and more raw material is bought with the proceeds. The ladies have sewing classes, instruction in cooking and dancing classes, and as a joint venture a Senior Citizens' Orchestra, and a Concert Party and Drama Group are in being which are most successful.

Re-employment bureaux

Many who work with older people have the firm conviction that lack of incentive, of interest and of occupation encourages the development of ill health and acts to produce invalidism. It is impossible to be complacent about the present situation because of the growing numbers of elderly people being admitted to mental hospitals.

There are innumerable part-time paid posts which these older people can fill with great personal satisfaction and perform a most useful duty for the community. Their life's experience in dealing with others makes them expert in dealing with the day-to-day personal problems of industry and commerce. They can provide politeness and courtesy in shops, hospitals and factories which are so sadly lacking in this modern society.

In the belief that there will always be some people who desire to work full-time until the age of 65 and will want to continue working even in retirement, an office was established in Glasgow in 1967 to arrange part-time paid employment for retired men and women who desired such occupations. This is staffed entirely by volunteers, themselves retired, and there is no charge made either to employees or employers. Over 3700 retired people who wanted such employment have been placed in jobs to their own and their employers' satisfaction. Men who have held senior executive posts realize that on retirement they cannot expect to find part-time jobs at the same level of responsibility. They want positions that will not give them worry. Some examples of posts obtained are: clerical work, handyman, companion-help, bookkeeper, clerks and clerkesses, and office messengers.

This project has helped to make life much more interesting for those placed in employment and has also given great satisfaction to those older people responsible for the success of the enterprise.

Retired employees' associations

This term appeals much more than pensioners' associations, as it avoids the idea of someone pensioned off and forgotten. These associations are formed by workers who have retired from the same firm. These people meet together usually in the canteen or lecture hall of the firm sponsoring the association and with the help of the personnel officer of the management. Usually an employee on retirement is automatically made a member of the Retired Employees' Association and the functions are:
1   Social activities.
2   Education.
3   Welfare.

4 Support for all voluntary organizations working for the benefit of old people.

Social activities. It is customary for many such organizations to send out a monthly newsletter and to arrange regular meetings usually held in the works' canteen or lecture room. Concert parties, travel films and lectures are arranged for these meetings.

Education. In addition to the courses provided by the Scottish Retirement Council (p. 13), experts in finance and education and doctors are brought to the factory to address the workers just before retirement, and a talk is given by the secretary of the Retired Employees' Association, who describes the difficulties he found in adjusting to retirement and by quoting examples from the experiences of his associates tries to reinforce advice given by the experts. One important point made is that the older workers are advised to plan their retirement in consultation with their wives.

Welfare. On his retirement each employee is given pre-paid addressed postcards. Should he become ill or find himself in difficulties he is requested to post one of these cards immediately. When the personnel officer of the firm receives this postcard, he visits the retired employee usually with another member of the Retired Employees' Association. This means that the old man is visited by one of his friends and by the personnel officer of the firm. To an elderly retired person this type of service means that he is never again lonely or isolated. The importance of this to the morale of old people is invaluable. Apart from the improvement in mental health which this service gives, it also means that if the old person is ill and has been advised to go into hospital, he knows that he has friends with continuing interest in his condition who will visit him during his illness. In addition, a sub-committee of this type of association also has a visitation list and arranges regular visits to those older people who are housebound.

Support for voluntary organizations working for the benefit of old people. Retired Employees' Associations can support work being done by voluntary organizations in the area for older people, and usually join the local Age Concern (Old People's Welfare Committee). This helps greatly in the integration of the services for older folk as the Old People's Welfare Committee can be informed of the people who are being visited regularly by members of the Retired Employees' Association. The fundamental importance of this type of work where older people are helping those still older and even more frail is immense. Many of the members of such associations are on different committees so that they are all deeply committed to the work of helping others: an outlook develops which is looking always towards assistance to comrades and not to constant concern with self and one's own problems.

All-day clubs, lunch clubs (with physiotherapy)

The provision of a cheap but good meal will entice many lonely, elderly people out of their houses and many varieties of such organizations exist. Older people can be encouraged to come together to prepare a lunch, doing all the cooking themselves, planning menus and washing up afterwards. This is a much more positive type of self-help than sitting at a table passively, while lunch already cooked and prepared by others, is served. Opportunity should be taken to interest the old people in attending the club's keep fit exercises and in dietetic instruction. Many other educational facilities can be provided.

Telephone reassurance schemes

Particularly in the United States of America much use has been made of the telephone by encouraging elderly chronically ill patients who may be in hospitals, or homes to telephone old people in the same neighbourhood who live alone. This gives the chronically ill old person a purpose in life and provides stimulus and help to the older individual who is by himself. This procedure boosts morale, demonstrates interest in the well-being of lonely people by others and can be arranged in many different ways.

Friendly visiting

There are many voluntary organizations who arrange for a visitor to go to an old person's house regularly and adopt, as it were, this old person. The advice given to such organizations is to have one friendly visitor per old person and not to overload the voluntary worker. This type of visiting can be organized through churches, women's organizations, rotary clubs and wherever friendly and interested people get together to help the elderly.

Sheltered housing

This has been the most significant social advance in the last 20 years filling the gap between independent housing and frail ambulant hostels and has important preventive, curative and continuing care implications.

Preventive implications. In sheltered housing the older person comes into a situation where the everyday activities are supervised unobtrusively. If any minor symptoms of illness develop these are picked up sooner than if the elderly individual had been living alone in her own home. In the latter case unless someone noted uncollected milk bottles, or just missed the old person or by chance a visitor called, the illness would not be detected. Early diagnosis means that many old people can be treated in their sheltered house by their own doctor and do not require to be admitted to hospital. By the provision of an intercommunication system whereby the older citizen can speak to the warden or caretaker of the group of housing, this in itself is a preventive measure as by the immediate response to a call, reassurance is given to the elderly individual living alone and the feeling of having someone at hand is most important to many elderly people. Such intercommunication systems can be installed into houses already built and by use of radio communication a central group of wardens can supervise a number of independent houses. In sheltered housing an additional preventive aspect is protection from unwanted callers and vandals.

Curative implications. Many old people who have lived unsupervised and alone are much improved physically and mentally by the knowledge that they are now in a protected environment and can receive help whenever it is required. Such housing allows much more freedom for the individual, encourages companionship and good neighbourliness, stimulates the elderly to plan and shop for themselves or others and yet in time of difficulty help is at hand. The old person can mix with her neighbours or keep to herself just as is desired. Relief of worry and anxiety has a wonderful effect especially following bereavement.

Continuing care. There are many old people who have been unwell and almost contrary to the expectation of their relatives and doctors have recovered and are now placed in continuing-care hospital geriatric units; many of these can manage well in sheltered housing. In addition there are some of the elderly in local authority or private homes for the aged who could care for themselves in sheltered housing. In such housing, people who are amazingly frail can find great happiness. Where the individual is living alone in such housing, with wide doors and freestanding baths, the possibility exists that the older person can return to this house, should any illness take place which means an admission to a hospital, to the extent of being able to live there in a wheelchair. In most schemes regular visits from social workers or health visitors are encouraged as well as the constant supervision of the caretaker. If the housing project is not too large and is well sited the elderly people can play a most active part in the local community.

In this type of housing modern warning systems can alert the warden should the older person be unable to perform the normal acts of daily living such as getting out of bed or using the toilet.

Homes for the physically or mentally frail

Physically or mentally frail individuals placed in such properly designed homes will in time improve, and it may well be that these homes should have built in their grounds a small group of sheltered housing. The care given in these particular homes for physically or mentally frail people is of such a quality that a therapeutic environment is created and older people previously thought to be frail but incurable can recover to an amazing degree. While this is not strictly a preventive measure, the point of importance here is that progress can be made by people thought to be beyond improvement if placed in a correct environment and that some progress should be made possible by the provision of sheltered housing so that the home for physically or mentally frail is not always regarded as an end point.

TV and radio programmes

The elderly greatly appreciate programmes specially designed for them and much health education can be provided in this way: keep fit exercises, advice on diet, best buys at the markets, fashions for the older lady; there are many ways to stimulate the interest and intellect of older people.

As preventive services evolve, more responsibility is now being placed on people themselves who must eventually play the major part in maintaining their own health. One example of this attempt is a booklet (Gray 1982) which contains practical recommendations on keeping fit as age advances.

Immunization

In the event of an approaching epidemic of influenza immunization in groups of elderly people with cardiovascular, pulmonary, hepatic disease or diabetes mellitus will reduce morbidity and mortality. The vaccine against influenza A viral infection is the most effective but it should not be administered to anyone with hypersensitivity to eggs or egg products. It is important to ensure that caring staff are also protected.

Polyvalent pneumococcal vaccine is also effective in preventing pneumococcal infection and one suggestion is that it should be given to all persons 45 years and over hospitalized because of chronic illness prior to discharge from hospital (Fedson & Baldwin 1982). There is no doubt that careful clinical judgement is required in the choice of elderly people suitable for immunization.

Ascertainment of illness

The self-reporting of illness is the basis of the accepted doctor–patient relationship. Ascertainment is concerned with the seeking out of disease and other care needs so that correct diagnosis and appropriate therapy may prevent disability and illness or at least lessen them. Many doctors working with the elderly have noted how much more they could have done if the patient had been seen at an earlier stage in their illness. A Consultative Health Centre for older people was established (Anderson & Cowan 1955) in an effort to secure earlier detection of disabling conditions and unsuitable social circumstances. People aged 55 and over were referred to the Centre by their own doctors for a complete clinical examination. The doctors were invited to refer those with a minimal or no complaint. The findings supported the idea of early intervention but it was realized that only those who could come to the Centre were being examined. Williamson (1966) coined the phrase 'the iceberg of unreported illness' and demonstrated that the old tend to attribute certain symptoms such as incontinence of urine or loss of balance to ageing and not to disease. A random sample of the elderly in their own homes revealed a marked increase in morbidity at 70 years and that those over 85 years required in the majority of cases some form of assistance to enable them to continue to live an independent life in their own homes (Akhtar *et al.* 1973).

From the examination of every fifth person 65 years and over in the Kilsyth area of Scotland it was found that at 70 years there was a marked increase in physical illness and that the medical problems were cardiac failure, anaemia, urinary symptoms, deafness and failing sight. In nearly every case a marked improvement in the quality of life resulted from therapy.

In any form of preventive medicine applied to the elderly the first essential is co-ordination of effort. The general practitioner, the local social service department, the hospital service and voluntary organizations must be integrated and work together. In this context the concept of health visitor, district nurse and social worker attachment to the health centre, individual general practitioner or group practice to enable a team effort to be made is of the greatest importance. The general practitioner can then co-ordinate the local services in his own community. The preventive outlook to illness in the elderly is rewarding and offers the main hope of reducing the demand on expensive and prolonged hospital care.

Experience has demonstrated that the older people especially at risk are:

The very old, i.e. those aged 85 and over.

The socially isolated.

The bereaved.

Those recently rehoused or discharged from hospital.

Kennie (1986), however, concluded that concentrating on the at-risk groups is not an efficient method of screening and that a more universal approach needs to be tried. Numerous methods of ascertaining the health of old people have been described using an age–sex register and having a clinical examination carried out by a member of the health care team or by the physician personally (Anderson 1981).

One way of maintaining the health of older people in a local district is for the general practitioner to ask the health visitor (community nurse) attached to the practice or health centre to pay a home visit to all the people 75 years and over with special regard to prevention. The health visitor is a health educator and from her training endeavours to preserve, as far as possible, the physical health of the individual visited, to maintain the mental health and to support the social circumstances. The trained nurse may not detect every minor impairment in physical and mental health but is usually capable of finding out the elderly person who should see a doctor. The visiting nurse can also observe the social health of older people by making recommendations with regard to the need for domestic help in the house, meals-on-wheels, or a change of environment. Powell & Crombie (1974) concluded that the use of a questionnaire by a health visitor provided a reliable, adequate screening procedure for the elderly in the community. They compared the health visitor's findings with those of a doctor and found them very satisfactory. The screening programme was found to be acceptable, of reasonable accuracy and as they stated, using a health visitor is less expensive than using a doctor. This study is in agreement with the study carried out by Williamson, Lowther & Gray (1966) whose correlation of findings were satisfactory with physical illness, but less so with psychiatric illness. Here also the individuals were seen by a health visitor and then examined by a doctor and in this instance by a psychiatrist also.

At 75 years there is sufficient physical, mental or social illness to justify a visit from a nurse, such as the health visitor who would obtain job satisfaction from her work. A nurse is regarded by some people as more appropriate than a doctor as in the elderly person's mind a physician is associated with illness and if a physician paid a home visit to people 75 years and over without being invited it would be difficult to sustain the idea that this visit was one concerned with health maintenance.

Barber (1982) has described a method of reducing the number of case-finding visits by mailing to a selected group of older people a series of simple questions regarding their health and social circumstances, e.g. Do you live alone? Who can you call for assistance? Are there any days when you are unable to have a hot meal? Are you confined to your home through ill health? Do you have difficulty with vision or hearing? An affirmative answer to any question or if the questionnaire is not returned is an indication for a home visit by the health visitor.

Early diagnostic health examination

This has been described above. The health visitor (community nurse) is able to detect by physical examination minor disabilities which may greatly handicap the old person, for example corns or bunions on the feet, the presence of obesity, or enquiry may reveal faulty nutritional habits. The dietitian has a part to play by visiting health centres or group practices and teaching all those concerned with the care of the elderly, for example doctors, social workers, health visitors, district nurses and home helps, about diet. Lowther *et al.* (1970) examined critically early diagnostic services for the elderly. Medical examination was offered to a high-risk group of old people; those living alone, or recently bereaved or just discharged from hospital, who were not necessarily known to their family doctor but were seen with his agreement. Clear evidence of improvement was found in one-half of patients who carried out the recommendations and this was attributed to earlier diagnosis than would have been achieved without the examination at the clinic in 42% of cases. Including all the patients examined, the proportion helped by early diagnosis at 18–30 months' follow-up was 23%. These authors concluded that the offer of a routine examination to a high-risk group was of benefit and was a form of medical practice which should be widely adopted. Only 3% of those seen were recommended for admission to geriatric units.

It is recommended that the health visitor/community nurse visit in the first instance those 75 years and over, as many elderly people fear disease and time given to elicit their worry followed by careful survey of their health forms a solid basis from which apprehension can be banished. On occasion, admission to the geriatric unit, of short duration, may be of great value, either to make a correct diagnosis or for treatment, for example of cardiac failure. The visiting nurse may play an important part in clearing out the drug cupboard of many elderly people who hoard medicines. Such an action may help to ensure that the old person takes the drugs recommended by the physician and may cut down the incidence of hospital admission from drug toxicity or overdosage. Home visiting, therefore, is of fundamental importance and Wilson (1970) has placed on record the feelings of the health visitor working among the elderly. Social isolation following bereavement can be prevented through support given at the time of greatest grief. The health visitor can overcome loneliness and encourage the intake of an adequate diet, while ensuring that the elderly person does not become completely cut off from family, friends and neighbours at that time of great risk. Wilson advocated that this preventive work could be rendered more effective if health visitors were notified automatically of all cases of terminal illness where the caring relatives were old people. This would call for better liaison between the hospital team and the community health team and would be of great advantage to the elderly.

The prevention of illness

At all ages diagnosis is the basis of good clinical medicine and the best gift that the physician can give the older patient is a correct one. In the elderly it is difficult and to differentiate between the 'normal ageing process' and the early presentation of disease requires expert skill obtained from good training and experience. The informed physician should be able to help in some way nearly every elderly person seen. Physical and mental disease are commonly intertwined and both aggravated by social circumstances. Two fundamental points must be made; the importance of knowledge about the home conditions and continuity of care.

Diet may require modification and information about the diet of the old in the area in which the physician is practising is useful, e.g. in the West of Scotland it has been shown by Dall and colleagues (1971) and by Judge & MacLeod (1968) that older people tend to select a diet which is low in potassium and therefore may have a borderline potassium intake.

Increasing calcium consumption and reducing that of alcohol, caffeine and protein and stopping cigarette smoking combined with taking more exercise are now stated to prevent bone loss and thus prevent osteoporosis.

Perhaps the greatest danger to health first realized by Dr Marjory Warren is the practice of unnecessary bed rest.

The range of 'normal' blood pressure in the very old is still a matter of debate and all patients must be judged individually but it is worth remembering that the old are susceptible to postural hypotension and perhaps to strokes through over-zealous therapy.

In any survey of older people's health osteoarthritis of the joints is commonly found. This condition, affecting knees or hips, is almost certainly aggravated by obesity and the prevention of this complication could cut down the incidence of osteoarthritis or at least delay its onset. Certainly a loss of weight in an obese individual will help the osteoarthritis. It is also likely that if joints were put through a fuller range of movement by the individual as he grows older this condition would not be so common. The wear and tear on one part of a bone would be spread more evenly over the weight-bearing surface. Mild exercises to give full range of movement of joints are worthwhile in an endeavour to prevent this condition developing as age increases.

Anaemia is another diagnosis frequently made among so-called healthy old people; frequently of iron deficiency type, more rarely due to lack of vitamin B_{12} (Addisonian anaemia). It is an insidious illness in the elderly as the symptoms are usually attributed to the process of ageing, or weakness, lethargy or, on occasion, oedema of the ankles are labelled as due to cardiac failure. Folic acid deficiency has also been shown to cause anaemia in apparently healthy older people. Estimation of the haemoglobin content of the blood is an essential part of the examination of elderly people and should there be symptoms of mental confusion or any suggestion of subacute combined degeneration, serum B_{12} and folate levels should be checked.

Chronic bronchitis, fibrositis and coronary artery disease were noted at the Rutherglen Consultative Health Centre and the usual therapeutic measures were recommended. The old people with these complaints can be kept active and out of hospital with careful supervision. Patients with symptoms of coronary artery disease can be taught to live within the tolerance of their heart and, if obese, weight reduction can be advised. If these measures fail and the patient becomes incapacitated by the symptoms, the advice of the cardiologist should be sought regarding surgical intervention.

Intermittent claudication seems on so many occasions to be a self-limiting illness. If the patient is not too severely disabled and can walk a reasonable distance then patience and attempts to avoid the pain will often result over the years in complete cure. If symptoms are severe the elderly person should be sent to a vascular surgeon.

Diabetes mellitus is often first discovered in old age, and in any screening examination must be excluded. Many cases in the elderly respond to dieting.

Gynaecological abnormalities, haemorrhoids and unsuspected hernias are among other findings commonly discovered in independent and healthy old people and life can be made much more pleasant if these conditions are remedied.

Corns and bunions are also of frequent occurrence and will be found on routine examination of older people. The attention of the chiropodist is of great value.

Many doctors prefer to examine older people themselves often after using some form of health ascertainment by, for example, postal screening. In assessing the elderly person regarding physical fitness, a complete physical examination is necessary and this should include a rectal examination. This is stressed for the obvious reason that some abnormality may be found and also for the more subtle one that when the patient discovers that this examination is to be performed he will often remember a history of constipation or of bleeding per rectum or, if a women, previous or present gynaecological troubles will be recalled. Elderly people are frequently unwilling to talk about troubles of this nature as they may regard them as unimportant or not relevant to the examination. The urine should always be tested for albumin and sugar and the haemoglobin and random sugar content of blood estimated and the chest x-rayed. A routine ECG should be taken and the results are frequently of value.

Oral hygiene must also be checked and the aim of a dental service should be to preserve oral health and routine examination of the elderly especially those over 70 is of value.

The eyes must be examined; conditions like cataract and glaucoma can cause blindness. McWilliam (1978) showed that it was after the age of 85 that vision started to fail and that if regular eye examinations are carried out the chances of blindness in old age are minimal.

The elderly require advice about hearing; some are deaf because of wax blocking their ear canals and the majority become unable to hear the higher notes and find difficulty in recognizing their friends' voices especially on the telephone. Older people require training in the use of hearing aids which amplify all sounds. These and other problems associated with the choice and care of deaf aids are discussed by Beswick (1987) and the differential diagnosis and treatment of tinnitus is detailed by Hickish (1987).

With increasing age mental health is commonly impaired; men are concerned about their physical health and older women find that living alone is a source of worry. Bereavement is a major problem for both sexes while the combination of poverty and adverse social conditions, not surprisingly, is a factor in promoting depression. The diagnosis of depression is difficult in the elderly as it is unusual for older people to complain that they are depressed. It is only after two or more interviews that the cause of the mental disorder may appear. Preventive measures include better education of medical students and physicians in the early detection of depression, the provision of promptly available primary care services and special attention to the social support of older people living alone. It is considered by some that the losses in physical, mental and social function observed in old age are not the result of disease but simply of disuse.

Whatever may be the conclusion of the value of ascertainment it must be of immense value to the general practitioner if as an older patient enters the consulting room a folder from the health visitor is produced giving an account of the patient's previous health history, the present social conditions and a brief report on the clinical problems.

Disease in the elderly results in deterioration in function. This embraces mobility, continence, mental state and the activities of daily living. Part of any caring support for older people must provide domestic, nursing and social services. This is essential to provide a protected environment and a feeling of well being.

One of the most difficult problems facing the general practitioner interested in preventive medicine is the all-too-common association between the elderly and bad social circumstances. The house in which the older citizen lives may be dirty, insanitary, without adequate lavatory facilities, or too large for his present needs. Any assessment of the elderly person's physical and social health must also include an accurate appraisal of his living conditions. As attempts are made to build up and maintain the fitness of the individual so the gradual building up of poor social circumstances should be encouraged. This may necessitate the temporary accommodation of the older person with relatives or in a home for the elderly until the house is cleaned and until adequate domestic help can be given. So frequently when this situation is found what is lacking is foresight. Looking ahead is the one method of preventing deterioration of the social circumstances of the old person. The possibility of re-housing is a real one if adequate warning is given to the housing department of the local authority. Many of the social difficulties can be anticipated and avoided by planning ahead but this can only be done if the patient's own doctor and others interested in his welfare consider the home life of the person as part of the individual's total existence.

REFERENCES

Akhtar A.J., Broe G.A., Crombie Agnes, Mclean W.M.R., Andrews G.R. & Caird F.I. (1973) Disability and dependence in the elderly at home. *Age and Ageing* **2**, 102.

Anderson F. (1981) Is health education for the middle-aged and elderly a waste of time? *Family and Community Health* **3**, 1.

Anderson W.F. & Cowan N.R. (1955) A consultative health centre for older people. The Rutherglen Experiment. *Lancet* **2**, 239.

Andrews G., Cowan N.R. & Anderson W.F. (1971) The practice of geriatric medicine in the community. In *Problems and Progress in Medical Care*, 5th Series, (Ed. McLachlan G.) London, Oxford University Press.

Barber J.H. (1982) The effect of a system of geriatric screening on general practice workload. *Health Bulletin* **40**, 152.

Beswick K.B.J. (1987) Today, there's none so deaf as can't be helped. *Geriatric Medicine* **17**, 55.

Dall J.L.C., Paulose S. & Ferguson J.A. (1971) Potassium intakes of elderly people in hospital. *Gerontologia clinica* **13**, 114.

Fedson D.S. & Baldwin J.A. (1982) Previous hospital care as a risk factor for pneumonia. Implications from immunization with pneumococcal vaccine. *Journal American Medical Association* **248**, 1989.

Gray J.A. Muir (1982) *Better Health in Retirement*. England, Age Concern.

Hickish G. (1987) How GPs can help tinnitus sufferers. *Geriatric Medicine* **17**, 37.

Judge T.G. & MacLeod Catriona C. (1968) Dietary deficiency of potassium in the elderly. *Proceedings of the 5th European Meeting of Clinical Gerontology*. Brussels, p. 295.

Kennie D.C. (1986) Health maintenance of the elderly. In *Clinics in Geriatric Medicine*, Vol. 2, No. 1 (Ed. Magenheim M.J.) Philadelphia, W.B. Saunders.

Lowther C.P., MacLeod R.D.M. & Williamson J. (1970) Evaluation of early diagnostic services for the elderly. *British Medical Journal* **3**, 275.

McWilliam R.J. (1978) Vision in the elderly. *Health Bulletin* **36**, 69.

Mehigan J.A. (1978) The doctor's life style. *Irish Medical Journal* **71**, 174.

Powell C. & Crombie Agnes (1974) The Kilsyth questionnaire: a method of screening elderly people at home. *Age and Ageing* **3**, 23.

Retirement Education in Scotland (1981), Scotland, Age Concern.

Rhee H.A. (1974) *Human Ageing and Retirement*. Geneva, International Social Security Association.

Scott C.J. (1976) Accidents in hospital with special reference to old people. *Health Bulletin* **34**, 330.

Sheldon J.H. (1960) On the natural history of falls in old age. *British Medical Journal* **2**, 1685.

Shephard R.J. (1987) Prescribing exercise. In *Geriatric Medicine Annual* (Ed. Ham R.J.) Oradell, New Jersey. Medical Economics Books.

Williamson J. (1966) Ageing in modern society. Paper presented to Royal Society of Health, Edinburgh, 9 Nov.

Williamson J., Lowther C.P. & Gray S. (1966) The use of health visitors in preventive geriatrics. *Gerontologica clinica* **8**, 362.

Wilson F.G. (1970) Social isolation and bereavement. *Lancet* **2**, 1356.

3
Problems in Diagnosis

Diagnosis in elderly people who are ill is the fundamental principle of geriatric medicine; it is difficult yet rewarding and interesting because of age-related changes.

The altered physiology of old people is only detected when stress is placed on an individual organ and then the diminished reserve of function becomes apparent. The symptomatology of disease in older people is, thus, changed. Illness comes on insidiously with less clamant symptoms than in the young and in an individual who may well already have many minor ailments.

Medical students listen to the favourite sayings of their seniors, perhaps today in a less believing way, and rightly in a more critical manner than heretofore. In dealing with the aged such long-held views and reflections by medical teachers are usually erroneous and worth careful re-examination.

History-taking

In medical school it is taught that the patient is the only person who knows what is wrong with him and if you allow him he will tell you. This presents certain difficulties in elderly people where history-taking becomes an art requiring the ability to separate wheat from chaff in a whirlwind manner. The information is there, the problem is how to obtain it. The previous history of illnesses or operations is vital and consultation with relatives, or in their absence with a friend or neighbour, is often essential. A warning note must be struck; the triangular conversation should be avoided at all costs, that is a three-part play where doctor, elderly person and relative are present together, and where reality tends to fly out of the window and a fascinating interplay of personalities occurs. While much intriguing family history may be revealed with skeletons falling out of cupboards one after the other, little of relevant value to the present illness will emerge. The old person and her relatives should at least on one occasion be interviewed separately. At another and very different interview when, after a period of hospital care the time comes for the older individual to leave hospital and to go home as planned, then the reverse is true. There should in fact be a three-cornered consultation between the relative, the doctor and the patient, so that there is no misunderstanding about the future plan or programme for the elderly individual. This procedure avoids the ping-pong game where the doctor is used as a ball to convey messages between patient and relative and relative and patient. During history-taking itself direct questioning is usually essential, and during this time it is necessary to complete at least one form of mental health (dementia) scoring system. This is invaluable, not only in diagnosis but in assessing progress. Time spent during history-taking should be used to build up the mental health of the patient by stressing any hopeful statement. The importance of asking a few leading questions after the history of the present illness has been taken must be emphasized. Inattention, deafness, confusion and the joy of reminiscing make for a long and tedious history-taking. The importance of maintaining the interest of the patient cannot be overstressed and the necessity for keeping the older person's mind on the business in hand is essential. Forgetfulness often means that some vital symptom is overlooked, and the innate modesty of some elderly women prevents them from complaining of embarrassing subjects or of affliction in awkward sites. Information should be sought regarding any previous hospital admission and direct questions asked about past important illnesses.

Tiredness, fatigue and general lassitude in a previously active old person demand investigation. These symptoms are frequently an early warning of incipient cardiac failure and merit among other tests the estimation of the haemoglobin content of the blood. Havard (1985) reviewed these symptoms. He stressed the importance of a clinical history, then of physical examination, often unhelpful, and the need to exclude depression and the importance of laboratory tests. These may reveal anaemia, osteomalacia, hypothyroidism or apathetic hyperthyroidism, uraemia, the macrocytosis and raised liver enzymes of alcoholism; hyperglycaemia may indicate diabetes mellitus. Patients with pernicious anaemia frequently present with oedema of the ankles and mild cardiac failure. Occasionally acute or subacute bacterial endocarditis will be discovered if the possibility of this diagnosis is kept in mind, and the elderly 'chronic bronchitic' may well be found to have tuberculosis. Weight loss in the elderly should not be attributed to advancing years. It is almost certainly true that in extreme old age people do lose weight but this occurs very slowly and is not noticed by the elderly or their friends. Any abrupt change in the usual functioning of the body demands attention, e.g. the sudden onset of loss of appetite or of constipation.

The fascination of geriatric medicine to the physician lies in the great difference in symptomatology between the elderly and the young. A middle-aged woman sustains an accident and fractures her femur. She is able to give a clear account of what happened, can define the injured area and has acute pain at the site of the fracture. An elderly woman gets out of bed during the night to empty her bladder, falls and may lie where she fell until morning. When help comes she may be confused and unable to give any history, the loss of the power in her leg may be noted and a diagnosis of cerebral infarct may be made. She may, however, remember what happened and complain only of weakness in the leg or of pain not in the affected hip but in the knee. This possibility of referred pain taught by the anatomist is worth recalling in dealing with the elderly; only careful examination and x-ray reveals the fractured neck of femur. Unless the occurrence of painless fracture is kept in mind mistakes are made. Such fractures are commonly missed but if a patient has a history of injury followed by a loss of function a fracture should be suspected; pain may not be a presenting symptom. Special care must be taken in the case of stroke patients who may have fallen as a result of the stroke and sustained a fracture of shoulder or hip. They may not be able to move their arm or leg on the paralysed side because of the stroke and any pain experienced may be attributed to the stroke. If there is any doubt x-ray examination should precede passive movements.

Pain

Medical teaching has always stressed that pain is a call for help, and this of course is generally true. But there is doubt about the value of the pain as a symptom in the elderly. It has been demonstrated clearly how infrequently pain is of diagnostic importance in myocardial infarction.

It has become commonplace to accept the 'silent' coronary and indeed an attack of myocardial infarction may present as a bout of breathlessness or a 'wee turn', a momentary fainting attack, or as a transient confusional state. Hildick-Smith (1984) described in detail the presentation of the 'funny turn'. She mentioned two main categories, those associated with impairment of consciousness and those without. The causes are numerous and hospital based investigations may be necessary to pinpoint the reason for the attacks. She concluded although a single cause for a patient's turns may not be identified, many patients improve with correction of the numerous abnormalities discovered by examination and investigation. A patient who continues to have turns is in danger of fractures or subdural haematoma. The natural sequelae of fear, loss of confidence and loss of mobility are common and bring with them their own dangers and a reduction in the person's quality of life. Thus every effort should be made to diagnose and treat the elderly patient with turns. Apathy, loss of appetite, desire to stay in bed or loss of mental alertness may be the first symptom of an acute infection such as pneumonia or pyelitis. Intra-abdominal disasters may occur in the absence of severe pain; constipation of sudden onset and atypical in that particular individual may indicate intestinal obstruction from one or other cause, and acute appendicitis may also be silent. Pain, when it does occur, may be felt in the wrong place and in the wrong organ. An elderly person may unwittingly baffle the physician by complaining of persistent pain in the back of the neck or in the chest when in fact the lesion is a benign ulcer of the lesser curvature of the stomach. In a previously well-adjusted person depression with apathy may indicate a painless peptic ulcer.

Posture

The control of posture becomes more difficult for the elderly person and thus falls are frequent. Complaints of vertigo, dizziness and unsteadiness are very common and are no doubt in part due to problems with posture. Once the older person feels a fall is imminent balance cannot be recovered quickly. It is important to treat the result of a fall in the elderly but it is even more important to try and discover why the old person fell in the first instance. A fall should be considered as a rash would be in an infant and careful attention must be given to try and discover what has caused the fall. Falls occur in the elderly in many different conditions; almost any serious illness can result in a fall and while drop attacks were stressed by Sheldon (1960) as the cause of about a quarter of falls in old people, a fall may also be the result of many illnesses, e.g. myocardial infarction, anaemia, heart block, latent chest infection and neoplasm. The fall may be precipitated by therapy as, for example, a hypotensive agent being prescribed with excessive zeal. The very useful phenothiazine derivatives may also cause postural hypotension and thus precipitate falls in older people. One immediate practice, where the patient complains of falls, is to stop all drug therapy and see what the result is. As people grow older, control of posture is helped by changing position slowly and the safe rule is to advise elderly people to change position by numbers as if they were in the army and to make the endeavour to avoid sudden movements especially of head and neck. Where no cause for unsteadiness on standing can be found, it is often of value to advise a few days complete rest in bed and then very gradual ambulation. On the first day the patient sits up in a chair for 10 minutes and behaves as if recovering from a severe illness with gradual increase in exertion over the period of a week.

Temperature

Temperature regulation becomes impaired in many elderly people and the value of temperature elevation as a pointer to infection is unreliable. Recording of the patient's temperature is still important and hypothermia is not too uncommon in the wintertime. Any illness when the older person remains immobile and exposed to a drop in temperature may, because of faulty temperature control, result in hypothermia, and the possibility of undiagnosed myxoedema should always be considered in patients with hypothermia.

Hyperpyrexia may be found when a patient with longstanding parkinsonism is transferred from his home to hospital. The exacerbation in the symptomatology of the illness is frequently associated with high temperature. This condition is so serious that if a patient with parkinsonism is being cared for at home and the relative desires correctly to have a holiday and the request is made for admission to a geriatric unit, the relative is always warned of the danger of transfer to hospital. This seems another example of the impairment of control of temperature regulation in ill old people.

The value of counting the respiratory rate has been stressed and this should always be recorded in the ill elderly patient. A rise in respiratory rate preceded the clinical diagnosis in lower respiratory tract infections.

There are different views as to the febrile response to infectious disease in the elderly but all are agreed that for some older patients the typical symptoms of an infective process are absent or non-specific and the illness is only detected if there is a high index of suspicion. Berman *et al.* (1987) noted that all patients with urinary tract infections had fever but frequently no urinary symptoms while approximately 13% of chest infections remained apyrexial and about one-quarter of them lacked the typical respiratory symptoms.

Thirst

The sensation of thirst appears diminished in elderly people as many come into hospital with a dry, brown tongue and take fluid immediately it is offered but seldom ask for a drink of their own accord. Such people are often suffering from faecal impaction and may have disturbance also of potassium balance. The need to restore correct quantities of water and electrolytes to the elderly person must be stressed.

Intra-abdominal disease

Intra-abdominal disease presents great difficulty in diagnosis and previous operations must be checked carefully. Few elderly people can remember the exact nature of the operative procedure. Bowel caught in an old scar either of anterior abdominal wall or in the opening of the posterior peritoneum from previous operations may cause an obstruction which takes a long time to become manifest and is almost unaccompanied by symptoms, except for constipation, until the illness has become extremely serious.

The most common cause of masses in the abdomen is faeces and thus repeated abdominal examination is essential. It is very easy to confuse an arteriosclerotic aorta pushed into prominence by compensatory lordosis of the lumbosacral spine for an abdominal tumour.

Rectal examination is always worthwhile in dealing with older people, and by performing this simple investigation the doctor avoids the common error of overlooking faecal impaction and in some instances of treating this with anti-diarrhoeal agents. The faecal-stained slime which leaks past the impaction can be mistaken for diarrhoea. A very high proportion of older people who come into hospital are faecally impacted on admission and this condition is an unpleasant, painful and, on occasion, very serious complication for the patient. When loss of appetite, unusual restlessness or left-sided abdominal pain are noted, faecal impaction should be excluded.

The differential diagnosis of diarrhoea must always include self-medication by the patient. Many older people not unnaturally dread constipation and take purgatives for many years. When questioned about intake of medicines the elderly patient always omits to mention any purgatives. Only the direct question: 'How do you regulate your bowels?' elicits the required information. Other common causes of diarrhoea in the elderly are dietetic indiscretion, especially if the diarrhoea occurs after a visiting day in hospital. It is important to warn older people not to eat fruit in large quantities at one time; so many of them do not buy this luxury food but tend to enjoy it too much when it is given to them as a present and eat thoughtlessly. Gastric carcinoma, uraemia and congestive cardiac failure are other causes of diarrhoea which serve to demonstrate that this is an important symptom in the elderly and if it lasts for more than 1–2 days should be investigated thoroughly. Constipation is another symptom frequently reported, and like diarrhoea, an attempt should be made to confirm objectively the complaint.

It has been said that the best cure for diarrhoea is to request a specimen of stool and it might be added that constipation should not be treated unless present. Constipation is a severe and distressing condition for an elderly person especially if associated with a poor myocardium and lack of power to expel hard faeces from the rectum. It must be emphasized, however, that this is a common symptom for the hypochondriacal and the depressed to choose, and a record of bowel movements combined with inspection of specimens of stool gives an accurate foundation for treatment. Faecal incontinence may be precipitated by diarrhoea or by faecal impaction and before any therapy for such incontinence is considered a rectal examination must be performed. Diverticulitis is one of the more usual causes of diarrhoea and should be treated energetically (p. 65). Marked improvements can follow therapy provided the diagnosis is correct.

An old person with an acute perforation of a peptic ulcer may collapse suddenly without pain and may mimic the onset of a silent myocardial infarction. In contrast unilateral abdominal pain may be the first sign of herpes zoster.

Mental state

In work with old people the importance of the mental health of the individual cannot be overstressed and a case was referred to the department where a man had become suddenly very depressed and talked of suicide. His wife reported this to the doctor and he was referred for investigation. This man of 70 was a retired labourer who kept saying: 'I cannot seem ever to get into a happy frame of mind', and who was found in fact to be deeply depressed. On investigation, a recent silent myocardial infarction was discovered and with bed rest there was a dramatic improvement in his mental state. There almost certainly was underlying endogenous depression, but this was a minor symptom compared with his mental state on admission. It is common to find mental illness associated with physical disease (Anderson & Davidson 1975).

The symptom of mental confusion nearly always precipitates a crisis in the patient's family especially if it develops suddenly, but medical advice is not always sought. As there are so many causes of this condition in the elderly (p. 233) this symptom should never be dismissed as part of the ageing process, particularly if of sudden onset. Nocturnal wandering many indicate cardiac decompensation and the re-establishment of the normal sleep rhythm is essential. A distended bladder in an old person may at first produce symptoms indicating the site of the pain, but as distension increases mental confusion may occur and only physical examination reveals the need for action. It is probably true that if the retention is acute and complete there may well be pain and a palpable bladder, but with chronic retention and overflow incontinence there is not always pain and the bladder is less easily felt. In older people constant care must be exercised to avoid missing a distended bladder. The only method of making sure that this is not overlooked is by examination of the abdomen followed by a rectal or a vaginal examination where there is any doubt. On rare occasions catheterization with the strictest aseptic precautions is the only way to confirm this suspected diagnosis. A lower abdominal swelling in an elderly female patient may be an ovarian cyst, but the probability of a gross distension of the bladder should be kept in mind. Sometimes this may be excluded by asking the elderly woman to stand even if needing support flooding will then occur as gravity helps to expel the urine and the diagnosis is confirmed.

An additional factor in causing mental confusion in old people is a change of surroundings, and this may be due to the diminished sensory intake of the elderly individual. Eyes do not see so clearly, hearing is dull, memory for recent events is poor so that the sequence of events leading to the new scene is forgotten. After admission to hospital, the physician, the nurse or the relative should always make sure that the old person understands who is present and to whom he or she is talking. The nurse should make herself known to the patient, identifying herself clearly and telling the old person the truth about her whereabouts and explaining to the patient that she is in hospital to get better and that she will soon become familiar with her surroundings. This may have to be done many times in order to establish contact between the old person and her new situation.

Some families rotate their elderly people round their houses, each taking mother for 3 months. This in time almost certainly leads to confusion as the old person grows older. The constant change makes it very difficult for the elderly person to realize that she has a home of her own, to build up a sense of belonging and to preserve in her mind the essential geography of the house in which she is living. Many people have thought that when an older person is admitted to hospital it would be helpful to allow her to take with her some object, for example, a photograph, with which she is familiar. This is to try and make some effort to overcome the hurdle of strange surroundings. There is no doubt that the old person recently admitted who on waking during the night in hospital may, because of diminished sensory intake, have no idea where she is and may become confused as the result of this lack of knowledge. The position of the patient's bed in the ward should not be altered during the initial period while the patient is becoming accustomed to her surroundings. Even a confused patient may notice some particular attribute about the bed in which she is placed and this link with reality may disappear if the patient's bed is moved.

Miscellaneous symptoms

Breathlessness may be the initial complaint when in fact a change of cardiac rhythm has developed and the onset of atrial fibrillation has occurred; this is often accompanied by the feeling of tiredness. Breathlessness with prostration found in thin, malnourished old men and often associated with a cough and blood-stained sputum should make one consider, as well as lung neoplasm and tuberculosis, Friedländer pneumonia.

Scurvy should be suspected when there is excessive bruising following minor trauma, especially in an old man looking after himself. The haemorrhages frequently occur round the knee or ankle and if the old person is edentulous there may well be no bleeding of the gums. Sheet haemorrhages are common; brawny haemorrhagic areas extending from the buttock to the popliteal space or round the ankle.

The presence of iron-deficiency anaemia should always provoke a search for neoplasm or hiatus hernia and the simple explanation, namely haemorrhoids, should not be overlooked (p. 132).

Backache in women is frequently the presenting symptom of osteoporosis, although the pain may radiate down the legs or to the front of the chest and abdomen. Rest relieves the pain while exertion aggravates it. It must be kept in mind that conditions like this may be associated with depression. The presence of organic disease in the body does not preclude or protect the individual from an affective psychosis; quite the reverse, and constant thought must be given to the question: 'Is this patient more depressed and anxious than her condition warrants?' 'Is she requiring therapy for this as a separate and different illness?' Many old people, apparently difficult to treat, constantly complaining and unappreciative of any effort made by doctors, nurses and relatives, are requiring psychiatric advice and treatment.

The difficulties in diagnosis abound, but two illnesses should never be far from the doctor's thoughts if there are symptoms of serious organic disorder in the central nervous system. The first is subacute combined degeneration and the diagnosis here is so important that any patient with symptoms of peripheral neuritis or unexpected leg weakness should be investigated specifically for this illness: undiagnosed this disease progresses relentlessly and the end result is paraplegia, bedsores and mental confusion. The second is the constant search for tumours of the coverings of the spinal cord, frequently benign. These do occur but perhaps are seen only once in a lifetime. A patient presenting with a slight but progressive weakness of limbs with no signs of cranial nerve or mental impairment should be investigated in the most thorough way. In any neurological case repeated physical examinations are required as it may be the change in signs which prompts the correct diagnosis.

The observation by an informed relative that the older person has aged suddenly is well worth noting and this is often explained by some remediable illness. A very sensible lady of 87 years was able to stand beside her bed without being able to walk. She noticed all was not well with her when she could no longer carry her history textbooks home from the library. On physical examination no abnormality was discovered apart from muscle weakness and it was thought that she had some metabolic disorder. When investigated in hospital she was found to have a profound potassium deficiency from inadequate nutritional intake and when this was remedied she was able to walk about in her usual manner and continue the activities of daily living. Illness such as potassium deficiency may make the task of the doctor very difficult indeed as the older person may only complain of a desire to remain in bed and not get up which is surely quite natural or so it seems in extreme old age. The sign of diminished mobility must be taken seriously and the causes range from the sudden onset as in stroke, fractured femur or silent myocardial infarction to those with gradual development as in hypothyroidism, Parkinson disease or depression.

A very elderly man was reported to have become 'mentally deteriorated' as he suffered from dribbling incontinence. The removal of a large stone from his bladder cured the incontinence and his relatives no longer complained about his mental state.

Disease in old age

Simpson (1974) discussed disease patterns in the elderly and described three groups of diseases:
1   Those illnesses in which the age incidence had shifted to include age groups beyond previously accepted age limits, but where the disease pattern remains true to type, for example pernicious anaemia, motor neurone disease, acute leukaemia and rheumatoid arthritis.
2   Diseases where previously accepted features, well known and recognized, may be lacking, or where the illness may take quite a different form when occurring in elderly subjects, for example tuberculosis, bacterial endocarditis, diabetes mellitus and thyrotoxicosis.
3   A number of new diseases, occurring mainly or entirely in older subjects, which have been described in recent years, and this includes illnesses such as polymyalgia rheumatica, cranial arteritis, pseudo-gout, Waldenström macroglobinaemia and accidental hypothermia.

The old, like the young, have a constant need for reassurance and an urgent need for a careful reappraisal of how the community regards the elderly individual. Newman (1969) has felt for many years that a proportion of elderly individuals with urinary incontinence had this symptom because they felt that they had been completely abandoned and neglected by society. They felt that no one cared for them any more and that there was no point in being continent, and they abandoned all pretence of being ordinary individuals. Certainly in looking at long-stay wards in other parts of the world, in the East, for example, where different moral and ethical codes prevail, incontinence does not seem to be so common as it is in the countries of the West.

The common occurrence of multiple pathology in the elderly must be kept in mind and this may make diagnosis extremely difficult, while an order of priority in therapy must be established and the doctor must not attempt to treat all diseases diagnosed at one and the same time. Simple medication ordered with clear instructions is the rule, with a close watch for any toxic drug effect essential. Many modern medicines are hallucinogenic, sometimes producing the most odd effects, and where such hallucinations are of recent onset, all drug therapy should be stopped immediately. It is important to remember that these older individuals would not have reached old age without having a certain soundness of structure in body and mind and they have an amazing aptitude for recovery.

It has been well said that no patient has a typical cerebral infarction and diagnosis of any illness should always be made only after thoughtful clinical investigation. Perhaps the greatest danger lies in labelling a patient with a diagnosis and then never re-assessing his case. Diagnosis is often only possible after a period of observation and one of the reasons for admitting patients to hospital is to secure accurate and continuous supervision. In such circumstances it is essential to perform repeated examinations. This applies also to long-stay patients where conditions may change dramatically and yet insidiously. Diagnosis in the elderly is difficult because illness may present atypically; more than one disease is commonly present and serious conditions may start in a quiet non-dramatic way. Better life-long health record-keeping is essential to ensure accurate knowledge of previous illnesses, operative procedures and immunization with a special note of any drug sensitivity. The art of diagnosis in the older patient is a time-consuming and mentally satisfying exercise but while a conclusion is being reached the patient should receive treatment designed to relieve pain and distress.

The good physician can help every patient he sees, and possibly even more those suffering from what are called in our present state of knowledge irremediable diseases. The presence of a cancer should not mean an end to rehabilitation. Once appropriate therapy has been applied, be it surgical or medical, then the patient requires attention to his physical, mental and social conditions. Only in the terminal state should there be a change in policy, and here again enthusiasm is essential. The effort must be made not to dull pain when it occurs but to prevent it. The anticipation of difficulties, mental and physical, the preparation of the relatives for the acceptance of the inevitable, and the maintenance of the patient's confidence in his doctor until the end; these are the duties of the physician.

REFERENCES

Anderson W.F. & Davidson R. (1975) Concomitant physical states. In *Modern Perspectives in the Psychiatry of Old Age* (Ed. Howells J.G.) New York, Brunner, Mazel.

Berman P., Hogan D.B. & Fox R.A. (1987) The atypical presentation of infection in old age. *Age and Ageing* **16,** 201.

Havard C.W.H. (1985) Lassitude. *British Medical Journal* **290,** 1161.

Hildick-Smith M. (1984) Don't dismiss the 'funny turn'. *Geriatrics for GPs* **14,** 20.

Newman J.L. (1969) The prevention of incontinence. 8th International Congress of Gerontology. *Proceedings* **2,** 75. Washington Federation of American Societies for Experimental Biology.

Sheldon J.H. (1960) On the natural history of falls in old age. *British Medical Journal* **2,** 1685.

Simpson R.G. (1974) Disease patterns in the elderly. *British Journal of Hospital Medicine* **12,** No. 5, 660.

4
Drug Therapy

The main interest of the patient is a speedy recovery from his illness. The treatment he is prescribed is of paramount importance to him. He will judge the physician not on his merits as a diagnostician but on his ability to relieve his symptoms and effect a cure. The faith that patients might once have had in foul or strong tasting medicines has now changed to a wish for medicines which are pleasant to take and attractively presented. No drug is completely free from risks but the doctor should prescribe the least toxic preparation available to produce the desired effect. Physicians should familiarize themselves completely with the drugs they prescribe. They should know the therapeutic dose, potential unwanted effects and any special precautions that are necessary. These principles are of special relevance when managing older patients.

Elderly people often benefit more from the doctor stopping drugs than starting them. As discussed before, diagnosis may be difficult and without a diagnosis treatment becomes haphazard. Multiple symptoms often lead to polypharmacy. A list of diagnoses should be made and a scheme of treatment priority planned to facilitate rational prescribing. In advising older people about the use of their medicines, great care should be taken to give clear instructions and explanations. Medicine taking should become a regular habit. Complex drug regimens should be avoided and instructions should be written down so that the patient and his carers are well aware of the treatment prescribed.

Ageing and drug action

The physician must be aware of changes in pharmacokinetics and pharmacodynamics that may occur with the ageing process or with diseases which commonly affect elderly people (O'Malley 1984).

Pharmacokinetics

Despite a variety of physiological changes with age, absorption of drugs given orally is not systematically changed. Substances administered at the same time may affect the absorption of drugs, e.g. the reduction of tetracycline absorption due to the formation of insoluble complexes if the patient is taking iron, calcium salts or antacids containing aluminium or magnesium.

Little is known about the effect of age on the distribution of most drugs. Old age is associated with reduced lean body mass, total body water and plasma albumin and a relative increase in body fat. As a result the distribution of water soluble drugs, e.g. paracetamol, may decrease and that of lipid soluble drugs, e.g. diazepam may increase. Many commonly prescribed drugs are bound to a greater or lesser degree to plasma albumin; only the unbound portion of drug is pharmacologically active. When two drugs are given at the same time and one has a higher binding capacity than the other, available binding sites may be saturated by the first drug leaving more of the second to exert its effects, e.g. aspirin a high binding drug may displace tolbutamide. An elderly diabetic who takes aspirin may be more susceptible to the hypoglycaemic action of tolbutamide.

Hepatic clearance of drugs may be diminished due to reduced hepatic blood flow, liver volume and a slower rate of hepatic metabolism (Stevenson *et al.* 1979).

The excretion of drugs is slower than in younger people as with age there is a reduction of renal capacity with impairment of both glomerular and tubular function. There is also the likelihood of co-existing renal tract disease, e.g. prostatism, chronic urinary tract infection or kidney disease. The elderly are therefore more susceptible to the adverse effects of potentially nephrotoxic drugs like the aminoglycosides.

Pharmacodynamics

In older people there is an increased sensitivity to some psychotropic agents, narcotic analgesics and coumarin anticoagulants. An apparent reduction in β-adrenergic receptors or an altered sensitivity is associated with a reduced response to the pharmacological effects of β-blockers.

Ageing can be accompanied by reduced efficiency of a number of homeostatic mechanisms. The elderly are often less able to compensate for the effects of many drugs. Altered baroreceptor function may be unable to cope with the effects of normal doses of antihypertensive agents and troublesome postural hypotension may result.

Adverse effects of commonly prescribed drugs

The elderly are more susceptible to the unwanted effects of drugs than their younger counterparts (Castleden & George 1984) and older people are frequently admitted to hospital as a result of side effects of prescribed drugs (Williamson & Chopin 1980). A number of factors may lead to the increase in adverse drug reactions (Table 4.1) (Caird 1985).

Table 4.1 Factors leading to increased drug reactions in old age.

Altered pharmacokinetics
Altered pharmacodynamics
Loss of reserve capacity
Reduced homeostatic control
Polypharmacy
Poor compliance

Adverse drug reactions are most often produced by diuretics, psycho-tropic drugs, digitalis glycosides, non-steroidal anti-inflammatory drugs and antiparkinson agents.

Diuretics are widely prescribed for the elderly at home and in hospital. Approximately one-third of the population over 65 years of age takes some form of diuretic. The main indications for diuretic therapy are heart failure and hypertension. Diuretics should be withdrawn when the current indication is no longer apparent (Williams 1985). Thiazides given orally act within 1 or 2 hours and the effect lasts for 12 to 24 hours. These agents have a flat dose response curve and increasing the dose produces little extra effect. Loop diuretics, e.g. frusemide or bumetanide, act orally within 1 hour and the action is complete within 6 hours. Intravenous doses produce a peak effect within 30 minutes. These drugs have a relatively steep dose response curve and increasing the dose produces an increased diuresis. Potassium sparing diuretics include amiloride, triamterene and spironolactone. They have a relatively weak diuretic action but they potentiate loop and thiazide diuretics and prevent potassium loss.

Older patients are particularly at risk from the unwanted effects of diuretics. All diuretics apart from potassium sparing agents produce a dose related hypokalaemia. This is most often mild and usually only important in patients with ischaemic heart disease, myocardial infarction or those on digoxin therapy. Cardiac sensitivity to digoxin may be increased and digoxin cardiotoxic effects may be promoted. The risks of potassium depletion due to diuretic treatment can be reduced by giving oral potassium supplements. These supplements may however be ineffective and elderly patients often fail to take them. A combination of loop or thiazide diuretic with a potassium sparing agent is more useful. Care must be taken in the presence of significant renal impairment or serious hyperkalaemia may result. Potassium supplements should not be pre-scribed with potassium sparing diuretics. Sodium depletion, hypovolaemia and dehydration may occur even with short-term usage of diuretics in otherwise fit, elderly people. The main clinical picture is of symptomatic postural hypotension and there may be evidence of lethargy and confusión particularly if the serum sodium falls below 124 mmol/l. Diabetes mellitus and hyperuricaemia can be induced by thiazide diuretics and urinary disturbances including incontinence or nocturia may be problems especially if the patient's mobility is compromised.

Long-term diuretic prescription in the absence of significant hypertension or cardiac failure may be inappropriate and of little value in most elderly people. Regular review of the need for a diuretic is important and these drugs should be discontinued whenever possible.

Mental confusion is readily induced by drug administration and any sudden change in an elderly person's mental state should indicate that adverse drug effects may be responsible. Attacks of transient cerebral ischaemia may be produced by antihypertensive agents especially if combined with diuretics. Any agent which lowers blood pressure can produce drowsiness, restlessness or confusion with or without neurological symptoms and signs. It is wise before prescribing hypotensive agents in elderly people to take the blood pressure in the lying and standing positions to avoid producing or aggravating postural hypotension.

The dangers of digitalis glycoside therapy in the elderly are well known (Dall 1965). Older people are more susceptible to the toxic effects of digoxin. Adverse effects include disorders of cardiac rhythm of practically every type but especially atrial and nodal tachycardia and A-V dissociation. Other unwanted effects may include refractory cardiac failure, mental confusion, severe anorexia and weight loss and gynaecomastia. Elderly patients on long-term maintenance digoxin therapy should be reviewed and in the absence of a known primary cardiac lesion an attempt should be made to withdraw digoxin.

The use of hypnotics in the elderly should be avoided whenever possible. Ideally these drugs should be reserved for short courses of treatment in the acutely distressed (British National Formulary 1987). The incidence of adverse reactions to hypnotics increases with age, the commonest being sedation leading to confusion, falls, urinary incontinence and hypothermia. There is considerable variation in the individual sleep requirements of old people. The elderly person takes longer to get to sleep, wakes up more frequently and spends less total time asleep during the night (Herbert 1978). Many people accustomed to sleeping for an uninterrupted 8 hours feel that anything less is undesirable and they may seek medical advice and become dependent on hypnotic drugs. An explanation of the normal age-related changes in sleep coupled with reassurance can relieve the patient's anxiety about not sleeping properly.

Sleeplessness in old people should be investigated. First it must be confirmed that the person is actually sleeping for less time or has a disturbed sleep pattern. The use of a sleep diary by patients, carers or nursing staff can clarify the situation. Disturbed sleep may be due to physical illness, e.g. pain of arthritis or angina or breathlessness due to left ventricular failure or chronic obstructive airways disease. Nocturia may be due to prostatic disease or the unwanted effects of long acting diuretics. Psychological causes of sleep disturbance include emotional stress, bereavement, depressive illness and confusional states.

When a diagnosis is made any underlying cause for insomnia should be appropriately managed, e.g. analgesia, diuretics for pulmonary oedema or antidepressant therapy. Leg cramps may respond to oral diazepam (Valium) 2 mg at night. A chronic persistent non-productive cough may be aggravated by a cold room and adjustment of the ambient temperature can immediately improve the situation and allow the patient to sleep.

When it has been established that there is no apparent primary cause for insomnia a number of simple measures can be adopted to improve sleep patterns (Table 4.2).

Table 4.2 Non-pharmacological management of insomnia.

Avoid before sleep	Advise
Alcohol	Regular exercise
Tobacco	Milky drinks
Caffeine containing drinks	Comfortable environment

Most hypnotic drugs belong to the benzodiazepine group. The elderly are more sensitive to the effects of these drugs and their elimination may be impaired. Tolerance and dependence may occur and a prolonged hangover effect is not uncommon. If however the cause of the sleep disturbance remains obscure or does not respond to simple measures hypnotics should be prescribed. The smallest effective dose should be given for a few days and then reviewed. Short courses will minimize the development of unwanted effects and the risk of dependence. Chlormethiazole (Heminevrin) 500 mg is generally a safe drug in the elderly. Longer acting benzodiazepines, e.g. flurazepam or nitrazepam, should be avoided. Lormetazepam (Noctamid) 500 µg is a medium acting drug which seems to be free from the rebound anxiety sometimes seen with short acting drugs such as temazepam and triazolam. Care should be taken that elderly people are fully aware of the recommended doses and they should make certain that the evening dose is not taken twice by mistake. The total quantity of hypnotics prescribed at the one time should be reasonable and large numbers of tablets should never be left in the patient's possession. When the physician is changing a prescription for insomnia he should ask his patient to return any remaining tablets of any previously prescribed hypnotics which have not proved suitable.

Sensible prescribing

The general rules of drug prescription in the elderly are based on the principle that old people are ill not because of age alone but because of disease processes. Multiple pathology is the rule rather than the exception. The first essential therefore is a correct working diagnosis or more often a list of diagnoses which should be placed in order of priority for treatment. The physician cannot always cure all of the disorders simultaneously and a rational approach to treatment is necessary. The majority of elderly people at home are responsible for taking their own medicines and as many as three-quarters of them will make errors. Underdosing is the most common problem (Table 4.3).

Table 4.3 Sources of error in drug compliance.

Underdosing
Overdosing
Taking out of date inappropriate drugs
Taking other people's medicines
Adding non-prescribed self-medication

A number of increasingly sophisticated devices have been developed to improve compliance (Davie & Wandless 1981) but very often real success can be achieved with a simple well-written card system developed by the patient and his carers in the home. This is basically an aide memoire to ensure correct dosage and frequency of prescribed medication. If drugs are not having the desired effect and compliance appears to be satisfactory then the prescription should be stopped or changed.

Before prescribing a drug the doctor must answer several important questions (Table 4.4).

The possibility of non-drug treatment should always be explored, e.g. realistic lifestyle changes or weight reduction if appropriate. Several drugs are of uncertain or no value in old age, e.g. cerebral activators, expectorants or antiobesity agents. They may have troublesome side effects and should therefore be avoided. Drug regimens should be simple and logical. The use of fixed combination preparations may improve the likelihood of compliance but they can create difficulties by reducing the flexibility of

Table 4.4 Questions before prescribing.

Is a drug required?
Is the chosen drug of proven benefit?
Can the existing regimen be simplified or reduced?
Are undesirable effects acceptable?
What is the likelihood of compliance?
Who will supervise the medication?

dosage. It is unwise to prescribe any drugs to a patient who has significant confusion and who is expected to supervise the taking of his own medicines. Carers should be properly instructed about prescribed drugs.

If the physician has taken the decision to prescribe a drug, then he should adopt some simple rules for prescription (Table 4.5).

Table 4.5 Rules for prescribing.

Choose least powerful drug available
Select appropriate formulation
Avoid potential serious drug interactions
Prescribe correct dose
Choose minimal dosage frequency
Select appropriate container
Ensure legible, sensible labels
Provide clear instructions
Decide on duration of drug treatment
Review all repeat prescriptions

If a diuretic is required a simple thiazide may be more appropriate than a powerful loop diuretic especially for maintenance therapy. Some elderly patients have difficulty in swallowing large tablets or lack manipulative skills because of arthritis or poor vision and cannot manage small pills or tablets. Liquid preparations may be preferred and many drugs can be taken as mixtures, solutions, elixirs or syrups. One major drawback of these liquid preparations however is that it is often difficult to measure an accurate dose of the drug.

Potential drug interactions between pairs of drugs are well documented (Hansten 1979). There are relatively few of these interactions which are clinically significant, however several are potentially fatal, e.g. spironolactone and potassium supplements could in combination produce life-threatening hyperkalaemia. Doctors must be aware of the more important potential interactions and avoid them in their elderly patients' drug regimens.

Compliance may be improved by prescribing drugs only in one or two doses a day rather than more often if this is feasible. Old people often have difficulty in removing drugs from their containers due to reduced manual dexterity, poor vision, confusion or complicated childproof mechanisms. Bottles should be large enough to be easily handled, have necks through which tablets easily flow and have tops which are simple to remove. Bubble packs should be avoided and where possible containers should be made of clear glass or plastic to ease identification of pills or tablets. Container labels should be legible and preferably typewritten in large print. Labelled instructions should be sensible and comprehensive. Instructions like 'as before' or 'as directed' should be avoided and exact dosage schedules should be employed.

Few drugs require life-long prescription and most can be taken in finite, short courses, e.g. antibiotics, hypnotics and dermatological preparations. Except in long-term maintenance therapy with, for example, hormonal replacement, oral hypoglycaemic agents or antiparkinson drugs all requests for repeat prescriptions should be reviewed carefully by the physician. Drugs should be discontinued whenever possible.

Doctors tend to under-report drugs prescribed to their elderly patients at home (Gilchrist *et al.* 1987) and this may be due to incomplete records, universal use of deputizing services and patients hoarding out of date or inappropriate medicines. We must emphasize the importance of both medical undergraduate and postgraduate training in drug sciences and practical prescribing in the elderly (Royal College of Physicians 1984). Efficient record-keeping, regular drug surveillance, rationalization of treatment and prompt removal of out of date or inappropriate medicines from patients' homes should be a routine part of management by the family physician who visits his elderly patients at home.

REFERENCES

British National Formulary (1987) No. 13 London British Medical Association and the Pharmaceutical Society of Great Britain.

Caird F.I. (1985) Drugs for the elderly. Copenhagen, World Health Organization Regional Office For Europe.

Castleden C.M. & George C.F. (1984) Prescription for the elderly. In *Clinical Pharmacology and Drug Treatment in the Elderly* (Ed. O'Malley K.) Edinburgh, Churchill Livingstone.

Dall J.L.C. (1965) Digitalis intoxication in elderly patients. *Lancet* **1**, 194.

Davie J.W. & Wandless I. (1981) Improving drug compliance in the elderly. In *Advanced Geriatric Medicine*, Vol. 1 (Ed. Caird F.I. & Grimley Evans J.) London, Pitman Books.

Gilchrist W.J., Lee Y.C., Tam H.C., MacDonald J.B. & Williams B.O. (1987) Prospective study of drug reporting by general practitioners for an elderly population referred to a geriatric service. *British Medical Journal* **294**, 289.

Hansten P.D. (1979) *Drug Interactions*. Philadelphia, Lea & Febiger.

Herbert M. (1978) Studies of sleep in the elderly. *Age and Ageing* Supplement 41.

O'Malley K. (1984) *Clinical Pharmacology and Drug Treatment in the Elderly*. Edinburgh, Churchill Livingstone.

Report of the Royal College of Physicians (1984) Medication for the elderly. *Journal of the Royal College of Physicians of London* **18**, 8.

Stevenson I.H., Salem S.A.M. & Shepherd A.M.M. (1979) Studies on drug absorption and metabolism in the elderly. In *Drugs and the Elderly* (Eds. Crooks J. & Stevenson I.H.) London, Macmillan Publishers.

Williams B.O. (1985) Use and misuse of diuretics in the elderly. *Prescribers' Journal* **25**, 51.

Williamson J. & Chopin J.M. (1980) Adverse reactions to prescribed drugs in the elderly: a multicentre investigation. *Age and Ageing* **9**, 73.

5
Gastrointestinal Diseases

As age increases the individual may notice impairment of the sense of taste and a gradual sluggishness of bowel habit. Studies of the alimentary tract in older people reveal increased frequency of disorder of oesophageal motility, the common occurence of achlorhydria and of the development of diverticula in various sites.

No attempt has been made to give a full account of disease of the gastrointestinal tract but rather to concentrate on those disorders which are common among older patients.

Mouth and salivary glands

The tongue in an elderly person may become smooth from atrophy of the filiform papillae, and if also pale these changes are suggestive of vitamin B_{12} deficiency; a shiny red tongue may be due to deficiency of iron, vitamins of the B group or folic acid. Sublingual haemorrhages may be noted in scurvy.

A common complaint among the elderly is of dryness in the mouth and this is sometimes associated with small ulcers, a frequent cause being the administration of the phenothiazine compounds. These preparations, especially in liquid form, are very liable to induce unpleasant drying of the tongue and mucous membranes and may require to be withdrawn because of this; the drug administered in tablet form may avoid this complication. Many other drugs may also produce redness and ulceration in the oral cavity, examples of these being emepronium bromide, the barbiturates, sulphonamides, iodides, phenacetin, phenolphthalein and salicylates. A dry mouth may also be a symptom of uraemia, diabetes mellitus or Sjögren disease. Aphthous ulcers are common, painful and often multiple. Treatment with pellets of 2.5 mg hydrocortisone (Corlan) is often effective, and if the ulcers are large and infected a tablet containing 250 mg of tetracycline and 250 000 units of nystatin (Mysteclin) is dissolved in water and used as a mouth wash 3–4 times a day. Choline salicylate paste may relieve the pain of small ulcers.

Recurring aphthous ulcers may be due to deficiency of iron, folic acid or vitamin B_{12} and the possibility of chronic blood loss or malabsorption due to small intestinal disease should be excluded. Unilateral mouth ulcers may also be found in herpes zoster while lichen planus, a skin disease with oral manifestations in the form of bilateral jagged ulcers on the buccal mucosa can occur.

Old people require dental attention very frequently. The edentulous should be supplied with dentures and ill-fitting dentures should be replaced; many need treatment and few try to obtain it (Smith 1979). Great benefit results from the provision of artificial teeth; the psychological effect can be dramatic as after proper dental attention the patient may look younger.

The most common tumours in the mouth are hyperplasias caused by chronic irritation, but squamous cell carcinoma can occur. Any ulcer not healing in 2 weeks is suspect.

Inflammation of the parotid or submandibular glands

This is commonly seen in patients with serious or terminal illness and should be treated with local heat and a course of penicillin. If no response occurs to this antibiotic the therapy may have to be changed; surgical drainage may be necessary if abscess formation occurs. Thrush may be found in old people and is treated with tablets of nystatin, 500 000 units three times daily. Local mouth lesions respond to nystatin pastilles (100 000 units) one four times per day. The pastilles should be sucked and it is advisable to limit fluids – nothing to drink 5 minutes before the pastille and for 1 hour afterwards. Painting with 0.5% gentian violet is an alternative treatment. The possibility of oesophageal thrush leading to intense dysphagia should be kept in mind. A complete examination of the oral cavity is necessary in the elderly as no complaint may be made even in the presence of ulcers or of new growth.

Leucoplakia

This is usually regarded as a precancerous condition which may occur in any mucous membrane but commonly involves the oral cavity. There is increased keratinization of the superficial layers of the epithelium with inflammation of the underlying connective tissue. The tongue is often the site, and syphilis, irritation, either chemical, thermal or bacterial, and smoking may be factors in causation. Men are more commonly affected than women. Treatment is concerned with the elimination of the oral irritation and with the therapy of the causative factor, e.g. syphilis.

The lesion should be observed regularly and if verrucous, fissured or eroded or if an area of hardness extends beyond the limit of the leucoplakia, a biopsy should be performed. If malignancy develops, treatment is by surgical excision or irradiation. If no malignancy is found, continued supervision of the patient is essential.

Dysphagia

The swallowing apparatus and mechanism of dysphagia were described by Croker (1982). Decreased amplitude of peristalsis with normal propagation rate may be a feature of ageing. Upper gastrointestinal endoscopy in elderly subjects with dysphagia is of great value (Gupta *et al*. 1987).

Dysphagia, or difficulty in swallowing, is commonly encountered in the elderly and should never be ignored. McMillan & Hyde (1969) describe dysphagia due to compression from the aorta and note that this condition may be helped by oesophagoscopy or bouginage or by operation in severe and persistent cases.

Diffuse oesophageal spasm with symptoms of dysphagia with pain made worse by emotional stress or hot fluids is common and may be confused with angina.

This is a disorder of motility and may occur due to conditions such as reflux oesophagitis, obstruction by malignancy, Parkinson disease, cerebrovascular disease, thyroid disease and diabetes mellitus. Isosorbide has been used with varying results as have calcium blocking agents, e.g. nifedipine, verapamil.

Benign peptic stricture is not uncommon and responds to active treatment by dilatation with Hurst bougies or Eder dilators.

Pharyngo-oesophageal obstruction

Painful diseases of the mouth and pharynx and external compression of the oesophagus must be excluded. Dysphagia due to pseudobulbar or bulbar palsy may be seen. The patient may make the peculiar observation that semi-solid food is easier to swallow than liquids. Dysphagia is unusual after a stroke of more than 1 week's duration unless there is impairment of consciousness or there has been a previous stroke affecting the opposite side. The Plummer–Vinson syndrome is found typically in a middle-aged woman who has dysphagia, iron-deficiency anaemia, chronic glossitis and diminished output of gastric hydrochloric acid. Treatment is that of the anaemia and consists of a course of oral iron; continuing observation is essential and this condition is considered premalignant by some. This syndrome may be associated with web formation in the pharynx and the passage of a bougie or cutting the obstructing membrane may be necessary. Oesophageal webs should be biopsied.

Post cricoid carcinoma of the oesophagus or an oesophageal pouch also causes upper oesophageal dysphagia; carcinoma of the larynx may also produce dysphagia of this type.

Dysphagia accompanied by dysarthria is occasionally seen due to dislocation of the tempero-mandibular joint complicating stroke (Wright 1985).

Mid-oesophageal obstruction

Obstruction of the middle-third of the oesophagus is commonly due to carcinoma. Other causes of dysphagia are external compression from aortic aneurysm, and enlargement of the mediastinal glands due to secondary neoplasm from such sites as bronchus, breast, stomach and pancreas. Scleroderma is a rare cause of dysphagia.

Carcinoma of the oesophagus

This should be suspected in any elderly patient who has noted increasing difficulty in swallowing usually associated with loss of weight, anaemia and regurgitation; on occasion the older patient is able to point to the site of the obstruction. The opinion of the surgeon should be sought immediately and radical treatment undertaken whenever possible. More active surgery is now often recommended. If this is not a practical solution, then a tube should be inserted to maintain an open passage. A modified Celeste tube may be inserted under intravenous sedation using a fibre-optic endoscope (Croker 1982). For those lesions that are inoperable because of site, e.g. at the level of the arch of the aorta or above, radiotherapy should be considered. This will often restore the patient's ability to swallow. Because oedema may follow radiotherapy it may be wise to dilate before starting and at the same time to pass a fine bore naso-gastric tube. In some cases dilatation of a stenosing carcinoma may be necessary and every step should be taken to enable the patient to obtain nourishment. Gastrostomy is rarely indicated and should probably be used only prior to a more radical operation. The patient should be kept free from pain by the use of adequate analgesic preparations such as morphine or pethidine combined with chlorpromazine or thioridazine. Carcinoma of the oesophagus occurs more frequently in people who eat extremely hot foods, and therefore irritation of the oesophageal mucosa should be avoided, especially by people with anaemia, oesophageal diverticula or the Plummer–Vinson syndrome.

Lower oesophageal obstruction

Dysphagia at this level is usually due to hiatus hernia, achalasia or carcinoma of the lower end of the oesophagus or cardiac end of stomach. Laser photocoagulation is the palliative treatment of choice for dysphagia due to oesophagogastric tumour and has been used in the frail elderly patient even when malignancy is at an advanced stage; this technique enables the patient to be managed in the community (Elizabeth *et al.* 1987).

Achalasia of the cardia

This is a chronic condition characterized by recurrent attacks of obstruction at the cardiac sphincter of the stomach and associated with dilatation of the lower end of the oesophagus. Balloon distension or endoscopic dilatation of the oesophagogastric junction under x-ray control is usually effective, but if the obstruction is not adequately relieved by this method, surgical treatment may be necessary. Operation such as the Heller operation in which the circular fibres of the cardia are cut may be helpful but is now much less used.

Oesophageal hiatus hernia

Two common varieties are seen:
1   *Oesophagogastric hernia*. Here the oesophagus and stomach herniate into the thorax and gastric reflux occurs. This is the more common type.
2   *Paraoesophageal hernia*. A knuckle of stomach can be seen herniating alongside the oesophagus, through the hiatus in the diaphragm; there is no disturbance of the sphincter mechanism and no reflux oesophagitis occurs.

It seems likely that with advancing age and laxity of muscles, increasing intra-abdominal pressure may precipitate these conditions. It has always seemed possible that the constipation which occurs in many people as they grow older is also a factor in the production of these anatomical changes, and it has been suggested that regular use of bran might help to prevent this condition.

Symptoms due to the hernia are more commonly found in the second type described. Retrosternal discomfort may be noted during a meal, relief being obtained by walking about. Symptoms due to reflux oesophagitis, more commonly seen in the first type, are heartburn and dysphagia. The heartburn is associated with a change of posture, e.g. bending down or lying down in bed at night. Bleeding may result in iron-deficiency anaemia, but if severe it is usually associated with an ulcer in the oesophagus. The heartburn may be so severe that myocardial infarction or angina pectoris is simulated. Localized pain can occur at the lower end of the oesophagus causing much discomfort and worry.

Weakness or incompetence of the lower oesophageal sphincter is found in reflux oesophagitis which can occur without a hiatus hernia.

Treatment

The patient should be taught to sleep in a semi-upright position with the head of the bed raised 23 cm (9 inches) in order to minimize the bathing of the lower end of the oesophagus by gastric juice, and instructed to avoid bending and exertion in that position. Traditionally a bland diet has been recommended but a high fibre diet may help bowel movement and reduce straining at stool; it can be made up in a low calorie diet for the obese. For the reflux oesophagitis antacids such as magnesium trisilicate should be given to relieve the heartburn or tablets of Nulacin or Gastrils may be sucked. A suspension of a local anaesthetic agent, oxethazaine with magnesium hydroxide and aluminium hydroxide gel (Mucaine) in 5 ml doses three to four times daily 15 minutes before meals and at bed-time may help. A mixture of alginic acid, sodium alginate, magnesium trisilicate, aluminium hydroxide gel and sodium bicarbonate (Gaviscon) two tablets after meals and on retiring is another useful remedy. This substance also contains sugar and this should be kept in mind when treating diabetic patients. Cimetidine (Tagamet) in a dose of 200 mg three times per day with 400 mg at night is effective. Rarely toxic confusional states in the elderly have been found. These respond to a reduction in dosage. Ranitidine (Zantac) has a similar action. Surgical operation for hiatus hernia should rarely be necessary in older people: advice from the surgeon should be sought if there is a history of recurrent bleeding either from the oesophagus or from the herniated portion of the stomach due to ulceration or a stricture of the oesophagus. If the pain is very severe an initial phase of rest in bed may be necessary. Anaemia may require correction with a course of oral iron. If obesity is present a reducing diet should be prescribed.

Bleeding oesophageal varices

This is associated with a higher mortality than from any other part of the gastrointestinal system. The symptoms and signs of chronic liver disease are usually present. Urgent endoscopy is essential; barium swallow can confirm the presence of varices but cannot demonstrate the source of the bleeding.

The first problem is the control of the immediate bleeding and resuscitation of the patient by blood or plasma as replacement fluids. Then if bleeding has ceased the surgeon may proceed to injection sclerotherapy. If bleeding continues then a continuous infusion of vasopressin may be used and if necessary balloon tamponade; surgeons now have other methods such as circular stapling devices. Many patients with oesophageal haemorrhage have other medical problems such as ascites, renal failure or neuropsychiatric disorders.

Candida oesophagitis

This may affect patients with malignant disease, diabetes mellitus and those treated with protracted courses of antibiotics or immunosuppressive agents. Treatment with 250 000 units of nystatin in watery suspension every 2 hours for 1 week is used initially and amphotericin, miconazole or ketoconazole are useful alternatives.

Stomach

The frequency of atrophic gastritis increases with advancing age while gastric acid production lessens.

Gastric ulceration

The history of the patient with a gastric ulcer may simulate closely that of gastric cancer. The older person with a gastric ulcer may have symptoms typical of this condition but not infrequently the site of the pain is misleading and delay in diagnosis is common. Persistent pain in the left side of the chest may be the only complaint and may be in any part of the abdomen, or confined to the lower part of either side of the chest or in the retrosternal region. In fact elderly people may have a gastric or duodenal ulcer without abdominal pain and this is often associated with the taking of non-steroidal anti-inflammatory drugs. Patients with unexplained anaemia, loss of appetite and weight and sometimes with depression might be worth considering for endoscopy and the benign nature of the ulcer confirmed.

Treatment

A preliminary period of medical treatment should be given but the patient should be kept under close observation.

The important lines of treatment are drugs that provide symptomatic relief, antacids, and agents that promote ulcer healing, e.g. H_2 receptor blocking agents, liquorice and bismuth preparations, bed rest and the avoidance of coffee, tea and alcohol with prohibition of smoking.

The antacids of choice are magnesium trisilicate or aluminium hydroxide and the dietary regimen should be devoted mainly to the frequent administration of non-irritating easily digestible foods in small quantities; the aim is to reduce to a minimum the stimulation of gastric secretion. The use of cimetidine in a dose of 200–400 mg three times per day and 400 mg at night given over a period of 3 months promotes the healing of gastric ulcers, and maintenance therapy usually prevents recurrence. In the case of the elderly cimetidine 800 mg at night is as effective as 400 mg twice per day and may be more convenient for older people. Ranitidine, a more recent H_2 antagonist is equally effective and possibly less likely to produce side effects such as mental confusion. The dose is 150 mg twice daily for at least 4 weeks and then a maintenance dose of 150 mg at night. The main problem is that there is a tendency for the ulceration to recur when maintenance treatment is discontinued; at present the appropriate length of drug therapy is not known. It is essential to remember that if a gastric ulcer does not heal with H_2 receptor blocking agents the patient may be suffering from gastric carcinoma and the symptoms may be relieved. Cimetidine inhibits the hepatic microsomal metabolism of some drugs and the increased plasma levels and the prolonged half life of warfarin and phenytoin are important. Tripotassium dicitrato bismuthate (De-nol) has been found to be of value; it should not be given to patients with renal disorders. This drug produces blackening of the tongue and stools. The deglycyrrhizinized liquorice preparation Caved-S in a dose of two tablets thrice daily after meals promotes healing of gastric ulcers in patients over 60 with no adverse effects. Some doctors have advised the administration of ascorbic acid 0.1 g daily.

Rest for many elderly people means admission to hospital and with a large gastric ulcer an initial phase of hospital therapy is advisable. Should anxiety be a feature, a sedative may be necessary. Benefit can be obtained from thioridazine 10 mg three times per day. Salicylates and other anti-inflammatory drugs should be avoided. These drugs may be necessary in the elderly and the risks must be calculated against the need for therapy of other diseases.

Duodenal ulceration

The symptoms are more typical of the disease as seen in middle-aged subjects and most patients respond to medical treatment. There is not the same difficulty in excluding carcinoma, and in the elderly there is probably less likelihood of bleeding than in gastric ulcer. Treatment with alkalis, as for gastric ulcer, may be tried and some find relief with compound antacids such as Asilone. Cimetidine and ranitidine promote healing and maintenance therapy usually prevents recurrence. Omeprazole acts selectively at the secreting surface of the parietal cell and produces sustained reduction of gastric acidity for 24 hours after a single dose. This drug is still being reviewed but a single dose of 10–30 mg daily appears promising (Prichard *et al.* 1985). Famotidine is a newer H_2 receptor antagonist which may be of value in the elderly as it is given in a once nightly dose. Sucralfate is a complex of aluminium hydroxide and sulphated sucrose and has a mucosal defence action and may be of use in maintenance therapy but its long-term effect is still being assessed as some aluminium may be absorbed. It is best used alone. The complications of perforation and pyloric stenosis are found as in gastric ulcer.

The consequences of gastric operations are seen not infrequently in the elderly and sometimes lead to a malabsorption syndrome.

Haematemesis

This is an ever-increasing problem in the elderly and is associated with a high mortality if the patient comes to surgery; two-thirds of the patients are now over 60 and one quarter over 80. Deaths are virtually confined to elderly patients. As for people of any age some estimate of blood loss must be made. Symptoms such as faintness, thirst and coldness and signs of pallor or sweating are suggestive of significant blood loss. Complete physical examination to exclude hepatic, renal, pulmonary or cardiovascular disease is essential. Repeated estimation of haemoglobin levels over a few hours gives guidance to the continuation of haemorrhage. Elderly people are at risk following a severe haematemesis; they may become confused and restless and a cerebrovascular accident or myocardial infarction may follow. Diagnosis is vital as it should never be assumed that a haematemesis is due to cancer. Haematemesis and/or melaena usually indicates a lesion proximal to the Ampulla of Vater. Enquiry about the ingestion of drugs, e.g. salicylates, non-steroidal anti-inflammatory agents and anticoagulants should always be made from the patient or a relative. Fibreoptic endoscopy should be performed wherever possible within 24 hours of admission to hospital.

Treatment

This depends on diagnosis but the first priority is resuscitation and evidence of blood-volume depletion indicates blood transfusion. Watch must be kept for circulatory overload and diuretics may be required. The introduction of a nasogastric tube may be helpful in following the progress of the bleeding process but should be avoided if oesophageal varices are suspected. In massive continuing haemorrhage laparotomy may be the only course of therapy. The elderly in the main are poor candidates for surgery, but there is much to be gained by seeking surgical advice early in appropriate cases; cimetidine has proved useful in gastric erosions.

Some have recommended special units staffed jointly by physicians specializing in gastroenterology and surgeons. Prognosis is poor where there is bleeding from oesophageal varices due to hepatic cirrhosis or from malignant neoplasm and where the quantity of blood required in transfusion exceeds 1500 ml.

Carcinoma of the stomach

This is a common illness in the upper age range; premalignant conditions affecting the stomach are chronic atrophic gastritis, pernicious anaemia and a previous partial gastrectomy. Those with blood group A have an increased risk. A patient complaining of dyspepsia who does not improve with bland diet and antacid therapy within 14 days should be investigated in order to exclude a diagnosis of gastric carcinoma. The administration of H_2 receptor blocking agents such as cimetidine should be avoided as the symptoms may disappear even in cases of gastric carcinoma. Diarrhoea after food or of persistent character is another mode of presentation, while an initial complaint of dysphagia may be noted; haematemesis or unexplained anaemia are other presenting signs. Particular attention should be paid to patients who have pernicious anaemia. Regular testing for the presence of occult blood in the faeces and barium meals at yearly intervals are recommended by some for such patients. Fibroscopy and barium meal examination are the most valuable routine diagnostic measures available. The repeated finding of positive occult blood tests in the faeces or the presence of blood in aspirated gastric juice may also be noted. Exfoliative cytology confirms the diagnosis if malignant cells can be obtained from gastric washings. The treatment is surgical and even in advanced cases a surgical opinion is essential. This is particularly so if there is pyloric obstruction with vomiting. A palliative operation should be considered as this may afford welcome symptomatic relief.

If there is any doubt about the diagnosis, laparotomy should be performed as the lesion may be shown to be benign. A careful follow-up is necessary of the patients who have had a partial gastrectomy and a close watch must be kept for the development of anaemia and malabsorption (p. 130). In patients who have received radiotherapy, radiation-induced malabsorption can occur. While chemotherapy has not been shown to prolong life, fluorouracil is the treatment of choice in patients with advanced disease who are symptomatic or have difficulty in coping with not receiving treatment (Clark & Slevin 1987).

Bowel obstruction

This condition, common in old people, is frequently due to faecal impaction from unrelieved constipation which is liable to take place if the elderly patient is put to bed for any reason. Care must be exercised in bed-ridden patients to prevent constipation. Faecal impaction constitutes a serious danger to the well-being of old people. It adds to the nursing difficulties and medical care of those with serious or other complicating illness. Should it occur, for example, subsequent to a myocardial infarction, it makes an already ill patient extremely uncomfortable. Any elderly person reduced to bed should be considered to be at risk and if inadequate bowel movement is occurring purgatives such as Senokot or bisacodyl should be prescribed. If a tendency to constipation is seen to be developing this must be treated promptly and adequately. A rectal examination is essential routinely in old people and attention should be paid to diet and to the intake of fluids.

Volvulus, neoplasm of large bowel, diverticulitis and hernias are all common causes of bowel obstruction and occasionally the same syndrome may be due to occlusion of a mesenteric vessel. Bowel trapped in a scar from a previous operation or a strangulated hernia may not be diagnosed as such because there may be no pain or tenderness at the site of the hernia itself; the pain may be of a generalized nature while vomiting may develop only at a later stage. Adynamic ileus can be induced by hypokalaemia from prolonged use of diuretics.

Acute mesenteric thrombosis

This occurs in elderly patients with evidence of vascular disease such as peripheral arterial insufficiency or coronary artery disease and is accompanied by sudden severe abdominal pain. This may be associated with blood-stained diarrhoea and signs of shock. Diffuse abdominal tenderness and rigidity are found and a straight x-ray of abdomen may reveal a dilated loop of bowel showing a fluid level. Treatment is surgical; however prognosis is poor.

Chronic small bowel ischaemia

This can cause weight loss and malabsorption in association with abdominal pain after eating. Widespread vascular disease is usually present; nutritional deficiency should be corrected and small and frequent meals may decrease the patient's pain.

Appendicitis in the elderly

The main clinical features in patients over 60 years may be similar to those under 60: there is a striking difference in operative findings; both gangrenous changes and perforation of the appendix occur more frequently in the older age group. Typical clinical findings may be absent and the time lag between symptoms of appendicitis before patients seek medical advice is longer in elderly patients than in the young. Loe (1969) quoted a perforation rate of 68% in a consecutive series of 44 patients 65 years and over with appendicitis. The most serious finding is the rapid progression of the disease and thus correct diagnosis must be made promptly in elderly people. The treatment of choice is appendicectomy.

Carcinoma of colon and rectum

Diseases of premalignant nature affecting the colon or rectum are adenomatous polyps and chronic ulcerative colitis and patients with these conditions should be kept under observation. Calkins (1964) states that any patient with chronic ulcerative colitis requiring continuous medical treatment for 7–8 years should have a colectomy and any patient with the same illness with pseudo-polyps formation that does not reverse itself within 2 years on medical therapy should have a colectomy. These patients should certainly have regular sigmoidoscopic examinations and barium enemata. The rectum is the most common site of cancer of the gastrointestinal tract in elderly people with involvement of the sigmoid, the caecum and ascending colon next in order of frequency. Carcinoma of colon and rectum seems to be associated with the western style of life and with a diet low in roughage and including highly processed foods. Carcinoma of the descending colon and rectum tend to produce obstruction while cancer of the ascending colon is usually associated with symptoms of toxaemia. Change in bowel habit or intermittent bouts of diarrhoea are common symptoms. In the early stages of carcinoma of the colon diagnosis may be very difficult. Diarrhoea of more than 3 days' duration or recurrent in nature, especially if associated with phases of constipation should indicate the need for investigation: rectal examination, colonoscopy and barium enema. Patients with rectal carcinoma may present with bleeding from the rectum, tenesmus with mucus in the stool and a change in bowel habit. They may have a feeling of being unable to empty the rectum completely. Cancer of the descending colon frequently produces abdominal pain with a change in bowel action. The pain is left sided and unrelated to meals and a few patients notice rectal bleeding. The first sign of this illness may be complete intestinal obstruction. Cancer of the caecum and ascending colon is usually silent in the early states. The patient is frequently anaemic when first seen and may complain of an aching pain at the right side, worse after food and associated with nausea. These symptoms may mislead the physician who may attribute them to a gastric lesion. Anorexia and tiredness then develop and not infrequently the patient may present with angina pectoris or even congestive cardiac failure secondary to the anaemia. Colonoscopy is a worthwhile investigation for colonic lesions which are doubtful following radiology.

The treatment of cancer of the colon or rectum is by surgical operation; every possible step should be taken to avoid the creation of a permanent colostomy. Careful preoperative preparation is essential including blood transfusion if indicated. If bowel cancer is to be detected at an early stage the slightest suspicion of bowel disturbance or an episode of rectal bleeding, especially in middle-aged or elderly patients, should indicate complete clinical and radiological investigation. The presence of haemorrhoids should not be allowed to rule out a diagnosis of cancer of colon or rectum and a rectal examination should always be performed followed if negative by a sigmoidoscopy.

Malabsorption

In older people there are several varieties of this condition:
1   It is found as one of the consequences of partial gastrectomy, which include iron-deficiency anaemia and postgastrectomy bone disease. It is now recognized that this procedure is responsible on occasion for low serum vitamin B_{12} levels which can result in megaloblastic anaemia and subacute combined degeneration of the cord, and in the absence of Paget disease or hepatic dysfunction a raised serum alkaline phosphatase in postgastrectomy patients is usually indicative of either overt or subclinical osteomalacia. It is essential, therefore, that patients who have had this type of operation should be kept under observation. It is recommended that routine endoscopy for such patients who have survived 20 years should be undertaken to exclude malignant change in the stomach.
2   The use of essential substances for the health of the body by abnormal intestinal flora, e.g. in the blind-loop syndrome, can cause malabsorption.

This abnormality can occur when a so-called blind loop is formed as a result of some operative procedure and under certain conditions a growth of bacteria in the blind loop leads to a form of megaloblastic anaemia associated usually with steatorrhoea, because the bacteria use up the cyanocobalamin and probably other substances. A similar deficiency may occur from multiple jejunal diverticulosis but the gross deficiency state associated with gastrojejunocolic fistula is probably due to invasion of the small intestine by colonic bacteria.

3   Radiation-induced malabsorption can occur.

4   Any operation that removes large parts of the intestine, e.g. surgical treatment of superior mesenteric thrombosis, may produce malabsorption.

After a fashion it might be considered that these groups of illness are examples of iatrogenic disease so that a special responsibility rests with the doctor to be on the outlook for them.

5   Generalized conditions such as skin diseases, e.g. psoriasis, dermatitis herpetiformis and scleroderma or diseases associated with arteritis, e.g. rheumatoid arthritis may sometimes lead to malabsorption and deficiency states.

6   A more usual cause of malabsorption in the elderly is idiopathic steatorrhoea (Coeliac disease). The classical symptoms are weakness and weight loss associated with diarrhoea, characterized by the passage of bulky, frothy, offensive, pale stools. Anaemia and sore tongue are also commonly found. In the elderly bowel symptoms are infrequently found. In the case of an older person who is eating well but failing to gain weight the possibility of a diagnosis of steatorrhoea should be investigated; or if he has a persistent feeling of weakness and especially if a macrocytic anaemia is also present. The diagnosis of these conditions may be difficult and depends on the complete radiological examination of the gastrointestinal tract by a barium meal follow through, and if necessary barium enema. Biopsy of the mucosa of the small intestine in selected cases may be of further value when other tests are inconclusive. Tests of absorption are usually employed and the simplest of these is to measure the excretion of fat. The patient is placed on an ordinary ward diet for 3 days and the stools are collected for that period. The fat in the stools is estimated and normally not more than 6 g of fat pass into the stools each day. The same stool can be used for estimating nitrogen to measure the absorption of protein. Radioactive isotopes can be used also to study absorption. While there are many other tests a plan of investigation is required for each case, these include: the estimation of fat in stool as described above, a full blood count with absolute values, glucose tolerance test, estimation of the levels in the serum of vitamin B_{12} folate, iron, proteins, urea, potassium, calcium, phosphorus and alkaline phosphatase; a radioactive vitamin B_{12} absorp-

tion test may be required. Other tests would only be performed to elucidate doubtful findings. In order to carry out these procedures the patient must be in a hospital with the necessary facilities for undertaking such investigations.

7   Chronic pancreatitis may be of unknown aetiology or due to abuse of alcohol or to gallstone disease leading to damage of the pancreas. This condition may be associated with abdominal pain often radiating to the back or shoulder, anorexia, steatorrhoea, diarrhoea and mild diabetes. The diagnosis is confirmed by finding greatly reduced pancreatic enzyme secretion following the Lundh test meal. This measures the pancreatic response to a test meal containing corn or soya bean oil, Casilan and glucose. The tryptic activity of the duodenal juice is measured after the ingestion of the test meal. The lower the level of trypsin activity the more severe the pancreatic disease. The test cannot differentiate between chronic pancreatitis and malignant disease of the pancreas. Ultrasonography is useful for assessing pancreatic size.

Treatment

If there are any local abnormalities of the gastrointestinal tract that are amenable to surgery they should be treated. The advice of a surgeon should be taken in any case where there has been a previous gastrointestinal operation. In patients with the malabsorption state accompanied by pain, laparotomy should be considered to exclude malignant disease of the bowel. Oral chemotherapy may be of value where the blind-loop syndrome is suspected. In many cases no remediable cause can be found and in such people a trial period of 6–12 months with a gluten-free diet should be instituted as for patients with idiopathic steatorrhoea. If this is of no value then a low-fat, high-protein diet should be prescribed and the deficiencies of vitamins and minerals corrected. If steatorrhoea has been present for some time, osteomalacia may be found and parenteral vitamin D may be necessary. The vitamin B compound tablet, strong, BPC is indicated in a dose of two tablets three times per day if glossitis or cheilosis is present; while if iron-deficiency anaemia is found ferrous sulphate 0.2 g three times per day should be administered orally. In those cases resistant to oral iron therapy, parenteral iron should be given. The megaloblastic anaemia, if present, usually responds to folic acid, 15 mg daily, but there may be evidence of cyanocobalamin deficiency and this, if so indicated, should be given as hydroxocobalamin intramuscularly in a dose of 1000 µg initially and then 1000 µg three monthly. The presence of a haemorrhagic tendency may indicate the need for the administration of vitamin K. Prednisone, 20 mg daily, may temporarily improve absorption, but it should be used with caution in the elderly because of its decalcifying action and other side effects.

For patients with chronic pancreatitis pain should be relieved and small frequent meals may help. If gallstones are found cholecystectomy is indicated. Alcohol intake should be discontinued and insulin may be necessary for control if diabetes mellitus is present. Pancreatic extracts are used to treat the malabsorption and recently cimetidine and pancreatic extracts combined have been tried. The diet should be low in fat, high in protein and carbohydrate with as required supplementation with calcium, fat soluble vitamins and vitamin B_{12}.

Acute pancreatitis

In most cases gallstones or alcoholism are the causes; more rarely viral infections, drugs, e.g. thiazides, metabolic or endocrine disorders, e.g. hyperparathyroidism, hyperlipidaemia are aetiological factors.

In most patients abdominal pain in the epigastrium with radiation to the back is the presenting symptom. Nausea and vomiting are common while fever is sometimes noted. The abdomen is tender and distended and bowel sounds are diminished or absent. A left-sided pleurisy with pleural effusion may develop. The patient is shocked with tachycardia and there is elevation of serum amylase; there is also a leucocytosis with a high serum lipase. Ultrasound may reveal pancreatic swelling.

Treatment

Pain relief by pethidine is important while restoration and maintenance of intravascular volume is essential by fluids, e.g. plasma, dextran or blood. Watch must be kept for respiratory or cardiac failure. Oral intake is stopped and nasogastric suction is usually prescribed. If there is evidence of a cholecystitis accompanying the acute pancreatitis antibiotic therapy is justified (Borda 1987). Consultation with a surgical colleague is recommended regarding the need for operative intervention.

Ulcerative colitis

This is a chronic inflammatory disease of unknown origin affecting the colon and occasionally only the rectum. Symptoms are as in young people and consist of diarrhoea and rectal bleeding. Endoscopic examination and biopsy confirm the diagnosis while barium enema will reveal the extent of the lesion. Complications include perforation, massive haemorrhage, abscess formation and carcinoma while arthritis, liver disease, eye and skin lesions can occur.

Treatment

Mild disease is limited to the rectum or rectosigmoid area and here rectal bleeding is the only symptom while diarrhoea is mild. Corticosteroid retention enemas or sulphasalazine or both will control symptoms. Enemas are given twice per day for 2 weeks and once daily for 6 weeks. Sulphasalazine 2–4 g/day is prescribed initially and when improvement occurs 2 g/day is continued for an indefinite period if necessary. If there is no improvement or complications appear 40 mg of prednisone daily may be substituted with a return to sulphasalazine as improvement occurs. The long-term use of corticosteroids is not advisable in the elderly. For those with abdominal cramps, fever, weight loss, anaemia and continuing blood-stained diarrhoea prednisone in 40–60 mg daily and if necessary the addition of 2–4 g of sulphasalazine orally. This treatment can be continued for months if necessary. On occasion steroid retention enemas may also be required and replacement of fluid, blood and electrolytes as necessary with the addition of haematinics. A milk-free diet may be of help or parenteral feeding may be necessary. Prednisone is gradually discontinued in remission but the sulphasalazine should be continued. For the most severe cases intravenous infusion of 300 mg/day of hydrocortisone and tetracycline 1 g intravenously per day is required with adequate fluid replacement – blood and electrolytes. Surgery is indicated if no clear improvement occurs in a few days. This involves a panproctocolectomy with formation of an ileostomy.

Diverticulosis: diverticulitis

Diverticula of the gastrointestinal tract are most commonly found in the colon and Manousos, Truelove & Lumsden (1967) discovered in healthy volunteers in the Oxford area an incidence of diverticulosis of one in every three persons above the age of 60 years. Below that age the condition was present in 7.6% of the population studied, and it was more common in women than men. Slack (1967) felt that about one-fifth of those with diverticular disease would develop symptoms. This condition when symptom-free is called diverticulosis. Diverticulitis means by definition inflammation of the diverticula and is diagnosed by the presence of discomfort in the left iliac fossa associated with tenderness but perhaps more commonly in the elderly by intermittent attacks of diarrhoea alternating with constipation. Some patients have vague indigestion, flatulence or a feeling of distension. On occasion, however, the abdominal pain may be so severe that it mimics appendicitis although occurring on the left side of the abdomen or the condition may be discovered because of a profuse haemorrhage from the rectum. The colon may be thickened and tender but the final diagnosis will be made following a barium enema.

Treatment

During an acute attack with fever, leucocytosis and raised ESR, bed rest, liquid diet or in severe cases a nasogastric suction tube and parenteral feeding may be required. Ampicillin or tetracycline may be necessary at first intravenously and then orally. Pethidine may be necessary to relieve the pain and an antispasmodic drug such as mebeverine hydrochloride may help as may heat applied to the abdomen. When the acute attack has subsided a high roughage diet is prescribed with the addition of bran and if necessary a high fibre bulk laxative. Complications of diverticular disease include abscess formation, perforation, obstruction, fistula and haemorrhage; bleeding usually responds to blood transfusion. If haemorrhage is persistent the diagnosis may be incorrect and angiography has been advised in such cases (Venables 1980). Surgical treatment was discussed by Wheeler (1981).

Ischaemic colitis

The most vulnerable part is the splenic flexure and an attack of ischaemic colitis is usually precipitated by a drop in blood pressure. The symptoms are left-sided pain in the abdomen with loose blood-stained stools. Abdominal tenderness and distension with loss of intestinal sounds may be noted. Confirmation of the clinical findings can be obtained by a barium enema which may show the thumb print and the saw tooth signs. Treatment is conservative with fluids and antibiotics.

Angiodysplasia of the colon

This has become recognized as a common cause of colonic bleeding which arises from angiomas usually in the ascending colon. These can be diagnosed by colonoscopy or arteriography. Treatment is by endoscopic coagulation or by surgical resection.

Constipation

This condition may be defined as the infrequent passage of hard stools and occurs in elderly people who take to bed; inactivity is thus a cause. Transit time in bowel varies from person to person and is also altered by the composition of the diet. Any recent change of bowel habit demands serious consideration. Colonic cancer is one of the most common malignancies in the elderly while diverticular disease often presents with alternating bouts of constipation and diarrhoea. Drugs such as aluminium hydroxide or codeine, myxoedema, depression or confusional states may cause constipation as may painful conditions of the anus, e.g. fissure or haemorrhoids. The common sequel to constipation in the elderly is faecal impaction. The treatment of constipation depends on the diagnosis but initially bowel action usually has to be obtained. If faecal impaction is present this requires to be cleared (p. 71). Otherwise an irritant purgative, e.g. a preparation of senna or cascara given orally, causes bowel movement if these drugs are not contraindicated by the diagnosis. When a lubricant alone is indicated dioctyl sodium sulphosuccinate (Dioctyl-Medo) acts by lowering the surface tension of the faecal mass and allowing absorption of water. The attempt should also be made to alter the diet by increasing the bulk of the stool with a high-residue regimen including bran so that purgatives hopefully are only necessary for a short time. Physical activity should be increased where possible and as some old people seem to have a poor sensation of thirst, fluid intake should be increased.

When elderly people complain of problems with their bowels, e.g. constipation or diarrhoea, it is always essential to try to examine a sample of stool.

Diarrhoea

The occurrence of diarrhoea is a constant source of worry in a geriatric unit and a strict nursing routine must be observed whenever this condition is detected. A specimen of stool must be sent to the laboratory and every effort made to avoid spreading of the illness to other patients. The most common cause of diarrhoea in the elderly is probably dietetic indiscretion, e.g. too much fruit following a visiting day. Education of the general public is essential here and a notice advising relatives that the patients are adequately fed and often on a specific dietary regimen may help. Visitors are asked not to be smugglers of food but rather to bring flowers to their relatives in hospital.

Diarrhoea is noted when there is a change in bowel habit with an increase in the frequency, fluidity or volume of the stools; it is particularly distressing for the elderly as it may be associated with faecal incontinence. This condition must be regarded as a symptom and a search made for the cause. History must be taken in detail with reference to recent dietary intake or a change in dietary habits, to drug intake including purgatives and to the involvement of other members of the family. Clinical examination must include a rectal examination and if the condition lasts more than a few days admission to hospital should be considered. Acute diarrhoea is commonly due to infections with *Salmonella, Shigella* or *Campylobacter* bacilli. It can be explosive with severe water loss and then admission to hospital is essential as acute renal failure may develop.

The diagnosis is confirmed by stool culture and should be suspected if more than one person in the same household or institution is affected. If there is an appropriate antibiotic it should be given if not then codeine phosphate 15–30 mg two to three times daily may help; diphenoxylate hydrochloride BP with atropine sulphate (Lomotil) is a useful alternative.

Bacillary dysentery must be treated promptly; the organism is usually *Shigella sonnei*, and in older people the diarrhoea may be mild and accompanied by a febrile illness with headache and muscle aching, so that it can easily be overlooked. If a case of this illness develops in a ward, rectal swabs should be taken at once in order to save time and the bacteriologist should be brought into consultation immediately. All further admissions to the ward should be stopped and rectal swabs taken from all members of staff and from the patients in the ward. Where it is possible the patient should be transferred to a fever hospital as the illness can spread in geriatric units with great rapidity. Food utensils and bedpans of all positive cases should be sterilized, and with the assistance of a bacteriologist a routine system of personal hygiene explained to the nursing staff. Before discharge home or transfer back to the geriatric unit it is desirable to obtain three negative bacteriological reports on specimens of faeces.

For patients with bacillary dysentery, an initial period of rest in bed is advised in most cases and tetracycline is usually administered, as most endemic strains of *Shigella* in this country have acquired resistance to sulphonamides. If a strain that is sensitive to sulphonamides is found to be present sulphadiazine is a satisfactory preparation. If diarrhoea is severe it is necessary to correct any disturbance of water and electrolytes, a watch being kept for potassium deficiency. Symptomless carriers should be given appropriate antibiotics. It is possible that the increasing use of disposable bedpans may help to reduce the incidence of this illness in geriatric units.

Chronic diarrhoea may be due to carcinoma of colon or rectum and in the latter tenesmus is a common symptom. Other causes are diverticular disease, ulcerative colitis and less commonly carcinoma of the stomach or Crohn disease especially of the rectosigmoid colon. Faecal impaction must never be forgotten as well as the need to ask older people in detail about the drugs being taken which may well include a purgative.

Faecal incontinence

Faecal incontinence is not as common as urinary incontinence, and constipation is often present, the rectum being loaded with faeces. This retention of faeces may extend into the colon for a considerable distance. When this happens liquid faeces often pass the scybalous masses and leak from the anus giving rise to incontinence and spurious diarrhoea. A rectal examination reveals the diagnosis. In the presence of faecal incontinence if impaction of the rectum is not found and diarrhoea is present the faeces should be examined for pathogenic organisms and the presence of occult blood.

Brocklehurst (1987) discusses the mechanisms which maintain continence while Parks (1985) describes the pelvic floor musculature.

Local causes

Constipation. Loading of the rectum causes spurious diarrhoea and is often associated with urinary incontinence; elderly patients who are confused are less aware of loading of the rectum. Rectal examination discloses a rectum loaded with faeces, which may be hard or soft.

Diarrhoea. An attack of diarrhoea may precipitate faecal incontinence and bowel infection with coliform, dysenteric or food-poisoning organisms is a common cause of diarrhoea, which may be associated with mucus, blood and pus. Dietetic indiscretion may cause bowel disturbance, and in this country this usually consists of excessive amounts of food or food which has been unsuitably prepared, e.g. too much fat, with consequent diarrhoea and incontinence. Rarely insufficiency of protein or vitamins especially the B group also produce diarrhoea and incontinence. Non-specific inflammatory diseases such as ulcerative colitis and diverticultis may also cause incontinence.

Neoplasms of bowel. These conditions are often accompanied by occult or frank blood in the stools and may be associated with loss of weight, occasional pain and obstructive symptoms.

Malabsorption syndrome. This can occur in the elderly from a number of causes (p. 61) and may produce diarrhoea with light-coloured, bulky and offensive stools.

General causes

Organic cerebral disease, especially when dementia is a feature, is a common cause of faecal incontinence in the elderly. When the brain disease is generalized with severe dementia and apathy there is a lessened appreciation of distension of the rectum with consequent faecal impaction and spurious diarrhoea.

In other cases with a more selective injury to the motor area of the cortex or its fibres, the rectum becomes hypertonic and contracts more quickly and frequently than normal. Lesions of the spinal cord may produce a rectum acting automatically under poor control, and if the cauda equina or sensory nerves are affected the rectum becomes atonic with a lax sphincter.

Serious illness may produce incontinence of faeces especially when delirium is a feature.

Physical disability causing difficulty in walking or clumsiness can be a cause of accidental incontinence.

Excessive doses of drugs such as aperients, iron, antibiotics and digoxin may produce diarrhoea and incontinence. Sedatives may also cause incontinence by reducing the cerebral awareness and control.

Diabetes mellitus can cause faecal incontinence as this disease may produce diarrhoea.

Investigation

1   A detailed history is taken with special reference to the type and duration of the incontinence, previous health and operations, the character of the stool, and the patient's attitude to his incontinence.
2   A complete medical examination including a rectal is performed, with a test of the mental state.
3   The incontinence is recorded with regard to the amount, the timing and the stool characteristics.
4   A fresh specimen of stool should be sent for culture or a rectal swab may be used if found more convenient. The stool must also be tested for occult blood. Occasionally estimations of the faecal fat may be required.
5   Special investigations may be required such as proctoscopy, sigmoid-oscopy, barium studies and laparotomy.

Treatment

In any effort to retrain patients with faecal incontinence it is essential to make sure that the colon is emptied before training is started. When rectal impaction with faeces is present, suppositories are the best initial treatment; bisacodyl (Dulcolax) or anhydrous sodium acid phosphate and sodium bicarbonate in an inert base (Beogex) are both satisfactory. If unsuccessful, a hygroscopic enema may be used such as the Fletcher enema containing sodium phosphate and sodium acid phosphate in a 128 ml disposable plastic container. If the faeces are very hard, an arachis oil enema of similar volume can be inserted in the evening and retained, and the hygroscopic enema given on the following morning. Occasionally manual removal of faeces from the rectum is advisable.

Following the initial clearing of the bowel, aperients can be given; bisacodyl tablets (Dulcolax) 5 mg as required alone or combined with the faecal softener dioctyl sodium sulphosuccinate 100 mg (Dulcodos); alternative preparations include senna in the form of Senokot tablets or a faecal softener such as dioctyl sodium sulphosuccinate 100 mg (Dioctyl-Medo) or a bulk laxative such as Normacol. Neostigmine bromide (Prostigmin) 7.5–15 mg initially once then two to three times daily by mouth may be given to stimulate peristalsis for a few days after the lower bowel had been cleared. It is worthwhile taking trouble to find the most effective drug and the correct maintenance dose for each patient, and this is usually best given in the evening if the patient has not had a motion that day.

Supervision of the diet is important, including the ordering of a suitable amount, the elimination of foods that disagree with the patient, and the correction of any deficiencies. If the patient is inactive the addition of bran to the diet may help to avoid constipation.

If a bowel infection is present with diarrhoea and a pathogenic organism is isolated, an appropriate antibiotic is indicated. If no pathogen is isolated, Kaolin Mixture is given or Lomotil (diphenoxylate hydrochloride with atropine sulphate) 5 mg four times daily. It is advisable to withdraw the kaolin after 2 or 3 days if the diarrhoea has subsided to avoid the danger of faecal impaction.

Surgical opinion should be sought if an organic lesion of the bowel such as neoplasm is found.

When dementia is thought to be the cause of incontinence, habit-training is of prime importance and the patient should be taken to the toilet after meals and also first thing in the mornings. The nursing measures detailed for incontinence of urine (p. 185) are essential, and it may be mentioned here that the incontinence of formed stools is usually due to dementia. For all elderly patients unable to go to the toilet, a commode is preferable to a bedpan and this may be helpful in incontinence especially if privacy can be provided. In those cases associated with a series of uninhibited contractions of the rectum and reflex inhibition of tone in the external anal sphincter, treatment with chalk and opium is often successful. If all else fails, the routine administration of enemata two or three times weekly may keep the patient clean or at least reduce the amount of soiling at other times. A full description of retraining the patient is given by Willington (1976).

When physical disability is a problem, thought should be given to the patient's distance from the toilet, the provision of a commode, and the dressing of the patient in suitable clothing.

Antidepressant drugs such as mianserin (Bolvidon or Norval) may be exhibited when a functional cause such as depression is thought to be present.

When a patient is having recurrent bouts of diarrhoea with incontinence and no cause can be found, the physician should assess the drug regimen carefully as many drugs can cause diarrhoea in the elderly, particularly those mentioned above. Older people seldom volunteer information about taking purgatives and the direct question requires to be asked.

LIVER DISEASE

With increasing age hepatic function declines slowly as the liver's size and blood flow decreases. This is not demonstrated by conventional tests. Serum bilirubin, alkaline phosphatase and transaminase levels do not change with increasing age and this applies also to conjugation mechanisms, i.e. sulphation and glucuronidation. Known microsomal enzyme activity (oxidation, hydroxylation and demethylation) is mildly impaired. Kenny and colleagues (1984) described elevated serum alkaline phosphatase in elderly patients with extrahepatic infection; this is not found in younger people and might reflect an age-related change. When disease of the liver does occur there is a marked decline in such features as protein synthesis or the clearance of foreign or toxic material. Any past history of jaundice, hepatitis, alcoholism or recent hospital admission should be sought. Any drugs prescribed must be detailed as even a medicament taken in the preceding month may be responsible for a drug reaction.

Chronic progressive jaundice with weakness suggests liver disease while acute rapidly increasing jaundice with pruritus is found in extrahepatic obstruction or in cholestatic drug reaction. Liver failure is manifested by severe mental changes, coarse flapping tremor and eventual coma. Tiredness, fever and wasting are commonly noted in liver disease while jaundice may not be present. Spider naevi, finger clubbing, Dupuytren contracture and the non-specific signs of ascites and peripheral oedema may be present. Liver enlargement is variable and splenomegaly is found in portal hypertension. Blood tests are often difficult to interpret, but if serum transaminase is elevated to a much greater extent than alkaline phosphatase disease of the liver is likely while if alkaline phosphatase is more elevated cholestasis is present. Serum gamma glutamyl transpepti-dase if elevated confirms cholestatic disease and helps to indicate that the raised alkaline phosphatase is due to hepatic or gall-bladder disease and not to bone disease.

Radio-isotope imaging is most useful in diagnosing intrahepatic disease and computed tomography is comparable to ultrasound and is rarely necessary except in evaluating the operability of tumours. Percuta-neous transhepatic cholangiography or endoscopic retrograde cholangiog-raphy can provide accurate information about the condition of the biliary tree. The value of a straight x-ray of abdomen should not be forgotten but the ultimate diagnostic tool, when indicated in parenchymal liver disease is liver biopsy.

Cirrhosis

A common cause of this condition is alcohol; more rarely it is due to car-diac failure or haemochromatosis; in many elderly patients it is not possible to find a cause. In the treatment of cirrhosis, alcohol should be avoided and if there is oedema and ascites present, a diet low in salt and high in protein is advocated. If diuretic therapy is required frusemide is used and potassium supplements are almost certainly necessary. By the addition of amiloride or spironolactone to the drug regimen additional potassium can be avoided. Mineral and vitamin supplements are advised especially thiamine, pyridoxine, vitamins A, D, C and K and folic acid. The onset of encephalopathy is an indication for a low-protein diet with the administration of lactulose usually 20 ml twice per day. Constipation should be avoided by the use of suppositories.

Chronic active liver disease

This term excludes alcoholic cirrhosis, biliary cirrhosis or haemochroma-tosis. It is uncommon in the elderly and the clinical and laboratory findings are indistinguishable from acute viral hepatitis but with an insidious onset. Hypergammaglobulinaemia is present and haematological abnormalities include anaemia, thrombocytopaenia, leucopaenia and a high sedimentation rate. Abnormalities in the serum noted are the presence of LE cells, antinuclear factor and antismooth muscle antibodies. Liver biopsy confirms the diagnosis. Treatment in younger people is with corticosteroids and azathioprine but prolonged therapy in the elderly is dangerous and treatment with these drugs is only recommended in cases with severe symptoms.

Primary biliary cirrhosis

This occurs usually in elderly women and the small interlobular bile ducts are destroyed by inflammation. There is a gradually increasing cholestasis with eventual development of cirrhosis and its complications. No treatment is recommended for asymptomatic patients but it is suggested that those with fatigue should have their thyroid function tested as hypothyroidism is common. Pruritus is often the main symptom requiring treatment and cholestyramine is of use. Nutritional deficiency takes place due to anorexia and malabsorption and supplementation with vitamins D, K and A are of help while restriction of fat intake to 40 g/day improves the steatorrhoea. Azathioprine may be of some benefit (Finlayson 1987).

Reactions to drugs

Drugs may cause either hepatitis, e.g. halothane, or cholestasis, e.g. chlorpromazine.

Tumours

Metastatic liver disease presents with weight loss and hepatomegaly and blood tests show elevation of alkaline phosphatase and γ-glutamyl transpeptidase, while a liver scan reveals multiple filling defects. Where essential, a liver biopsy establishes the diagnosis and detects potentially curable lymphomas.

Primary liver carcinoma usually occurs in a liver damaged by alcohol, hepatitis B virus infection or haemochromatosis.

GALLSTONES

The main problem is to give advice to elderly people in whom a gallstone is found as part of a routine physical examination during investigation for some other illness. In one series gallstones were found on autopsy in 29% of 1057 patients over the age of 80 years. The advice then was that in those over 70 years the stone should be left unless severe symptomatology was present (Amberg & Zboralske 1965). Since then the gallstone if found by chance under certain conditions can be treated medically. Chenodeoxycholic acid or more recently ursodeoxycholic acid dissolves gallstones provided:

1 They are small cholesterol stones in a functioning gall-bladder.
2 The treatment is taken regularly for a prolonged period.
3 During therapy watch must be kept for alteration in liver function.

The dose of chenodeoxycholic acid is 15 mg/kg body weight per day. Thus three to five capsules are taken daily for up to 2 years. Diarrhoea is common and usually responds to anti-diarrhoeal agents. This drug is contraindicated in inflammation of the gastrointestinal tract or of the liver or biliary system and also in severe kidney impairment. Ursodeoxycholic acid is given in a dose of 8–10 mg/kg, i.e. three to four tablets of 150 mg per day. The appropriate dose is taken in two administrations after meals. Treatment may last 2 years and is contraindicated in similar conditions to chenodeoxycholic acid.

The recently developed technique of extracorporeal shock wave lithotripsy may be a useful addition to chenodeoxycholic acid and ursodeoxycholic acid in the treatment of solitary gall-bladder stones up to 30 mm in diameter (Sackmann *et al.* 1988).

An entirely different approach should be in mind for the patient who has had an attack of jaundice or recurrent bouts of biliary colic or cholecystitis. Such incidents almost certainly become more frequent and the patient's condition deteriorates. Chronic and recurrent biliary disease leads to liver damage, and at an optimum time operation is indicated.

Acute biliary disease

Tweedie (1987) reviewed the diagnosis and treatment of acute biliary diseases. The complications of calculous biliary disease in the gall-bladder are biliary colic, acute and chronic cholecystitis, carcinoma; in the bile ducts, obstructive jaundice, acute pancreatitis, acute suppurative obstructive cholangitis and in the intestine, acute intestinal obstruction.

Biliary colic

Bile duct stones are common in patients with gallstones in the gall-bladder. The classical presentation is of biliary colic, jaundice and cholangitis, but in the elderly pyrexia of unknown origin, septicaemic shock, pancreatitis, jaundice suggesting malignancy or abnormal liver function without jaundice may occur.

In this condition the first essential is the relief of pain and for this pethidine by slow intravenous infusion is useful; if vomiting is a feature fluids must be given intravenously and nasogastric intubation will be necessary. Investigations will be required as soon as possible to determine the diagnosis.

Acute and chronic cholecystitis

This illness presents with anorexia, nausea, vomiting, fever and pain in the right hypochondrium where there is marked tenderness. If jaundice is present it may indicate calculous obstruction of the common bile duct. If obstruction at the gall-bladder persists the organ may become filled with pus producing an empyema of the gall-bladder and this affects mainly the elderly.

Rarely in cholecystitis no calculi are demonstrated. Routine investigations include blood count, amylase estimation, urine analysis, chest x-ray and ECG. If jaundice is present, serum alkaline phosphatase, transaminases and bilirubin should be estimated. Other important investigations as necessary include straight x-ray abdomen, ultrasonography, scintigrapy, percutaneous transhepatic cholangiography. Endoscopic retrograde cholangiography as well as providing a diagnosis can remove common bile duct stones by sphincterotomy or in obstruction due to carcinoma allow an internal drainage catheter to be passed to provide a palliative surgical bypass.

Treatment

Conservative management with antibiotic treatment supported by intravenous fluids and analgesia is now being superseded by good preoperative preparation and surgery as promptly as is possible; the aim is cholecystectomy. The elderly person with jaundice due to stones in the common bile duct should be managed by endoscopic sphincterotomy and gallstone removal.

Jaundice in the elderly

In the elderly jaundice is most commonly obstructive in type; the most common cause of obstruction is malignant disease with calculi next and the toxic effects of drugs the least common. Hepatocellular damage is found even less commonly and haemolytic jaundice is rare. Everyone agrees that painless jaundice in the elderly is frequently due to a stone in the common bile duct. Drugs such as chlorpromazine, phenylbutazone, methyltestosterone, norethandrolone, thiouracil, and sulphonamides can cause jaundice due to biliary canalicular stasis, and enquiry about the administration of drugs should be made in all patients with this sign. The diagnostic difficulty lies mainly in those with jaundice due to hepatocellular damage. Laparotomy in the presence of viral hepatitis carries the danger of hepatic failure; surgical advice should be sought as soon as possible.

REFERENCES

Amberg J.R. & Zboralske F.F. (1965) Gallstones after 70. *Geriatrics* **20**, 539.

Borda I.T. (1987) Drug treatment of gastro-intestinal disorders. In *Clinical Pharmacology in the Elderly* (Ed. Swift C.G.) New York, Marcel Dekker, Inc.

Brocklehurst J. (1987) Disorders of the lower bowel. In *Practical Geriatric Medicine* (Ed. Exton-Smith A.N. & Weksler M.E.) Edinburgh, Churchill Livingstone.

Calkins W.G. (1964) Premalignant gastrointestinal lesions. *Geriatrics* **19**, 707.

Clark P.I. & Slevin M.L. (1987) Chemotherapy for stomach cancer. *British Medical Journal* **295**, 870.

Croker J.R. (1982) Dysphagia. *Geriatric Medicine* **12**, 71.

Elizabeth J., Barr H. & Krasner N. (1987) Oesophago-gastric tumour in old age: palliative treatment by laser photocoagulation. *Age and Ageing* **16**, 234.

Finlayson N.D.C (1987) Treatment in primary biliary cirrhosis. *British Medical Journal* **295**, 867.

Gupta S.D., Petrus L.V., Gibbins F.J. & Dellipiani A.W. (1987) Endoscopic evaluation of dysphagia in the elderly. *Age and Ageing* **16**, 159.

Kenny R.A.M., Hodkinson H.M., Prendiville O.F., Hayes M.C. & Flynn M.D. (1984) Abnormalities of liver function and the predictive value of liver function tests in infection and outcome of acutely ill elderly patients. *Age and Ageing* **13**, 224.

Loe R.H. (1969) Acute appendicitis in senior citizens. *Postgraduate Medicine* **45**, 179.

McMillan I.K.R. & Hyde K. (1969) Compression of the oesophagus by the aorta. *Thorax* **24**, 32.

Manousos O.N., Truelove S.C. & Lumsden K. (1967) Prevalence of colonic diverticulosis in general population of Oxford area. *British Medical Journal* **3**, 762.

Parks Sir A. (1985) The physiology and pathophysiology of the pelvic floor musculature. In *Principles and Practice of Geriatric Medicine* (Ed. Pathy M.S.J.) Chichester, John Wiley & Sons.

Prichard P.J., Rubinstein D., Jones D.B., Dudley F.J., Smallwood R.A., Louis W.J. & Yeomans N.D. (1985) Double blind comparative study of omeprazole 10 mg and 30 mg daily for healing duodenal ulcers. *British Medical Journal* **290**, 601.

Sackmann M. *et al.* (1988) Shock wave lithotripsy of gall bladder stones. *New England Journal of Medicine* **318**, 393.

Slack W.W. (1967) The pathology of diverticular disease of the colon. *Hospital Medicine* **1**, 1095.

Smith J. (1979) Oral and dental discomfort – a necessary feature of old age? *Age and Ageing* **8**, 25.

Tweedie J.H. (1987) Management of acute biliary disease. *British Journal of Hospital Medicine* **37**, 53.

Venables C.W. (1980) Gastrointestinal bleeding; advances in the management of gastrointestinal bleeding. *British Journal of Hospital Medicine* **23**, 338.

Wheeler M.H. (1981) Acute gastrointestinal bleeding. In *Acute Geriatric Medicine* (Ed. Coakely D.) London, Croom Helm.

Willington F.L. (1976) *Incontinence in the Elderly*. London, Academic Press.

Wright A.J. (1985) An unusual but easily treatable cause of dysphagia and dysarthria complicating stroke. *British Medical Journal* **291**, 1412.

6
Heart Disease

Heart disease is the most important single cause of death in old age in both sexes worldwide. Over the age of 65 years heart disorders account for more than 70% of all cardiovascular deaths in many countries. The most important form of heart disease is ischaemic heart disease. There has been a recent fall in the mortality from ischaemic heart disease in men and women over 75 years of age, although the incidence of ischaemic heart disease does rise dramatically with age and women develop myocardial infarction about 10 years on average after men.

Many surveys of elderly population groups have noted a high prevalence of heart disease (Kennedy *et al.* 1977). In relatively fit elderly subjects living at home 40% in the age group of 65–74 years and 50% in the age group of 75 years and over have undoubted evidence of heart disease. Evidence of ischaemic heart disease is present in 20% of men and 12% of women over the age of 65 years, and hypertensive heart disease is present in 8–13% of men and 12–16% of women over the age of 65 years. Rheumatic heart disease and pulmonary heart disease are relatively uncommon in elderly populations. Electrocardiographic abnormalities are commonly found in symptomatic and asymptomatic elderly subjects.

The prevalence and the incidence of cardiac failure increases with age and heart disease is a major contributory factor to a loss of independence in disabled elderly subjects living at home.

Pomerance (1981) has observed that many pathological changes are present in the majority of elderly subjects, e.g. coronary atheroma, but these should be regarded as diseases and not normal age changes. The incidence of most cardiac disorders and especially ischaemic heart disease increases with age and a variety of heart diseases, for example senile primary cardiac amyloidosis, calcific degenerative disease, primary mucoid degenerative valve disease and non-bacterial thrombotic endocarditis occur predominantly or exclusively in the old.

Diagnosis

The analysis of cardiac symptoms in elderly patients is often made difficult by a lack of an accurate history owing to mental confusion or failing

78

memory. As in diseases of the respiratory system, the symptoms are often insidious and may be attributed by both patient and doctor to the age process itself. The most striking symptom of heart disease is often not breathlessness but lethargy. Many elderly subjects admit to breathlessness on close questioning, but this may not be a commanding symptom due to restricted exercise tolerance from arthritis or neuromuscular disorders. Episodic breathlessness at night is suggestive of paroxysmal nocturnal dyspnoea and underlying left heart failure. Cardiac pain is usually less commanding or even absent in elderly patients with ischaemic heart disease. Angina may be less likely due to reduced activity or reduced exercise tolerance, but the reasons for the reduced incidence of cardiac pain in old age are not clear. Ankle swelling may be due to the oedema of congestive heart failure, but by itself is more likely to be due to poor venous return or hypoproteinaemia.

Careful clinical examination can detect abnormalities of cardiac rhythm, evidence of valvular disease and clinical signs of heart failure. Sclerosis of the radial and brachial arteries have no special clinical significance. The slow rising pulse of severe aortic stenosis and the collapsing pulse of aortic regurgitation may be identified although the former may be masked by an age-related increase in the rate of the arterial upstroke due to increased stiffness of the vessel wall. The blood pressure should be measured in both the lying and standing positions or the lying and sitting positions. A drop of 20 mm or more in the systolic pressure should be taken as evidence of significant postural blood pressure drop and symptoms may occur particularly if the systolic pressure falls below 110 mm Hg on assuming the erect position. The venous pulse is often easier to detect in the elderly due to atrophy of the skin and subcutaneous tissues. Obstruction of the venous return in the left innominate vessel is often present, and this is due to elongation and unfolding of the aorta, a phenomenon that disappears on deep inspiration. Praecordial palpation usually helps to detect enlargement of the ventricles and identify abnormal pulsations, e.g. left ventricular dyskinesia. The apex beat may be displaced by chest deformities due to kyphoscoliosis or by left ventricular enlargement. The character of the apex beat is more important than the site, and it is forcible in left ventricular hypertrophy but diffuse in left ventricular dilatation. Severe right ventricular hypertrophy is rare in old age, but a palpable exaggerated right ventricular impulse at the left sternal border can be detected in pulmonary hypertension which is usually due to rheumatic mitral valve disease or occasionally atrial septal defect.

Systolic murmurs show an increased prevalence with age and are more common in women. They may be detected in as many as 60% of otherwise cardiovascular normal elderly subjects. Most are due to multiple aortic or mitral minor valve abnormalities usually due to calcific degenerative change. Diastolic murmurs are always abnormal and are usually due to mitral stenosis or aortic regurgitation. It is often difficult to differentiate on auscultation between aortic and mitral valve murmurs due to kyphoscoliosis and the elderly patient's difficulty in breathholding. Aortic systolic murmurs are usually ejection or non-pansystolic and heard at the second right intercostal space with radiation to the right carotid artery and left sternal border but they may be louder at the apex. Mitral systolic murmurs are usually pansystolic, best heard at the apex and radiate to the left axilla but they may be atypical and be best detected at the base of the heart.

Cardiac investigation

Chest radiograph

Although there are difficulties in interpreting chest radiographs in elderly patients, evidence of cardiac enlargement, pulmonary oedema or congestive heart failure may be observed. Unfolding of the aorta is often associated with an age-related prevalence of calcification particularly in elderly women and calcification in the cardiac valves is evidence of significant valvular disease. Lateral radiographs may help identify areas of calcification particularly in the presence of costal cartilage or tracheobronchial calcification.

Electrocardiogram (ECG)

There is an increased incidence of ECG abnormality with advancing age (Fisch 1981). There is little evidence that ECG abnormalities are normal age-related variants in old age or that a different coding for normality should be defined. The ECG is of greatest value in elucidating dysrhythmias and may be of assistance in the diagnosis of metabolic disorders including hypothyroidism, potassium and calcium imbalance. Significant changes include Q/QS patterns, ST–T patterns including T wave flattening, left ventricular hypertrophy in association with ST–T changes, left-bundle branch block and right-bundle branch block. Continuous telemetric ECG monitoring may be helpful in diagnosing transient dysrhythmias in elderly patients with intermittent symptoms.

Echocardiogram

Echocardiography is a useful non-invasive technique for investigation of the left heart including structural changes in the valves, valvular movement, cavity dimensions and thickness of the wall. Cardiac tumours, pericardial changes (calcification, effusion and fibrosis) and the valvular vegetations of infective endocarditis may be visualized.

Cardiac scintiscan

Radio-isotope scanning using Technetium or Thallium is relatively non-invasive. This technique gives reliable measurements of cardiac chamber volumes, regional myocardial perfusion and indices of ventricular performance, e.g. ejection fraction and regional wall motion.

More invasive investigation techniques, for example cardiac catheterization and angiocardiography, should only be considered in elderly cardiac subjects when surgical intervention is proposed, as for example, in myocardial revascularization procedures or valve replacement, when a proper assessment of the coronary vessel circulation and left ventricular function is necessary before operation.

Cardiac dysrhythmias

The resting heart rate alters very little with age although there does appear to be an age-related fall in maximum heart rates on exercise. The resting cardiac output does not fall with age alone and the cardiac output can rise considerably with stress due to increases in the stroke volume and the heart rate. The ageing myocardium is more vulnerable to biochemical insults which produce irritability, for example hypoxia or hypokalaemia.

Ectopic activity (extrasytoles)

These are the most common cause of an irregular rhythm. Occasional atrial or ventricular ectopic beats are present in almost half of the apparently healthy elderly population and they are of little clinical significance, but frequent ectopic activity is less common and may be due to cardiac disease, metabolic disorders, hypoxia or digoxin toxicity. The elderly person who becomes aware of palpitation for the first time should be examined with care and have an electrocardiogram. Tobacco, excess tea or coffee and even a heavy meal on retiring may be associated with ectopic beats, and if relevant these factors should be eliminated as part of a rational regimen. Underlying causes of frequent ectopic activity may require separate treatment.

Supraventricular dysrhythmias

Sinus bradycardia with a heart rate of less than 60/min may be physiological, but causes can include hypothyroidism, obstructive jaundice, myocardial infarction or sino-atrial dysfunction (the sick sinus syndrome). Other possible causes include digoxin or β-blocking drugs. Treatment of sinus bradycardia is required during acute myocardial infarction or when symptoms of reduced cardiac output are present. Precipitating causes must be removed or treated and atropine or isoprenaline may be required as a temporary measure. Long-term drug therapy is rarely useful and cardiac pacemaking may be required. Sinus tachycardia with heart rates of over 100 beats/min may be due to extracardiac causes like fever, infection, anxiety, pulmonary embolism, anaemia, hyperthyroidism, metabolic upsets, hypoxia, hypovolaemic states and cardiac causes, for example acute myocardial infarction or heart failure. Treatment is usually restricted to management of underlying causes.

Atrial fibrillation

This condition is the most frequent dysrhythmia after multiple ectopic beats observed in old age. The presence of atrial fibrillation constitutes an unfavourable prognostic feature in congestive cardiac failure, but the dysrhythmia does not, however, carry the same serious significance as in the young in the absence of clinically demonstrable heart disease. The dysrhythmia may be temporary, paroxysmal or chronic and the temporary form is often associated with acute illnesses like myocardial infarction or infections. Rheumatic heart disease is an unlikely cause of atrial fibrillation in the elderly, but this dysrhythmia in response to hyperthyroidism occurs almost exclusively in elderly patients. Lone atrial fibrillation without evidence of heart disease carries an increased risk of thromboembolism and stroke (Brand *et al.* 1985). Elderly patients with atrial fibrillation may be asymptomatic or they may suffer from palpitation or breathlessness, confusion, syncope or manifestations of peripheral arterial embolization. The irregular radial pulse may be associated with a pulse deficit, a singular jugular venous wave, variable intensity of the first heart sound and the ECG is diagnostic.

Treatment

In atrial fibrillation with a normal ventricular rate and no adverse haemodynamic consequences no treatment is necessary. Fast ventricular rates require treatment and spontaneous reversion to sinus rhythm may occur if underlying causes, for example infection, are controlled. Fast atrial fibrillation with or without cardiac failure requires urgent treatment, and it is in patients with atrial fibrillation and congestive cardiac failure that the action of digoxin is seen to its best advantage. The aim is to maintain the heart rate between 60 and 80 beats/min. Digoxin is absorbed rapidly after oral medication and therapeutic serum levels are reached within 1 hour and are maintained for 6 hours or more. Parental digoxin is rarely justified unless the patient has dysphagia or compliance is a problem. Intramuscular digoxin is painful due to muscle necrosis, but intravenous administration may be indicated in life-threatening circumstances. An oral loading dose of 0.75 mg or 0.5 mg with 0.25 mg maintenance daily should produce serum digoxin concentrations within the therapeutic range without the risk of toxicity within 48 hours when renal function is normal or near normal. If renal function is impaired a loading dose of 0.5 mg followed by maintenance with 0.125 mg daily should be appropriate. A maintenance dose of 0.0625 mg is rarely adequate for the elderly. Constant watch must be kept for toxic effects on the one hand and for escape from the effects of the drug on the other. Most of the toxic effects of digitalis therapy occur in elderly patients with advanced heart disease and atrial fibrillation who are receiving injudicious maintenance dosage. Toxicity is more likely in the presence of poor renal function, severe hypokalaemia, hypercalcaemia, hypothyroidism or after acute myocardial infarction. The value of plasma digoxin concentrations, particularly for the diagnosis of toxicity has been questioned. Severe anorexia and other gastrointestinal symptoms may predominate in the elderly, particularly in females. Confusion may be the major presenting feature and gynaecomastia and xanthopsia are rare. Cardiac dysrhythmias are common manifestations of digitalis toxicity in the elderly. Most dysrhythmias or degrees of atrioventricular block can occur, although the most common cardiac toxic manifestation is of ventricular bigeminy. Multifocal ventricular ectopic activity may occur and paroxysmal atrial tachycardia is typically associated with atrioventricular block. Patients on long-term digoxin should be reviewed regularly, and unless there is good reason for continuing the drug it should be stopped. This is particularly the case when atrial fibrillation has been precipitated by an acute cause such as pneumonia and spontaneous reversion to sinus rhythm has occurred. Digoxin should never be given in hospital practice until the prescribing physician is satisfied that the patient has not received the drug outside and until the previous dosage is clarified. If digitalis intoxication is suspected, the drug must be withdrawn, potassium supplements administered to correct hypokalaemia and dysrhythmias should be managed appropriately. Lignocaine or phenytoin can correct ventricular tachyarrhythmias and supraventricular tachycardia will respond to β-blockade.

Poor control of the ventricular rate in atrial fibrillation by digoxin may suggest underlying thyrotoxicosis or cardiac amyloid disease and the addition of a β-blocking agent, e.g. propranolol 40–160 mg daily in divided doses, may improve ventricular rate control. If no primary cause for the dysrhythmia has been found and digoxin fails to control the ventricular rate other drug options should be considered. A number of agents can be given alone or in combination with digoxin. Disopyramide, verapamil, flecainide and amiodarone can control the ventricular rate or, in some cases, restore sinus rhythm. Disopyramide tends to have side effects particularly in elderly males. Amiodarone can adversely affect thyroid and liver function and induce a slate grey skin pigmentation. It should only be used when other drugs prove ineffective. The combination of digoxin and quinidine should be avoided as long-term treatment can induce a marked increase in the serum digoxin level with an increase in toxicity.

Electrical cardioversion should be limited to atrial fibrillation of recent onset. Before cardioversion heart failure should be controlled and oral anticoagulants should be given to prevent thromboembolism. The long-term success of cardioversion is limited if the atrial fibrillation has been present for more than 6 months or if there is marked cardiac enlargement, heart failure, significant valvular disease or underlying thyrotoxicosis. The recurrence rate of atrial fibrillation is high in the elderly.

Atrial flutter

This condition has a similar aetiology to atrial fibrillation in the elderly. The dysrhythmia is usually associated with underlying organic heart disease and although it usually produces a heart rate of 130–170/min, different degrees of heart block and varying heart block can result in ventricular rates as low as 50/min or a totally irregular rhythm clinically indistinguishable from atrial fibrillation. The diagnosis can only be confirmed with the help of an electrocardiogram. Treatment is usually digitalization and the flutter rhythm may be converted to sinus rhythm or atrial fibrillation. If digitalization fails to control the rhythm then other useful drugs include β-blocking agents or verapamil. If drug therapy is ineffective electroconversion or atrial pacing may be indicated.

Paroxysmal supraventricular tachycardia

The paroxysmal tachycardias are characterized by a rapid heart rate and the patient may give a history of sudden onset of palpitation, which may be associated with faintness or occasionally with convulsions. The heart rate is usually between 130 and 180/min. The dysrhythmia is usually associated in elderly patients with ischaemic heart disease, digoxin toxicity, the Wolff–Parkinson–White syndrome or malignant disease of the thorax. Paroxysmal supraventricular tachycardia is not well tolerated in the elderly and it may precipitate heart failure or symptoms of myocardial ischaemia. Treatment includes vagal stimulation using carotid sinus massage or the valsalva manoeuvre. Digitalization may be necessary. If the dysrhythmia is life-threatening direct current cardioversion may be a successful treatment. Paroxysmal atrial tachycardia with 2–1 or 3–1 atrioventricular block is usually due to digoxin toxicity, but it can occur in some forms of organic heart disease. If the dysrhythmia is digoxin associated then the digoxin therapy must be stopped and any existing potassium depletion must be corrected slowly. If further treatment is required then β-blocking drugs or phenytoin may be effective. If digoxin therapy is not the cause then digitalization is indicated.

Sino-atrial disorder

This condition, often named the sick sinus syndrome, is common in old age and occurs in two main forms with either predominant bradyarrhythmias or alternating tachycardia and bradycardia with long periods of asystole following termination of the tachycardia. Clinical features may include no symptoms but the condition can present with unexplained falls, bradycardia, atrial fibrillation with a slow ventricular response or Stokes–Adams attacks. The natural course of this disorder is not clear, but it is likely to be a relatively benign condition and permanent cardiac pacemaking is only required if symptoms are particularly troublesome.

Ventricular dysrhythmias

Ventricular tachycardia is usually a complication of acute myocardial infarction, and if it is producing disturbance of consciousness or cardiac failure it should be treated with synchronized electrical shock and correction of any co-existing metabolic acidosis. If the ventricular tachycardia is recurrent a number of drugs may be useful including phenytoin or disopyramide, but the latter agent is contraindicated if congestive cardiac failure or gross cardiomegaly are present as the profound negative inotropic effect of disopyramide may depress atrioventricular conduction, aggravate hypotension and heart failure.

Primary ventricular fibrillation is a complication of acute myocardial infarction in 4% of the elderly treated in Coronary Care Units (Williams *et al.* 1976). This life-threatening dysrhythmia must be treated with urgent unsynchronized electrical shock in full doses.

Conduction defects

Disorders of cardiac conduction are common in the elderly population and treatment is generally directed to the management of associated causes or if symptoms occur.

Bundle branch block

Right-bundle branch block is more common than left-bundle branch block in old age. Bundle branch blocks are not usually associated with symptoms in themselves, but symptoms of co-existing cardiac disease may be present and the conduction disorder may progress to complete heart block with Stokes–Adams attacks.

Atrioventricular block

This condition is usually defined in three degrees or grades.

1   First-degree or latent heart block is an ECG abnormality where the PR interval is prolonged beyond the upper limit of normal which is 0.22 seconds. Although this conduction defect may be found in 2% of ECGs of otherwise healthy old people, in most cases the cause is unknown and its prognostic significance is doubtful.

2   Second-degree heart block may be associated with a progressively lengthening PR interval until a ventricular beat fails to occur, or it may be associated with a constant PR interval and occasional dropped beats.

3   Third-degree or complete heart block occurs when there is no conduction between the atria and ventricles, and this condition is usually associated with chronic degenerative or ischaemic heart disease.

Symptoms of acute or chronic heart block are due to bradycardia when the heart rate falls below 40 beats/min. Stokes–Adams attacks are characterized by transient syncopal episodes associated with ventricular asystole, bradycardias or supraventricular or ventricular tachycardias. The objectives of treatment of complete heart block or lesser degrees of block are to increase the ventricular rate to minimize the risk of Stokes–Adams attacks, prevent cardiac failure and to reduce the likelihood of life-threatening ventricular dysrhythmias. In acute complete heart block an isoprenaline intravenous infusion may increase the ventricular rate in a dosage regimen of 0.02–0.10 µg/kg of body weight/min. The effect of oral isoprenaline in chronic states is unpredictable and often ineffective. In these circumstances a trial of transvenous endocardial pacemaking is indicated with implantation of a permanent pacemaker as required. The decision to pace the asymptomatic elderly patient with complete heart block is a difficult one. It is probably not necessary to advise permanent pacing if the ventricular rate accelerates with atropine or exercise. A common clinical problem is that of the elderly patient with a chronic confusional state and complete heart block. Chronic complete heart block can cause an ischaemic encephalopathy resulting in dementia and this may sometimes remit with the use of permanent cardiac pacemaking. A trial of pacing is indicated in these circumstances, but the trial must continue for at least 1 week to determine if permanent pacemaking is required.

ISCHAEMIC HEART DISEASE

Angina pectoris

Anginal pain is often less severe in the elderly than in middle-aged patients. This may be due to a reduction in normal physical activity or an altered pain perception. The pain is usually effort induced but can occur at rest or in bed. Physical signs may be absent but clinical features of left ventricular dysfunction, anaemia, hypothyroidism or aortic valve disease may be present.

Management should include weight reduction where indicated, avoidance of cigarettes and regular exercise. Glyceryl trinitrate 0.5 mg is the drug of choice and tablets can be chewed and allowed to lie in the buccal mucosa until the pain is relieved and then swallowed. Failure of pain control with nitrates is an indication for the use of β-adrenergic blocking drugs and propranolol may be administered orally in divided dosage in a total of 40–480 mg daily. Nifedipine, a vasodilator and calcium antagonist, is useful in the treatment of intractable angina in the elderly. This drug should be administered orally in doses of 10 mg thrice daily. Verapamil is well tolerated in the elderly and this drug should be given in a total daily dose of 120–360 mg in divided doses. Constipation may be a troublesome side effect. Failure of medical treatment to control angina may be an indication for coronary angioplasty or aorta-coronary bypass surgery in the elderly. Advanced age should not exclude a patient from consideration for myocardial revascularization procedures. Coronary artery bypass surgery performed for angina in the elderly gives long-term results that are satisfactory and comparable with the results obtained in younger patients (Rahimtoola *et al.* 1986).

Acute myocardial infarction

The clinical features of acute myocardial infarction may be extremely variable in the elderly. Although the classical presentation with chest pain and breathlessness is quite common, atypical presentations are more frequent in the elderly than in younger patients (MacDonald 1984). Painless infarction is common (Bayer *et al.* 1986). Major presentations may include breathlessness, exacerbation of heart failure or neurological manifestations (Table 6.1). Less common symptoms include palpitation, vomiting or sweating.

Table 6.1 Presentation of acute myocardial infarction in the elderly.

Chest pain or tightness
Dyspnoea
Exacerbation of heart failure
Acute confusion
Stroke
Syncope
Giddiness
Sudden death

Acute myocardial infarction should be suspected in any elderly person who has a sudden unexplained change in behaviour, poor cerebral perfusion or unexplained abdominal pain or hypotension. The diagnosis is based on the history and physical examination and confirmed by ECG and cardiac enzyme evidence. Clinical signs may include hypotension, left ventricular enlargement, a fourth heart sound and a transient pericardial friction rub. A soft pansystolic mitral murmur may be due to papillary muscle dysfunction or left ventricular dilatation.

Most elderly patients with acute myocardial infarction have dysrhythmias or conduction defects, but only a minority of these are of any clinical significance. The severity of myocardial infarction increases with age and the complications of conduction defects and atrial fibrillation and flutter are more common in old age as are the shock picture, pulmonary oedema and congestive cardiac failure.

Management

The majority of elderly survivors of uncomplicated acute myocardial infarction are probably best managed at home, but hospital admission is indicated if the patient continues to have symptomatic bradycardia, an unstable cardiac state after 3 hours, heart failure, hypotension, or has been resuscitated from a cardiac arrest. Social factors are very important and the patient may prefer to stay at home or the home circumstances may be unsuitable for domiciliary medical and nursing care. Rapid pain relief should be achieved with morphine 5–10 mg or diamorphine 2.5–5 mg intravenously. In the anxious patient general sedation may be achieved with diazepam 2–5 mg in the short term. Bed rest is necessary for a few days only and in mild uncomplicated cases the patient should normally be up and about by the end of the first week. Prolonged bed rest should be avoided to avoid problems of constipation, venous thrombosis, hypostatic pneumonia and impairment of the normal physiological regulating mechanisms with cardiovascular deconditioning and postural hypotension.

In selected elderly patients with acute myocardial infarction in coronary care units the risk of mortality can be reduced with the early intravenous use of the thrombolytic agent streptokinase (Italian Group, 1986) or the β-blocking agent atenolol (ISIS–1 Collaborative Group, 1986).

Routine anticoagulant therapy may protect the elderly patient against thromboembolism and short-term parenteral heparin therapy should be given to high risk elderly patients after severe infarction, in prolonged bed rest, with obesity or where a previous history of venous disease is elicited. Anticoagulant regimens can be stopped when the patient is fully ambulant but contraindictions to therapy include active ulceration of the gastro-intestinal tract, severe renal or hepatic disease, anaemia, pericarditis, acute stroke or significant systemic hypertension. Bladder care may be a particular problem in the male. Urinary retention may be promoted by the use of potent diuretics, atropine and enforced bed rest. The risk of constipation and faecal impaction can be reduced by the use of a daily oral laxative and diets should be in a soft, digestible form. After the initial period of medical treatment the aim of rehabilitation in the elderly coronary patient is to return him to the activities normal for his age and avoid unnecessary invalidism. The elderly patient and his relatives are often unduly pessimistic about recovery chances and the older infarct patient tends to have an increased degree of disability, especially of anxiety, depression, dyspnoea and fatigue (Peach & Pathy 1979).

Secondary prevention of myocardial infarction in the elderly is still controversial. In one study a reduced reinfarction rate and mortality rate was noted over a 2-year period in a selected elderly patient group treated with long-term oral anticoagulant therapy (Sixty Plus Reinfarction Study Research Group 1980). The role of β-adrenergic blockers as long-term prophylaxis in elderly infarct patients is not yet clear. In a recent study using timolol 10 mg twice daily there was a reduction noted in the mortality and the reinfarction rate in men up to the age of 75 years (Norwegian Multicenter Study Group 1981). There is no good evidence that aspirin in conventional or lower dosage reduces mortality after myocardial infarction and as yet there are no firm recommendations for the use of aspirin or similar platelet antiaggregant agents as secondary prevention measures in the survivors of acute myocardial infarction.

Age is a major adverse prognostic factor in acute myocardial infarction, but the elderly benefit as much as their younger counterparts from admission to Coronary Care Units (Williams *et al.* 1976), and haemodynamic monitoring in the Coronary Care Unit has led to a significant reduction in mortality in old age (Marchionni *et al.* 1981), and the long-term survival of elderly infarct patients is better relative to their natural expected mortality than younger patients. In elderly patients who survive the first 3 months after an acute myocardial infarction the expected survival at 3 years is 71% (Pathy & Peach 1981).

VALVULAR HEART DISEASE

Rheumatic heart disease

Rheumatic fever is uncommon in the elderly but it may be recurrent, and it may be characterized by a prolonged course associated with a slight fever and a very low incidence of cardiac damage. Acute rheumatic fever should be considered as a diagnosis in elderly patients with tachycardia, unexplained fever, joint symptoms, cardiac signs and a poor response to digoxin if atrial fibrillation is present. The prevalence of rheumatic heart disease in the elderly population in hospital is of the order of 3–4% (Kennedy *et al.* 1977). Mild or moderate chronic rheumatic heart disease in the elderly is usually associated with minimal valvular lesions associated with breathlessness and cyanosis. The mitral valve is most often involved, the aortic valve next, and other valves are rarely affected.

Mitral valve disease

In elderly patients with rheumatic heart disease the dominant lesion is mitral stenosis and half of these patients have evidence of aortic valve involvement. Clinical features are the same as in younger patients as are the electrocardiographic and radiological findings. The echocardiogram permits assessment of the thickness of the mitral leaflets and the degree of left atrial enlargement, and two-dimensional echocardiography can give a quantification of the degree of mitral valve stenosis. Atrial fibrillation is a common complication and is often associated with heart failure. Infective endocarditis is an occasional complication.

Rheumatic mitral regurgitation is not usually associated with symptoms unless heart failure or other complications supervene. Infective endocarditis is especially common, even if the valve lesion is minimal.

Mitral regurgitation may occur in the elderly as a result of mitral annulus calcification which is more common in females, mitral cusp mucoid degeneration or papillary muscle dysfunction. Papillary muscle dysfunction should be suspected in the elderly coronary patient who develops a late or pansystolic murmur during or after recovery from acute myocardial infarction.

Surgery of the mitral valve

Mitral valve surgery should be considered in selected cardiac patients if medical management has not produced satisfactory control of symptoms. Mitral valve replacement has become safer in recent years in elderly patients (Jolly *et al.* 1981), but the elderly tolerate mitral valve replacement less well in cases of mitral regurgitation than in mitral stenosis.

Aortic valve disease

Aortic valve stenosis in the elderly is usually due to fibrosis and calcification, and only a minority of cases are due to rheumatic heart disease. Aortic stenosis occurs in about 4% of the elderly (Kennedy *et al.* 1977), and it is more frequent in men under the age of 80 years and in women over the age of 80. All forms of aortic stenosis have similar clinical findings. The main diagnostic difficulty is in differentiating aortic sclerosis from aortic stenosis, but in the latter the murmur is louder and is associated with left ventricular hypertrophy and reversed splitting of the second heart sound. In systolic murmurs that are difficult to elucidate in the elderly phonocardiography and carotid systolic time interval tracings are helpful in excluding severe aortic stenosis.

Aortic regurgitation

Chronic aortic regurgitation in old age is commonly due to calcific disease and less commonly due to congenital or rheumatic heart disease or after infective endocarditis, syphilis or ankylosing spondylitis. Aortic regurgitation acquired in early life is compatible with survival into very old age, but symptoms of reduced exercise tolerance and breathlessness may be associated with the development of cardiac failure. Classical signs of aortic regurgitation may be present.

Isolated aortic incompetence in the elderly is of unknown cause and it appears to be related to dilatation of the aorta with increased aortic ring circumference and no major disorder of the aortic valve. The condition is usually asymptomatic, the pulse and pulse pressure are normal and left ventricular enlargement is not evident. The outlook for this condition is good and cardiac failure is an unusual complication.

Surgery of the aortic valve

Surgical treatment for aortic stenosis can be very effective in selected elderly patients whose symptoms are troublesome; although emergency surgery greatly increases operative deaths, the operative mortality for aortic valve replacement in patients over 65 years of age is the order of 2.5–18%. Late survival can be excellent and as many as 86% of operative survivors after valve replacement for aortic stenosis are alive at a mean follow-up period of 43.5 months (Canepa-Anson & Emmanuel 1979). The indications for proceeding to aortic valve surgery in the elderly are the same as in any other age group.

Percutaneous valvuloplasty of the aortic valve is a therapeutic option in patients with symptomatic severe calcific aortic stenosis who are otherwise considered to be unfit for valve replacement (Jackson *et al.* 1987).

Anticoagulants in rheumatic valve disease

There appears to be an increased risk of systemic embolization in rheumatic valve disease in the elderly, especially if atrial fibrillation is present. There is a good case for long-term oral anticoagulation in all patients with more than minimal mitral stenosis regardless of the cardiac rhythm, but the known increased risk of haemorrhagic complications in the elderly tends to produce a great reluctance in physicians to prescribe long-term anticoagulants for them. There are as yet no clear recommendations for the long-term use of anticoagulants in elderly patients with cardiac disease.

Pulmonary heart disease

Pulmonary heart disease is an unusual finding in the elderly and it usually occurs in elderly males. This condition is frequently associated with other forms of heart disease and is usually found with chronic obstructive airways disease and less often with pulmonary fibrosis or kyphoscoliosis. Cardiac failure most often develops over a few days following an acute respiratory infection. Central cyanosis, warm peripheries and a regular tachycardia may be associated with signs of congestive cardiac failure, and other helpful evidence may include hypoxaemia associated with hypercapnia and the electrocardiogram shows evidence of tall pointed

P pulmonale, a vertical heart and evidence of right ventricular hyper-trophy. In the management of cor pulmonale attention should be directed at preventing or treating intercurrent respiratory infections and cardiac failure. Pulmonary heart disease is usually a manifestation of the end stage of a natural history of chronic obstructive airways disease and although considerable improvement can be achieved in exacerbations the disease is progressive and incurable.

Pulmonary embolism

Venous thrombosis and pulmonary embolism is a frequent cause of death in elderly hospital in-patients. Certain groups of patients have a much higher risk of developing pulmonary thromboembolic disease. These include the obese, patients with anaemia, cardiac failure, immobility, fractured femur, chronic venous disease in the legs and hemiplegia.

Prevention

Various methods have been devised to reduce the risk of thromboem-bolism in high risk patients. Low dose heparin (5000 units twice daily subcutaneously) may cause a significant reduction in deep venous thrombosis and pulmonary embolism after elective abdominal surgery but it is not as effective after orthopaedic lower limb surgery. Warfarin may reduce venous thrombosis after hip replacement. Long-term use of heparin for more than 6 months may induce or aggravate osteoporosis.

The prevention of venous thrombosis and pulmonary embolism relies on early ambulation both in acute illness and after injuries or operations. Passive movements should be performed as early as possible in bed by the physiotherapist and active movements of the patient should be en-couraged. The legs should be frequently examined for signs of venous thrombosis and these may include swelling, calf tenderness, the Homan sign, dilated superficial veins and increased temperature in the affected lower limb. Massive fatal pulmonary embolism occurs when more than half of the pulmonary circulation is obstructed by emboli. The patient may be shocked and extremely breathless and cyanosed, although less severe forms may be asymptomatic or associated with varying degrees of breathlessness, haemoptysis, pleuritic chest pain or fever. Clinical signs may include an increased respiratory rate, unexplained sinus tachycardia, atrial fibrillation or flutter of sudden onset, a pleural friction rub, segmental lung collapse or consolidation or pleural effusion. The ECG may be normal or it may have the classical $S_1 Q_3 T_3$ pattern. Increasing clockwise rotation of the heart may occur in association with an RSR pattern in leads V_1 and V_2. The chest radiograph may be normal, but there may be evidence of a linear or wedge-shaped shadow in association with a pleural effusion. Arterial blood–gas analysis may show evidence of hypoxaemia and hypocapnia with reduced gas transfer. Pulmonary arteriography and isotope lung scanning are useful aids in diagnosis. Characteristic disturbances of regional lung perfusion and ventilation may be demonstrated.

Treatment

Anticoagulation is the treatment indicated for venous thrombosis with or without pulmonary embolism. High-dose intravenous heparin by constant infusion pump should be commenced in a dose of 20 000 units in 24 hours or by intermittent intravenous doses of 10 000 units every 4 hours and oral warfarin should be commenced at the same time. The elderly are more susceptible to the effects of heparin and maintenance dosage must be adjusted to maintain the whole blood clotting time at two or three times the pre-treatment value. Heparin should be given for at least 48 hours until the warfarin has taken its effect. Warfarin should be commenced in doses of 5 mg once a day for 3 days and maintenance dosage is more difficult to control in elderly patients but where possible treatment should be continued for a period of 3 months.

Infective endocarditis

Although infective endocarditis is an uncommon illness it has increasingly become a disease of the elderly and often in patients with no known valvular disease. The peak incidence now occurs in the sixth and seventh decades and the mean age of affected patients continues to rise (Moulsdale *et al.* 1980). It is likely that the changing pattern of infective endocarditis reflects the use of antibiotics, the decline of rheumatic fever and increased survival of the elderly in the population. The most common infecting organism is still *Streptococcus viridans*, but many other bacteria may be implicated and non-bacterial forms may be due to fungi such as *Candida* and *Aspergillus*. A source of infection is only detected in a minority of elderly patients, and dental procedures are less likely to produce infective endocarditis than urological intervention or surgical treatment of the gall-bladder or colon. Even pressure sores may be the source of infection. Cardiac factors that predispose to infective endocarditis include calcific disease of the valves, rheumatic valve disease, mucoid degeneration of the mitral valve, pacemaker wires and prosthetic valves. The largest single group of elderly patients with infective endocarditis have previously normal valves.

The diagnosis of infective endocarditis is often difficult to make in elderly patients as the classical features are often absent. Most elderly patients present with generalized ill health associated with weight loss, anorexia, and weakness. Fever is present in the majority but the murmurs may be intermittent, soft or absent. Neuropsychiatric disturbances are quite common and one-third of affected patients have neurological signs most commonly coma or acute hemiplegia. If heart failure intervenes the outlook is considerably poorer for the elderly patient.

Echocardiography can help to confirm the site of valve lesions and may be useful in visualizing the vegetations in infective endocarditis. The diagnosis usually rests on bacterial examination of blood cultures, which should be taken on four to six occasions during 1 or 2 hours. Treatment should begin as soon as cultures have been taken because valve destruction may occur very early in the course of this disease. Parenteral therapy is indicated and intravenous infusion using a central subclavian line is preferred especially if muscle wasting makes intramuscular injections difficult for the elderly patient. Most cases respond to penicillin-G in doses of 10 grams in 24 hours combined with gentamicin 80 mg thrice daily. Changes in antimicrobial therapy depend upon bacteriological advice. Treatment should be continued for a minimum of 3 weeks and rehabilitation should commence when the fever and tachycardia have settled and when the ESR has normalized.

Infective endocarditis should be prevented in susceptible elderly subjects by administering prophylactic antibiotic therapy before dental or urological procedures. A single 3 g dose of amoxycillin 1 hour before surgery effectively prevents the bacteraemia which is associated with dental extraction.

Thyroid heart disease

Hyperthyroidism is relatively uncommon in the elderly, but the incidence of cardiac involvement increases with age. There is a high incidence of atrial fibrillation and 50% of elderly patients revert to sinus rhythm when they are rendered euthyroid. Hyperthyroidism may be associated with sinus tachycardia, a raised systolic blood pressure, left ventricular hypertrophy and cardiac failure. The treatment of choice for elderly hyperthyroid patients with atrial fibrillation is radio-iodine therapy, but half of those elderly patients require more than one dose and there may be an undue delay in control of symptoms with radio-iodine. In these circumstances a swift therapeutic response may be achieved with antithyroid preparations, for example carbimazole 15 mg four times a day or propranolol 40 mg four times a day.

Although bradycardia is traditionally associated with hypothyroidism it only occurs in the minority of affected patients. Myxoedema is associated with cardiac enlargement, hypertension, ischaemic heart disease and pericardial effusion. The hypothyroid state is associated with a significant increased risk of the development of ischaemic heart disease and cardiac failure. The ECG shows evidence of low voltage complexes and flat or inverted T waves, which usually revert to normal after replacement with thyroxine. Great caution must be exercised in the administration of thyroxine replacement therapy in the elderly as their cardiovascular systems appear to be particularly sensitive to the effects of the hormone.

Cardiac amyloidosis

This condition is rarely diagnosed or suspected in elderly patients during life. The diagnosis is usually made at post-mortem and the disorder ranges in severity from microscopic deposits to a diffuse extensive amyloidosis with associated extracardiac deposits. There are no associated clinical abnormalities with the milder forms, but the clinical picture may include atrial fibrillation, cardiac enlargement and cardiac failure.

Heart failure

The prevalence of heart failure increases with age and in most cases heart failure in old age is associated with a multiplicity of cardiac pathology. Left heart failure and pulmonary oedema are usually associated with ischaemic heart disease, hypertension or aortic or mitral valve disease and symptoms include effort dyspnoea, paroxysmal nocturnal dyspnoea and orthopnoea. Physical signs include tachycardia, pulsus alternans, gallop rhythm and bronchospasm associated with bilateral lung crepitations. Congestive cardiac failure is usually due to right heart failure but it may complicate chronic pulmonary disease or multiple pulmonary emboli. Congestive heart failure should be diagnosed only when there is dyspnoea, elevation of the jugular venous pressure in all phases of respiration, basal crepitations in the lungs, hepatomegaly and bilateral ankle or sacral oedema. Elevation of the venous pressure or ankle oedema by themselves are not evidence of cardiac failure.

Treatment

Heart failure is a syndrome and where possible the underlying cause or precipitant should be identified and managed, for example respiratory infection, cardiac dysrhythmia, myocardial infarction or pulmonary embolism. Heart failure may be precipitated or aggravated by fluid retention due to salt excess or to a variety of drugs including steroids or non-steroidal anti-inflammatory preparations.

Acute left heart failure should be treated as a medical emergency, and the management is based on the use of intravenous loop diuretics, for example frusemide 40–80 mg or bumetanide 2 mg. Bronchospasm may be relieved by parenteral bronchodilators, for example aminophylline 250 mg, and high-flow humidified oxygen should be administered by a face mask if the elderly patient has no evidence of chronic obstructive airways disease and if he can tolerate the procedure. Morphine 10 mg subcutaneously is a useful sedative and controls breathlessness.

In elderly patients with congestive cardiac failure bed rest or chair rest with elevated legs is an important part of the management. Diuresis is promoted if exercise is restricted and the elderly patient should not walk until oedema free. Oxygen therapy is indicated if it can be tolerated, but stringent restriction of fluid or salt intake are not necessary when the patient is receiving diuretic therapy.

High-efficacy diuretics, for example frusemide or bumetanide, should be administered in the early stages of treatment of moderate or severe heart failure, but maintenance therapy or treatment of milder cases can be achieved with medium-efficacy thiazide diuretics. Low-efficacy diuretics, for example potassium-sparing triamterene or amiloride or the aldosterone antagonist spironolactone, should be used in combination with high- or medium-efficacy diuretics. Adverse effects of the diuretics may include urinary incontinence or retention, postural hypotension, reduced glucose tolerance or biochemical abnormalities including hypokalaemia and hyperuricaemia.

All diuretics apart from potassium-sparing agents or aldosterone antagonists may produce hypokalaemia, and this may be associated with an increase in the cardiac sensitivity to digitalis, postural hypotension or muscle weakness. The elderly are more susceptible to the hypokalaemic effects of diuretics and potassium depletion should be avoided by providing oral potassium supplements or combining high- or medium-potency diuretics with spironolactone or potassium-sparing agents. Digoxin therapy is indicated in patients with congestive heart failure associated with atrial fibrillation, but the value of digitalis compounds in the treatment of patients with cardiac failure in sinus rhythm is controversial. In patients in sinus rhythm digoxin has a short-lived inotropic action, and it may improve cardiac function on exercise but maintenance digoxin probably confers no lasting benefit. Most elderly patients in sinus rhythm on maintenance digoxin can have the digoxin withdrawn, particularly if the plasma digoxin level is less than 0.8 ng/ml.

Vasodilator agents can improve cardiac performance in patients with acute and chronic heart failure. Most of these drugs either reduce the preload, that is the venous capacitance is increased and the intracardiac blood volume is reduced, or the afterload, that is the arteriolar resistance is reduced. Sublingual nitroglycerin is short acting but useful in acute left heart failure and sublingual isosorbide dinitrate may be useful in maintaining a preload reduction. Oral hydrallazine reduces the afterload and long-term therapy with this agent may be combined with nitrate.

Inhibition of the angiotensin-converting enzyme system is now an established approach to the treatment of moderate or severe chronic heart failure. Both captopril and enalapril are effective in producing short-term and long-term haemodynamic and clinical improvement and they may reduce the mortality rate (Leading Article 1987). Captopril (Capoten) is well tolerated in the elderly (Murphy *et al.* 1986). The initial dose can cause marked hypotension within the first 3 hours in patients taking diuretics or a low sodium diet. Side effects may also include persistent dry cough, loss of taste or proteinuria, agranulocytosis, neutropenia and hyperkalaemia which are more common in patients with renal impairment. Treatment should be supervised in hospital and the starting dose should be 6.25 mg by mouth and thereafter the dose should be titrated gradually to a maximum of 25 mg three times a day in addition to existing therapy with diuretics and digoxin where appropriate. Enalapril (Innovace) has similar potential unwanted effects and should be administered with similar precautions in a starting dose of 2.5 mg increasing to a maximum of 40 mg daily in divided doses.

Elderly patients in cardiac failure should first be managed with diuretic therapy, digoxin where appropriate and early institution of vasodilator therapy may have a gentler effect on preload and afterload than full doses of diuretics and digoxin. In heart failure that does not respond to standard therapy and if no haemodynamic monitoring facilities are available then a mixed preload–afterload reducing agent, for example captopril or enalapril, should be administered.

Resistent heart failure in elderly patients requires a review of the diagnosis. Underlying hyperthyroidism and anaemia must be excluded. Pneumonia and pulmonary emboli must be treated and chloride or potassium depletion, uraemia or hypoproteinaemia must be corrected. Digoxin toxicity should be ruled out by electrocardiogram or serum levels.

During treatment of cardiac failure the patient should be weighed daily if this is possible, and this gives a good indication of the patient's diuresis and this technique is of much greater value than that derived from charts of urinary output in incontinent patients. Once heart failure is controlled as shown by the disappearance of oedema and a fall to normal of venous pressure, the patient should be mobilized gradually being allowed to walk a few yards at first and then by increasing amounts until fully ambulant within 10–14 days. During this period of rehabilitation the previous treatment should be maintained unaltered and careful watch kept for evidence of recurrent heart failure. This is first noticed by a gain in weight. Thereafter the treatment regimen should be modified and simplified to the minimum compatible with control of failure. This usually requires a medium-efficacy diuretic, for example bendrofluazide 5 mg daily, with potassium supplements or potassium-sparing combination. It is often possible to discontinue the treatment of cardiac failure altogether, particularly in patients whose heart failure had a major precipitating cause, such as a chest infection, anaemia or recent myocardial infarction. Digoxin maintenance therapy should be continued in patients who remain in atrial fibrillation.

REFERENCES

Bayer A.J., Chandra J.S., Farag R.R. & Pathy M.S.J. (1986) Changing presentation of myocardial infarction with increasing age. *Journal of the American Geriatric Society* **34,** 263.

Brand F.N., Abbott R.D., Kannel W.B. & Wolf P.A. (1985) Characteristics and prognosis of lone atrial fibrillation. 30 year follow-up in the Framingham Study. *Journal of the American Medical Association* **254,** 3449.

Canepa-Anson R. & Emmanuel R.W. (1979) Elective aortic and mitral valve surgery in patients over 70 years of age. *British Heart Journal* **41,** 493.

Fisch C. (1981) The electrocardiogram in the aged. In *Geriatric Cardiology* (Ed. Noble R.J. & Rothbaum D.A.) pp. 65–74. Philadelphia, Davis.

ISIS–1 (First International Study of Infarct Survival) Collaborative Group (1986) Randomised trial of intravenous atenolol among 16 027 cases of suspected acute myocardial infarction. *Lancet* **2,** 57.

Italian Group for the Study of Streptokinase in Myocardial Infarction (1986) Effectiveness of intravenous thrombolytic treatment in acute myocardial infarction. *Lancet* **1,** 397.

Jackson G., Thomas S., Monaghan M., Forsyth A. & Jewitt D. (1987) Inoperable aortic stenosis in the elderly: benefit from percutaneous transluminal valvuloplasty. *British Medical Journal* **294,** 83.

Jolly W.W., Isch J.H. & Shumacker H.B. (1981) Cardiac surgery in the elderly. In *Geriatric Cardiology* (Ed. Noble R.J. & Rothbaum D.A.) pp. 195–210. Philadelphia, Davis.

Kennedy R.D., Andrews G.R. & Caird F.I. (1977) Ischaemic heart disease in the elderly. *British Heart Journal* **39,** 1121.

Leading Article (1987) Consensus on heart failure management? *Lancet* **2,** 311.

MacDonald J.B. (1984) Presentation of acute myocardial infarction in the elderly – a review. *Age and Ageing* **13,** 196.

Marchionni N. *et al.* (1981) Intensive care for the elderly with acute myocardial infarction. *Journal of Clinical and Experimental Gerontology* **3,** 47.

Moulsdale M.T., Ekyn S.J. & Philip I. (1980) Infective endocarditis, 1970–1979 – a study of culture positive cases in St Thomas' Hospital. *Quarterly Journal of Medicine* **49,** 315.

Murphy P.J., Van der Cammen T. & Malone-Lee J. (1986) Captopril in elderly patients with heart failure. *British Medical Journal* **293,** 239.

Norwegian Multicenter Study Group (1981) Timolol induced reduction in mortality and reinfarction in patients surviving acute myocardial infarction. *New England Journal of Medicine* **304**, 801.

Pathy M.S.J. & Peach H. (1981) Change in disability status as a predictor of long term survival after myocardial infarction in the elderly. *Age and Ageing* **10**, 174.

Peach H. & Pathy M.S.J. (1979) Disability in the elderly after myocardial infarction. *Journal of the Royal College of Physicians of London* **13**, 154.

Pomerance A. (1981) Cardiac pathology in the elderly. In *Geriatric Cardiology* (Ed. Noble R.J. & Rothbaum D.A.) pp. 9–54. Philidelphia, Davis.

Rahimtoola S.H., Grunkemeier G.L. & Starr A. (1986) Ten year survival after coronary artery bypass surgery for angina in patients aged 65 years and older. *Circulation* **74**, 509.

Sixty Plus Reinfarction Study Research Group (1980) A double blind trial to assess long term oral anticoagulant therapy in elderly patients after myocardial infarction. *Lancet* **2**, 989.

Williams B.O., Begg T.B., Semple T. & McGuinness J.B. (1976) The elderly in a coronary unit. *British Medical Journal* **2**, 451.

7

Disorders of Blood Pressure

Arterial blood pressure does not necessarily rise with age but in Western Societies there is a tendency for most people's systolic blood pressure to rise until the age of 75. Diastolic pressures tend to remain more stable. There is no apparent rise in pressures in more primitive cultures.

Hypertension

Hypertension defined as a systolic blood pressure of 160 mm Hg or more, a diastolic blood pressure of 95 mm Hg or more, or both, is present in more than half of the elderly population over the age of 60 years. High blood pressure is an important risk factor for cardiovascular morbidity and mortality in both sexes at any age (Koch-Weser 1979). Isolated systolic hypertension is associated with a significant risk.

Most elderly patients with hypertension are essential hypertensives and only a small number have secondary hypertension; most of these individuals have chronic renal disease. Drug-induced hypertension may occur as a result of therapy with sympathomimetic amines or non-steroidal anti-inflammatory preparations.

Assessing the elderly hypertensive

The majority of older hypertensives are asymptomatic. Marked blood pressure lability occurs in the elderly and casual measurements of pressure are particularly unreliable. The presence of hypertension should be confirmed with three blood pressure readings at separate visits. Blood pressures should be recorded by the same person preferably at the same time of day in the patient's right arm after 5 minutes of quiet rest. Phase V readings should be accepted as the diastolic pressure. The blood pressure should be measured in the erect and supine positions. Most elderly hypertensives have mild or moderate hypertension and the malignant form is rare in old age.

Investigations should normally include the serum urea and electrolytes and creatinine, thyroid function tests, random blood sugar and serum uric acid. Chest x-ray and electrocardiogram may show evidence of possible

101

hypertensive heart damage and urine analysis will exclude proteinuria or evidence of urinary infection. There is little justification for specialized investigations if there is no clear evidence of a likely primary underlying cause. Intravenous urography and more advanced renal function tests are only indicated if renal artery stenosis is suspected and only in patients who would otherwise be fit for surgical intervention.

Treatment

Recent evidence would suggest that lowering the blood pressure in elderly hypertensives will confer benefits in terms of reduction of cardiovascular mortality and morbidity (Amery *et al.* 1986; Coope & Warrender 1986). The problem of isolated systolic hypertension is however a difficult area although the risks of systolic hypertension are well established and the condition is common. There is as yet no evidence to support the use of antihypertensive treatment in elderly patients with a normal diastolic blood pressure. Guidelines for the treatment of hypertension in the elderly are shown in Table 7.1.

Table 7.1 What levels of blood pressure should be treated?

60–80 years
1   Uncomplicated hypertension: treat if standing blood pressure >160/95 mm Hg
2   Target organ damage: treat if blood pressure persistently >160/90 mm Hg

>80 years
1   Uncomplicated hypertension: treat if standing blood pressure >180/100 mm Hg
2   Target organ damage: treat if blood pressure persistently 160/95 mm Hg

Patients with evidence of target organ damage such as left ventricular hypertrophy and strain on the electrocardiogram, proteinuria or with a history of myocardial infarction, angina or stroke are at increased risk of acute vascular events. The threshold for treatment of such patients should be lower than for those with uncomplicated hypertension.

Each elderly person should be considered individually for antihypertensive treatment. Factors to be assessed must include the level of blood pressure, presence of postural hypotension, age, intellectual state, motivation, associated medical conditions and any other long-term drug therapy. It is very important to assess whether the hypertensive patient will actually tak the medicines prescribed.

Adverse reactions to antihypertensive drugs have been reported to be more common in the elderly (Williamson 1979) but a significant reduction in blood pressure may be achieved gently and gradually without major side effects. If the decision to treat established hypertension has been made then the elderly person should be advised to reduce cigarette consumption, moderate any alcohol intake and avoid extra salt at meal times. Dietary weight reduction might be indicated in obese subjects.

Antihypertensive agents should be started in the lowest available dosage and increased gradually. The aim should be to reduce the standing blood pressure to 140–160/85–95 mm Hg while avoiding side effects including significant postural hypotension. The adrenergic neurone-blocking agents such as guanethidine and bethanidine should be avoided and reserpine is contraindicated in the elderly due to its tendency to produce depression. Generally the first line of treatment should be a thiazide diuretic, a β-blocking agent or a combined preparation of both drugs. Low doses of a thiazide such as bendrofluazide 2.5 mg or hydrochlorothiazide 25 mg should be used to minimize the risks of glucose intolerance, frank diabetes mellitus, gout and hypokalaemia. The thiazides produce a blood pressure reduction of 10–15 mm Hg. Urinary potassium loss in the elderly may be reduced by using a thiazide combined with a potassium-sparing agent, for example hydrochlorothiazide and amiloride or hydrochlorothiazide and triamterene. Elderly patients often have contraindications to the use of β-blockers, such as cardiac failure, chronic obstructive airways disease or peripheral vascular disease. These drugs can however be given to selected elderly hypertensives without contraindications. They are particularly useful in patients who also have angina. Several preparations are available and once daily dosage is usually satisfactory to control blood pressure and maintain patient compliance. A cardioselective agent such as atenolol 50 mg or metoprolol 200 mg should be prescribed daily. A fixed combination preparation of β-blocker and diuretic, for example pindolol 10 mg with clopamide 5 mg may be effective.

Calcium ion antagonists are effective and well tolerated in the elderly. Long acting preparations, for example nifedipine retard 10 mg twice daily may be useful options as antihypertensive monotherapy in the elderly. Side effects are usually mild and transient and are associated with vasodilatation. They include headache, flushing, nocturia and gravitational oedema.

If the blood pressure is inadequately controlled with a single agent, a second agent may be added. Alternatively some patients will respond well to the substitution of a drug with a different mode of action. Only in exceptional circumstances should a triple drug regimen be required in the elderly.

Other antihypertensive agents may be used if thiazides, β-blockers or calcium ion antagonists are contraindicated or ineffective. Methyldopa has many potentially serious side effects but this drug may still be effective if prescribed in small doses for example 125 mg thrice daily. Prazosin is an α-1 antagonist which should be started in a low dose, for example 0.5 mg twice daily because of the uncommon but real risk of first dose serious postural hypotension. Angiotensin converting enzyme inhibitors such as captopril and enalapril are effective antihypertensives but cannot yet be recommended as first line therapy in the elderly.

Patient supervision

The elderly hypertensive should be supervised particularly carefully in the first 2 or 3 months of therapy to ensure a gentle reduction in the blood pressure with the minimum of unwanted effects. Erect and supine blood pressures should be checked at each visit. When target blood pressures are achieved, monthly checks should be performed and an annual assessment of the serum urea, electrolytes, creatinine, uric acid and random blood sugar should be done if the patient is prescribed a diuretic. In some elderly hypertensives who have been on therapy for months or years the blood pressure may continue to fall and therapy can be stopped. Many of these patients may have normal pressures for long periods of time after cessation of therapy and this may be partly due to a resetting of the baroreceptor system. The blood pressure may however rise again and treatment may be required.

Postural hypotension

Postural blood pressure drop is usually defined as a fall of 20 mm Hg or more in the systolic blood pressure on standing but symptoms of postural hypotension are usually only present when the systolic pressure falls below 110 mm Hg. In practice, patients with dizziness and a fall in systolic pressure of more than 10 mm Hg on standing should be investigated for possible causes of postural hypotension. Postural blood pressure drop is common in the elderly and its prevalence increases with age. This condition has been observed in up to 24% of old people living at home (Caird *et al.* 1973).

Blood pressure control

The normal response to standing up is for the blood pressure to fall and this stimulates the baroreceptors and the autonomic nervous system to promote an increase in the peripheral vascular resistance and an increase in the heart rate and myocardial contractility to maintain the erect blood pressure and protect the cerebrovascular blood supply. Normal ageing may be accompanied by impaired baroreceptor reflexes, reduced ability of resistance vessels to vasoconstrict and increased venous pooling on standing. When potentially hypotensive drugs are prescribed or an acute illness occurs, some patients develop symptomatic postural hypotension.

Causal factors

There are many possible causes of postural hypotension in the elderly (Table 7.2).

Table 7.2 Causes of postural hypotension.

Immobility or prolonged bed rest
Acute illness or metabolic upset
Chronic illnesses or conditions
Drugs

Prolonged bed rest may produce a degree of cardiovascular deconditioning and difficulty in maintaining the erect blood pressure. Acute conditions may aggravate a tendency to postural blood pressure drop, for example infections, myocardial infarction, dehydration, blood loss, hypovolaemia, hyponatraemia or hypokalaemia. Chronic disorders may be implicated, for example parkinsonism, cerebrovascular disease, spinal cord lesions, polyneuropathy, diabetes mellitus, hypothyroidism, anaemia, renal failure, cardiac failure and varicose veins. Idiopathic orthostatic hypotension is relatively uncommon in the very old. Many drugs may interfere with the circulatory reflexes and together they constitute the most common cause of symptomatic postural hypotension in the elderly (Lennox & Williams 1980). The drugs most commonly involved include sedatives, antihypertensives, diuretics, antidepressants, levodopa, antihistamines and alcohol.

Clinical features

Many elderly people with postural blood pressure drop have no symptoms. Problems are more likely to occur when there is a failure of cerebral autoregulation and resultant reduced cerebral blood flow (Wollner *et al.* 1979). Symptoms may include dizziness or lightheadedness in the mornings on getting out of bed and confusion, tremor, weakness, pallor and cyanosis may occur. Other problems may include poor balance, falls, syncope and urinary incontinence. Symptoms may only occur after a few steps have been taken on assuming the standing position. In any elderly patient in whom postural hypotension is suspected it is mandatory to measure the blood pressure in the lying and standing or sitting and standing positions to confirm the diagnosis.

Investigation

It is important to take a detailed drug history and a full blood count, plasma glucose concentration, blood urea and electrolytes, urine culture, electrocardiogram and chest radiograph should be carried out. More detailed tests of autonomic function (White 1980) may assist in detecting the underlying mechanism.

Management

Elderly people with asymptomatic postural blood pressure drop require no specific treatment but care should be taken to avoid prescribing drugs that might aggravate the condition as they are at an increased risk of developing symptomatic postural hypotension. If these people develop any acute illness or require potentially hypotensive drugs, for example diuretics for heart failure or levodopa compounds for parkinsonism then they should be monitored carefully for the development of symptomatic postural hypotension.

When symptoms are a problem, careful modification of drug regimens may restore the standing blood pressure to an asymptomatic level. Antihypertensive agents should be stopped. Sedatives should be reduced and discontinued where possible. Diuretics should be stopped if there is no current indication for them. Reduction of diuretic dosage under supervision may be possible in patients with a history of cardiac failure. A gradual reduction in levodopa compounds may be attempted in parkinsonian patients.

Underlying causes should be treated appropriately. Dehydration, anaemia and biochemical disorders should be corrected and diabetes mellitus should be adequately controlled. Rarely postural hypotension may be due to primary autonomic failure as in the Shy–Drager syndrome and these patients require referral for specialist investigation and management.

Some patients may have persistent postural hypotension despite full investigation and treatment of correctable conditions. These patients should be advised to avoid sudden changes in posture especially when getting out of bed in the morning. They should sit at the edge of the bed with their feet on the floor for a few minutes before standing up. These patients should avoid standing in one position for long periods of time to prevent venous pooling. Post-prandial postural hypotension may be prevented by ingestion of a caffeine-containing drink such as tea or coffee immediately after eating.

Postural training

In some subjects, baroreceptor function can be improved by tilting the head of the bed and daily increasing the angle of tilt. The patient may then progress to a Buxton chair, which can be tilted to varying degrees from horizontal to upright.

Improving venous return

Venous pooling can be reduced by the use of adequately-fitting long elastic stockings or a custom-fitted counter-pressure support garment.

Drug therapy

Only a minority of elderly patients with symptomatic postural hypotension will require specific drug therapy. Fludrocortisone acetate promotes fluid retention, increases intravascular and extravascular volumes and has a mild vasoconstrictor effect. Oral dosage should start with 0.1 mg daily and should be increased by 0.1 mg increments daily each week until symptoms are controlled, a total daily dose of 1 mg is reached or adverse effects of oedema or hypokalaemia become troublesome.

Vasoconstrictor drugs such as ephedrine, amphetamine and phenylephrine are not very effective. Monoamine oxidase inhibitors which block noradrenaline breakdown are not indicated in the elderly because of potentially dangerous side effects. Dihydroergotamine may reduce venous pooling on standing but the therapeutic effects of oral preparations are variable and supine hypertension may be a problem.

Prostaglandin synthetase inhibitors have been used with varying degrees of success in patients who have disabling idiopathic postural hypotension that does not respond to other measures. These drugs inhibit prostaglandin induced vasodilatation and promote fluid retention. Indomethacin can be given orally in divided doses of 75–150 mg daily but gastrointestinal side effects may be particularly troublesome in the elderly.

β-Blocking drugs with intrinsic sympathomimetic activity may in some cases produce an increase in vascular tone. Propranolol and pindolol may have some limited value in resistant postural hypotension.

Cardiac pacemaker

Atrial pacing may be of value in elderly patients who have troublesome postural hypotension in association with bradyarrhythmias.

REFERENCES

Amery A. *et al.* (1986) Efficacy of antihypertensive drug treatment according to age, sex, blood pressure and previous cardiovascular disease in patients over the age of 60. *Lancet* **2,** 589.

Caird F.I., Andrews G.R. & Kennedy R.D. (1973) Effect of posture on blood pressure in the elderly. *British Heart Journal* **35,** 527.

Coope J. & Warrender T.S. (1986) Randomised trial of treatment of hypertension in elderly patients in primary care. *British Medical Journal* **293,** 1154.

Koch-Weser J. (1979) Treatment of hypertension in the elderly. In *Drugs and the Elderly* (Ed. Crooks J. & Stevenson I.H.) pp. 247–262. London, Macmillian Publishers.

Lennox I.M. & Williams B.O. (1980) Postural hypotension in the elderly. *Journal of Clinical and Experimental Gerontology* **2,** 313.

White N.J. (1980) Heart rate changes on standing in elderly patients with orthostatic hypotension. *Clinical Science* **58,** 411.

Williamson J. (1979) Adverse reactions to prescribed drugs in the elderly. In *Drugs and the Elderly* (Ed. Crooks J. & Stevenson I.H.) pp. 239–246. London, Macmillan Publishers.

Wollner L., McCarthy S.T., Soper N.D.W. & Macey D.J. (1979) Failure of cerebral autoregulation as a cause of brain dysfunction in the elderly. *British Medical Journal* **1,** 1117.

8

Respiratory Diseases

Although total lung volumes do not change, gross examination of the lungs shows that they appear to become lighter and fluffier with age. There is no loss in the total number of alveoli although there appears to be some increase in the size of the alveoli with age. The thickness of the alveolar wall is reduced and there are fewer capillaries present. There is a fall in the ventilatory capacity mainly due to muscular weakness and chest wall stiffness. The vital capacity (VC) and the forced expiratory volume in 1 second (FEV_1) fall with age, but the rate of decline in the VC and FEV_1 appears to slow after the age of 65. Lung compliance increases with age due to diminished elastic recoil and there is a known decline in the diffusing capacity, which is of little clinical significance. The alveolar–arterial oxygen difference increases but the arterial carbon dioxide pressure does not alter.

Some changes in the ventilation and perfusion of the lungs have been noted in elderly men. This appears to be due to a reduced uniformity of ventilation and this is associated with some increase in the blood flow to the upper zones.

On clinical examination many elderly patients have a moderate degree of dorsal kyphosis and the chest expansion is usually reduced. On auscultation crepitations may be heard at the lung bases in patients who have been confined to bed for long periods. These may also be found in pneumonia, pulmonary oedema due to left ventricular failure and in bronchiectasis. The complete elucidation of physical signs depends on the history, inspection of the sputum, electrocardiograph and chest x-ray. The clinical examination of a patient is never complete without a chest x-ray; physical examination of the chest is not a reliable method of excluding disease.

Other investigations of value include FEV_1 VC and the peak expiratory flow rate (PEFR), which is measured by the Wright Peak Flowmeter. The FEV_1 and VC are useful in patients suffering from airways obstruction who are receiving treatment. Their response to treatment can be observed by serial FEV_1 and VC measurements. The PEFR is a useful bedside measurement and is of value in elucidating the cause of dyspnoea. Severe dyspnoea in a patient with a PEFR of 250 l/min or more is unlikely to be due to airways obstruction; a cardiac cause is more likely. Arterial blood gas analysis is of value in patients with pneumonia, infective exacerbations of chronic bronchitis and acute or chronic asthma. The carbon dioxide partial pressure of the arterial blood is important in deciding the amount of oxygen that can be given to a patient without inducing dangerous hypercapnia. It is also of value as a base-line measurement in patients with chronic bronchitis suffering from an infective exacerbation. If treating the infection significantly lowers the arterial carbon dioxide tension, the prognosis is better than if it remains high. Radio-isotope lung scans and pulmonary arteriography may be of value in the diagnosis of ventilation perfusion defects and pulmonary embolism.

Pneumonia

In the general population the maximum morbidity and mortality associated with pneumonia is in the eighth and ninth decades (Austrian 1981). Pneumonia is a complex of an acute inflammatory disorder of the lung of diverse causes. Classical lobar pneumonia may occur in the elderly but it is uncommon compared with the incidence of bronchopneumonia.

It has become customary to divide the pneumonias into two main groups: (1) specific pneumonias, and (2) aspiration pneumonias.

The specific pneumonias

This type of pneumonia is due to a specific aetiological agent and may be caused by bacterial, viral, mycoplasmal or rickettsial infection. Of bacterial pneumonias that due to the pneumococcus is the most common, but other causative organisms include *Staphylococcus pyogenes, Klebsiella pneumoniae* and *Mycobacterium tuberculosis. Staphylococcal pneumonia* sometimes follows influenza and often has the appearance on chest x-ray of small multiple cavities within an area of consolidation. *Klebsiella pneumoniae* infects the lungs of the elderly more frequently than those of young people and watch must be kept for tuberculosis in elderly males.

Legionnaire disease is caused by the bacillus *Legionella pneumophila.* This illness starts with influenza-like symptoms and the clinical picture develops with fever, chills and prostration. Diarrhoea is often present and acute confusion may be severe in the elderly.

The aspiration pneumonias

In old age individuals often bear the trauma of previous illness, such as suppurative pneumonia leading to bronchiectasis, disease of the heart, kidneys or cerebal vessels, and these people are particularly liable to retain mucous secretion. This type of pneumonia is due to a breakdown in the pulmonary defence mechanism and is often caused by an accompanying disease. Coma due to cerebrovascular disease or uraemia, malnutrition, shock, heavy sedation or even immobilization may by impairment of the coughing reflex precipitate the onset of such a pneumonia. Dysphagia is another cause, and results in the aspiration of food. The organisms responsible for this type of pneumonia are commonly the mixed bacteria normally resident in the upper respiratory tract. These include pneumococci and haemophilus influenzae.

These pneumonias are commonly of lobular distribution and are sometimes called bronchopneumonias. Hypostatic pneumonia is a variety of this group which occurs in elderly bedridden patients too weak to cough effectively; secretions accumulate and the lungs become infected.

Diagnosis

Any of the classical features of pneumonia that occur in younger patients may occur in the elderly, but the clinical features are usually much less dramatic so that the illness is often insidious in its onset, and it may present as a non-specific deterioration of health in much the same way as many other acute illnesses present in old age. Fever and other features of acute infection may be absent. The sudden onset of mental confusion, the worsening of the cardiac invalid, the deterioration in the condition of the hemiplegic, are some of the suggestive symptoms of this illness. A fall or the refusal of a previously active person to get out of bed, generalized weakness or faintness are other indications. The unexpected failure of a rational line of therapy, devoted to the treatment, for example, of cardiac failure, should arouse suspicion of pneumonia, as a complicating factor. The physical examination of the patient may reveal dehydration, tachycardia and increased respiration rate without any or much rise in temperature. Movement of the chest is impaired on the affected side and percussion note duller. On auscultation bronchial breath sounds may be heard and fine or coarse crepitations. If some degree of collapse is present, air entry is diminished. Repeated attacks of pneumonia on the same side, or a history of recurrent febrile bouts should suggest the more serious underlying diagnosis of bronchial malignancy. Sputum should be cultured but it is often difficult to obtain sputum from the elderly patient with a chest infection. In this situation laryngeal swabs, blood cultures or cultures of pleural fluid (if an effusion is present) may be helpful in providing a bacteriological diagnosis. Immunofluorescent techniques may give a rapid diagnosis in some viral infections. Serum antibody titres may be raised significantly if the first sample is taken within 7 days of the onset of the illness but usually paired sera taken 10 days apart are necessary to confirm viral infection. The chest x-ray confirms the presence of patchy consolidation or lobar pneumonia. Arterial blood gas estimations should be carried out especially in a patient who develops a pneumonia as a complication of chronic obstructive airways disease.

Treatment

The elderly patient should be treated at home if possible, but if domestic conditions are unsatisfactory hospital admission should be sought promptly. The patient should be managed in a warm room with a temperature that remains constant night and day. The elderly patient is usually more comfortable propped up and supported by a backrest. The physiotherapist has a cardinal role to play and the patient should be encouraged to cough up as much sputum as possible and a disposable' sputum cup should be placed where the patient can easily reach it. Copious fluids should be prescribed and a careful assessment of fluid balance should be maintained. If oral fluids cannot be tolerated then intravenous fluids may be necessary and 2 litres of fluid are usually required in the first 24 hours. Attention to the skin is essential with regular movement of the patient to avoid bedsores and the heels should be protected and a bed cage provided to avoid weight on the feet. A constant watch should be kept for the development of contracture of the knees. Home nursing of the elderly patient is greatly assisted by the provision of a urinal or a bedside commode. The avoidance of constipation is an ever present task in managing elderly patients, and the risk of deep venous thrombosis in the pelvic or leg veins must always be kept in mind. In patients with a history of previous deep venous thrombosis, prophylactic anticoagulant therapy should be considered; active and passive movements of the lower limbs are of value as a preventive measure. The diet should be light and easily digested and assistance with feeding may be required during the early stages of management. The patient may get out of bed when any tachycardia or pyrexia have settled and his general condition seems satisfactory.

Antibacterial treatment should be started as soon as a clinical diagnosis has been made, but preferably after sputum or blood cultures have been taken. Parenteral therapy is required in patients who are severely ill. The initial choice should be a broad spectrum antibiotic to combat a variety of micro-organisms. Ampicillin should be given in a dose of 1 g 6 hourly or amoxycillin in a dose of 500 mg 8 hourly provided that the patient has no known allergy to penicillin. In situations of penicillin allergy co-trimoxazole may be given in a dosage of two tablets 8 hourly or cephalexin 250–500 mg 6 hourly.

A course of 7–10 days of antibiotic treatment is usually sufficient, but longer courses may be required for patients with widespread consolidation or lung abscess.

If within 48 hours there has been no clinical response to the first antibacterial agent, and depending on the results of the sputum and/or blood cultures, the diagnosis may require to be reviewed and other possibilities such as pulmonary infarction or bronchial carcinoma should be considered. Staphylococcal infections are liable to occur in hospital and they are likely to affect patients suffering from chronic bronchitis or other respiratory infections. Flucloxacillin 250–500 mg 6 hourly should be added to the regimen if staphylococcal infection is suspected. Pneumonia due to *Klebsiella* and other Gram-negative organisms such as *Enterobacter*, *Escherichia coli* and *Proteus* require intravenous infusion therapy with gentamicin in a dose of 80 mg 8 hourly. Blood levels of gentamicin must be monitored to prevent the problems of nephrotoxicity or ototoxicity especially if treatment is required for more than 5 days or if renal failure is present.

Legionnaire disease can be identified in sputum by immunofluorescent techniques or by serological methods. In previously healthy subjects this form of pneumonia usually resolves spontaneously but it may be much more severe in the elderly especially in patients with previous chest disease. The infection usually responds to erythromycin given initially intravenously and followed by oral maintenance treatment in a dose of 2–4 g per day in divided doses for 3 weeks. Non-bacterial infective causes of pneumonia may respond to erythromycin or tetracyclines. Expert bacteriological advice should be sought.

Hypoxia may be a complication of pneumonia due to occlusion of the bronchi by inflammatory exudate, pulmonary consolidation and localized atelectasis. Oxygen therapy is therefore an important part of treatment. In the gravely ill patient it may be life saving. In patients who do not have a history of chronic bronchitis where oxygen therapy is unlikely to produce a significant increase in the arterial carbon dioxide tension it is advisable to give oxygen in high doses. This can be achieved by using a polymask. In patients with advanced obstructive airways disease less concentrated flows of oxygen are required in view of the problems associated with hypercapnia. Oxygen should be prescribed by Ventimask or Edinburgh mask at a flow of 4 l/min. Nasal cannulae may be better tolerated by elderly patients.

Bronchospasm may be a problem in patients who develop pneumonia on a background of chronic bronchitis, and this can be relieved by intravenous injection of aminophylline in a dose of 250–500 mg or by nebulized inhalation of salbutamol or terbutaline. Chest pain may be relieved by simple analgesics like paracetamol with the local application of heat, but more commanding pain may require the parenteral use of opiates, for example 10 mg of morphine. If a troublesome non-productive cough is present it can be relieved by codeine or pholcodine mixtures. Most analgesics and cough suppressants can depress respiration and should be used with caution.

The elderly patient who is troubled with confusion and sleeplessness during the toxic stage of the illness may well require a mild sedative or hypnotic, for example chlormethiazole 500 mg two or three times a day. If the patient becomes more confused, restless and noisy a worsening of hypoxaemia should be suspected. This may be due to sedation or to the accumulation of bronchial secretion. Monitoring of the arterial blood gases is helpful in the circumstances and sedation should be avoided if drug effects are implicated.

Some elderly patients continue to deteriorate and become hypotensive despite adequate oxygen and antibiotic therapy. A trial of high dosage intravenous corticosteroids, e.g. hydrocortisone 0.5–2.0 g 6 hourly, may produce benefit as the inflammatory response may be suppressed and the circulation supported until more specific measures take effect.

Heart failure is not an uncommon complication of pneumonia and appropriate treatment will be required.

Pneumonia may be complicated by pleural effusion. The effusion is quite frequently sterile but may well be missed if this complication is not kept in mind. Pleural effusion in association with pneumonia should always be aspirated. If the appearances of the aspirate are those of an empyema, it must be aspirated to dryness and, if possible, a pleural biopsy taken. While a bacteriological report is awaited, 1 mega unit of benzyl penicillin may be introduced into the pleural space. It is essential that an empyema is diagnosed while it is acute and can be removed by simple needle aspiration. If this is not done, the empyema becomes chronic and the thicker consistency requires open drainage by means of a Malecot catheter, or even open drainage by rib resection for its evacuation. Finally, where a delayed resolution of the pneumonia occurs, further investigation to eliminate tuberculosis and bronchial carcinoma may have to be undertaken.

Acute bronchitis

Acute bronchitis may occur very suddenly and the patient may be seriously ill. In the elderly it is more common in those who have chronic bronchitis and the treatment would be as for an acute exacerbation of chronic bronchitis.

When the attack of acute bronchitis comes on suddenly and unexpectedly, with a dry cough, wheezing respiration and many dry sounds in the chest, the patient is put to bed in a warm room. The temperature of the room should be kept as constant as possible, as cold air is liable to provoke paroxysms of coughing. Hot drinks are important in promoting expectoration and the patient should be forbidden to smoke. If the bronchitis is severe an antibiotic should be administered even if fever is absent. Codeine linctus or pholcodine linctus in a dose of 5 ml may be of use but should be stopped when the cough becomes productive, while if there is a dry painful cough associated with thick sputum difficult to bring up, hot drinks or the inhalation of steam three or four times a day may be given. If there is retrosternal soreness then local applications of heat, e.g. by an electrically warmed pad, to the chest are useful. A close watch must be kept for the sudden development of pneumonia which produces a marked deterioration of the patient's condition. Accurate diagnosis is important as the onset of an acute bronchitis-like syndrome may be the first sign of cardiac decompensation in the elderly. Breathlessness associated with bronchospasm should be treated as for the same symptom under chronic bronchitis.

Chronic bronchitis and chronic airflow obstruction

Chronic bronchitis is associated with chronic bronchial hypersecretion. Chronic airflow obstruction denotes predominantly irreversible airflow obstruction and in some cases this will be due to emphysema. In most patients chronic bronchitis and chronic airflow obstruction are caused or aggravated by cigarette smoking.

Chronic bronchitis is a progressive disease with a variable course which generally ends in considerable disability due to exertional dyspnoea due to chronic airflow obstruction. It usually starts in early middle age with repeated attacks of winter cough productive of mucopurulent sputum. As the disease advances the patient has a productive cough all year round. The diagnosis of chronic bronchitis is based on a history of chronic cough, recurrent chest colds with mucopurulent sputum, increasing dyspnoea and a history of heavy cigarette smoking. During an infective exacerbation, the chronic bronchitic may be gravely ill due to respiratory failure. He may be deeply cyanosed, dyspnoeic at rest, confused and he may develop muscular twitching. Retinoscopy may reveal fundal vein engorgement and in some cases papilloedema. Arterial blood gas analysis shows a low oxygen tension and a raised carbon dioxide tension, which may be as high as 80 mm in some cases.

Treatment

In an attempt to reduce irritation of the bronchial mucosa it is worthwhile trying to persuade the patient to stop smoking although this advice will rarely be heeded. If the old person is overweight a reduction diet should be recommended.

The most likely pathogens in the sputum in an acute exacerbation of chronic bronchitis are *Streptococcus pneumoniae* and *Haemophilus influenzae*. In most cases routine bacteriological culture of the sputum is unnecessary but it will be indicated in atypical clinical presentations or if the sputum remains purulent after a week's course of antibiotics. Infective episodes will usually respond to a 10-day course of oral ampicillin 250–500 mg 6 hourly or amoxycillin 250–500 mg 8 hourly. Possible alternative antibiotics include trimethoprim, co-trimoxazole or erythromycin. The first antibiotic used may require to be changed on the basis of bacteriological advice or if there is no clinical response. A patient who has been in hospital or who has suffered an episode of influenza may have sputum containing *Staphylococcus aureus* and this organism is usually sensitive to flucloxacillin.

Cough suppressants and mucolytic agents are unlikely to be effective in the treatment of chronic bronchitis (Thomson 1987) but codeine linctus or pholcodine linctus may be helpful in some patients with a troublesome, unproductive nocturnal cough.

Chronic airflow obstruction

The presence of predominantly irreversible airflow obstruction should be assessed using an inhaled bronchodilator. The response to a dose of bronchodilator at 10–30 minutes or after several weeks of treatment can be assessed by measuring base-line and serial peak expiratory flow rates using a peak flow meter. A 20% increase in the peak expiratory flow rate above the base-line level usually denotes a significant response to the bronchodilator, but a trial of steroids may be necessary to assess the full extent of the reversibility of the airflow obstruction. These tests will identify patients with undiagnosed asthma with reversible airflow obstruction.

Even patients with predominantly irreversible airflow obstruction may benefit from the use of bronchodilator drugs. The selective β-2 adrenoceptor stimulants include salbutamol, terbutaline, fenoterol and rimiterol. These drugs can be administered by pressurized aerosol inhalers. Side effects are relatively uncommon. It is very important that the patient is properly educated in the use of his inhaler but if an inhaler is contraindicated because of compliance difficulties, oral bronchodilator therapy may produce a satisfactory response. The anticholinergic bronchodilator ipratropium bromide may promote some bronchodilation in patients with chronic bronchitis and airflow obstruction who fail to respond to the selective β-2 adrenoceptor stimulants. This drug is administered by aerosol inhalation and anticholinergic side effects are uncommon.

Corticosteroids may reduce the chronic limitation of airflow caused by inflammation and bronchoconstriction and they may be useful in acute exacerbations of chronic bronchitis when severe wheezing fails to respond to bronchodilator treatment. The response to steroids is less likely to be satisfactory in chronic cases particularly if there is co-existent significant emphysema. Most responders will respond by the eighth day of treatment. A trial of steroids is reasonable for the chronic bronchitic with predominantly irreversible airflow obstruction who remains breathless despite treatment with maximum doses of bronchodilators (Rudd 1984).

Severe acute exacerbations of chronic bronchitis

Patients who are gravely ill with an infective exacerbation are best treated in hospital. Antibiotic treatment should be started as soon as a specimen of sputum, if available, has been sent for culture. Arterial blood gas analysis should be performed and controlled oxygen therapy started. Physiotherapy may help some patients. Regular encouragement should be given to the patient to cough up sputum but if this is not successful, tracheal suction may be necessary. A polythene tube should be passed into the trachea and the airways should be sucked clear of secretions. This procedure requires direct laryngoscopy and local anaesthesia of the mucosa of the tongue, pharynx and larynx. The patient should be fasting for at least 4 hours before tracheal suction to avoid vomiting and aspiration of food into the lungs.

Acute on chronic respiratory failure is frequently associated with carbon dioxide retention. Respiratory stimulation may be indicated and doxapram hydrochloride may be given as an intravenous infusion of 2 mg/ml 5% dextrose at a rate of 0.5 mg/min to 4 mg/min dependent on the response of the patient. Sedation can be extremely dangerous because of likely further depression of ventilation but if hypoxia has been corrected and night sedation is required, this can be achieved using one or two tablets of dichlorphenazone. Bronchodilators, if indicated, are best administered by nebuliser and steroids should be given for severe wheezing not responding to maximal doses of bronchodilators. Prednisolone 30–40 mg orally daily should be given until the desired effect is achieved, usually within 1 week. The daily dosage is thereafter gradually reduced until the steroids are withdrawn.

Resuscitative measures including intermittent positive pressure ventilation should only be undertaken when there is a reasonable prospect of
success. Care must be taken not to render elderly people uncomfortable or
mentally distressed because of overenthusiastic or unrealistic treatment.

Prevention

There are no clear recommendations for the prescription of long-term low
dose antibiotics for the prevention of exacerbations of chronic bronchitis.
A supply of antibiotics may be provided for the patient or a carer with the
instructions that the antibiotics should start as soon as the symptoms of an
exacerbation occur. Appropriate antibiotics in these circumstances might
include ampicillin, amoxycillin or co-trimoxazole.

There are no definite indications for the universal use of annual
influenza immunization in elderly chronic bronchitics but it is reasonable
to offer this form of protection to patients with severe airflow obstruction
in an attempt to reduce the likelihood of winter exacerbations.

Chronic pulmonary emphysema

Chronic pulmonary emphysema usually occurs in association with
chronic bronchitis. The clinical diagnosis of this condition is difficult,
unless the chest x-ray shows the presence of multiple bullae, big lungs
with low flat diaphragms or large hilar arteries with peripheral attenuation
of the vessels. The presence of chronic pulmonary emphysema aggravates
the symptoms of chronic bronchitis. The patient becomes increasingly
dyspnoeic due to the destruction of lung tissue and abnormalities of
ventilation/perfusion ratio.

Pulmonary hypertension, due to the destruction of the vascular bed
and arteriolar constriction resulting from hypoxia, may lead to congestive
cardiac failure. Occasionally chronic pulmonary emphysema may occur
by itself, with little or no associated chronic bronchitis. The prognosis of
these patients is generally poor and progressive dyspnoea is the main
symptom.

Treatment

It is assumed that antibiotics have been given as for chronic bronchitis;
bronchodilators may also be of value. As pulmonary ventilation is
mechanically inefficient in this state, breathing exercises directed to correct
faulty methods of respiration are sometimes of value. They may overcome
the inco-ordination usually present as bronchitic patients with emphyse-

ma often contract the abdominal muscles when inspiring. They also enable the patient to relax and may improve the ventilation of patient's lungs. The patient who is very distressed on exertion may find a portable oxygen apparatus enables him to go from his bed to the lavatory and so make life less unpleasant. Unfortunately this apparatus is somewhat heavy and only a few patients can obtain benefit from this. Oxygen given by inhalation for a few minutes after washing or defaecation may give relief to a patient in severe respiratory distress.

When a patient with chronic bronchitis and pulmonary emphysema develops an acute respiratory infection, the treatment is the same as for chronic bronchitis without emphysema.

Bronchial asthma

This condition can occur for the first time at any age and may be episodic, with periods of freedom between attacks, or chronic. The cause of bronchial asthma is incompletely understood, but factors such as allergy and psychological disturbance appear to play a part. Adult onset disease is generally of the intrinsic or non-allergic type and attacks are usually precipitated by respiratory infections, exercise, exposure to non-specific irritants or emotional factors. Asthmatic attacks may be induced by drugs including the β-adrenergic blocking agents, aspirin and indomethacin. The diagnosis of episodic bronchial asthma is usually not difficult and is made by a carefully taken history. The patient complains of attack of wheezing, which may last for days at a time, with variable periods of freedom between attacks. During an attack the patient is distressed by wheeze and dyspnoea. Clinically there is cyanosis and on auscultation high and medium pitched rhonchi are heard over both lungs. During a severe attack the chest may be remarkably silent, air entry is reduced and rhonchi may not be much in evidence. As the patient improves, the velocity of airflow through the bronchi increases and, for a time, the patient begins to wheeze loudly.

Treatment

The treatment of the acute paroxysm depends on its severity. Asthmatics often control minor attacks without sending for their doctor. An aerosol inhaler, e.g. salbutamol, terbutaline, fenoterol or rimiterol is useful for this purpose. A patient who has had a severe wheeze for many hours or days is in status asthmaticus and should be treated in hospital. This is a serious medical emergency requiring urgent treatment. Arterial blood gas analysis generally shows a very reduced oxygen tension, but the carbon dioxide tension is usually normal or is only slightly raised. Oxygen can therefore be given with safety and must be administered as soon as possible. Aminophylline, 0.25–0.5 g in 10–20 ml of water, should be given intravenously. This injection should be given slowly over about 5 minutes. An alternative treatment is salbutamol 250 μg by slow intravenous injection. In addition to a bronchodilator, hydrocortisone should be administered in a dose of 200 mg intravenously. Most cases admitted to hospital require corticosteroids. There are no contraindications to the short-term use of these drugs, which are often life saving. Prednisolone, 10 mg four times a day, should be given for a week, after which it can be gradually withdrawn, provided the response has been satisfactory. In some instances up to 2 weeks of treatment may be necessary. As acute asthma is often precipitated by respiratory infection, an oral antibiotic, such as ampicillin, should be given in every case. The possibility of acute pneumothorax should always be considered and a chest radiograph should be performed.

Chronic bronchial asthma can be very disabling and may closely resemble chronic bronchitis. There are, however, certain important points of difference. The chronic asthmatic is rarely a heavy smoker. Quite often he is unable to smoke because of the respiratory distress it produces. The sleep of the chronic bronchitic is usually undisturbed, but the chronic asthmatic is frequently wakened during the night by wheeze. The ventilatory capacity of the chronic bronchitic as measured by the PEFR or the forced expiratory volume in 1 second, is not usually significantly increased by bronchodilator drugs; that of the chronic asthmatic commonly is.

The chronic asthmatic is usually admitted to hospital because of increasing wheeze. Clinically such a patient may be in status asthmaticus and should be treated in the same way as acute asthma. Once the patient improves, the question of long-term treatment arises. A carefully taken history is essential before a decision can be made. If symptoms are mild and do not interfere with the patient's life, a simple bronchodilator like terbutaline 2.5 mg three times a day or sustained release aminophylline 225 mg twice a day is sufficient. An aerosol inhaler may also be prescribed to be used as required. Regular use of the anticholinergic bronchodilator ipratropium bromide by aerosol inhaler may be useful in preventing asthamatic attacks. It is essential that the patient be shown how to use the inhaler correctly, as many elderly patients find it difficult to breath in and discharge the aerosol at the same time. They must also be warned that excessive use of the inhaler may be dangerous. If wheeze has seriously interfered with the patient's everyday life, or has prevented adequate sleep for long periods, treatment with long-term corticosteroids must be considered. Such a decision should not be taken lightly and must be based on objective evidence of corticosteroid responsiveness of the broncho-spasm. Steroid aerosol inhalers using beclomethasone or betamethasone up to 12 puffs daily may be effective and they are relatively free from un-wanted effects. Sodium cromoglycate may be administered as a powder using a special spinhaler. This agent stabilizes the mast cells, and it may be a relatively effective preventive therapy for allergic or exercise-induced attacks of bronchospasm, but it is of no value for the treatment of established bronchospasm; it is not a bronchodilator and it must be used regularly to be an effective prophylactic. It is generally ineffective, however, as a prophylaxis in older patients with intrinsic asthma.

Carcinoma of the bronchus

This disease accounts for approximately 9% of male and 2% of female deaths over the age of 65 in Scotland (Scottish Health Service 1981). Many older people present clinically with symptoms due to secondary deposits. Howell (1965) found the common sites in those over 60 years for such deposits were mediastinal glands, liver, suprarenals, spleen, superior vena cava and kidney in that order of frequency. In his subjects over the age of 80 years, however, widespread metastases were not found. This illness may present as in younger people with dry persistent cough, haemoptysis, weakness, loss of weight, breathlessness or pain in the chest. On occasion symptoms due to secondary deposits in the brain are the initial manifes-tations of the disease. It is essential that any patient who has the symptoms and signs of a brain tumour should have an x-ray of chest as a routine. This illness is sometimes discovered in patients who were thought to be suffering from an acute bronchitis or pneumonic consolidation. Non-metastatic manifestations may include neuromuscular disorders like polyneuropathy, proximal myopathy, a myasthenia-like syndrome, spino-cerebellar degeneration and dermatomyositis. Bronchial carcinoma may present with a variety of syndromes due to the secretion of polypeptides with hormone-like properties, for example Cushing syndrome, inappro-priate ADH secretion causing hyponatraemia, gynaecomastia due to hyperoestrogenism, hypercalcaemia due to a parathormone-like sub-stance and a carcinoid syndrome producing flushing. Painful joints may be the presenting symptom of hypertrophic pulmonary osteoarthropathy and on occasion the patient with carcinoma of bronchus may start as polyarthritis resembling rheumatoid arthritis.

Treatment

The treatment with the best chance of a cure is surgical excision of the can-cer when possible. Surgery is however contraindicated in most patients because of the site of the tumour, intrathoracic spread, metastatic disease or co-existing serious illnesses and the operative mortality rate is high in elderly patients. Bates (1970) reviewed 100 patients who were aged 70 and over and who had undergone thoracotomy for bronchial carcinoma. A mortality of 24% was found among those who had undergone pneumonectomy, but the mortality for lobectomy was much less at 13%. Bates concluded that if a bronchial carcinoma can be adequately removed by lobectomy or segmental resection, these operations should be performed even in the old. It is, however, difficult, to know preoperatively if lobectomy will remove the tumour and pneumonectomy will not be necessary. For this reason the decision to subject the elderly patient to thoracotomy requires careful consideration. Every effort must be made to discover distant metastases, and if these are found surgery is contraindicated. The supraclavicular fossae must be carefully examined for enlarged glands. If found, a gland biopsy under a local anaesthetic may prevent needless surgery. Ventilatory function tests, the forced expiratory volume in 1 second and the vital capacity, must be carried out in every case. The effort tolerance of the patient should also be assessed by making him walk up one flight of stairs at a normal pace. If this makes him too out of breath to carry on a conversation, he is unlikely to stand the removal of a lung. The presence of important respiratory disease excludes surgery. The diaphragms should be screened for phrenic paralysis and a barium swallow done at the same time for evidence of mediastinal glands indenting the oesophagus. If no contraindication is found, the patient should be bronchoscoped and the vocal cords inspected for recurrent laryngeal nerve paralysis. If at bronchoscopy the tumour is found to be too near the main carina, surgery is not possible.

The finding of a small rounded opacity in the periphery of the lung field on a chest x-ray, the coin lesion, presents a special problem. Deciding the aetiology of such a lesion may be difficult. A chest x-ray taken a year or more previously, if available, is of great value. If the opacity has remained unchanged it is less likely to be a carcinoma; tomography and the tuberculin test are sometimes useful. Satellite lesions or the presence of calcium in the opacity are suggestive of tuberculosis. Processes radiating outward that are continous with the lesion are highly suggestive of carcinoma.

The role of radiotherapy in the elderly patient with carcinoma of the bronchus is almost entirely palliative. Superior vena caval obstruction, compression of the trachea, recurrent troublesome haemoptysis, involvement of the chest wall and painful skeletal secondaries, are the main indications for palliative radiotherapy. Dyspnoea, cough, malaise and fatigue without local symptoms cannot be helped by radiotherapy. This is therefore not indicated if these are the patient's only complaints, except in the case of right upper lobe lesions where the prevention of superior vena caval obstruction may call for radiotherapy in the absence of other symptoms.

Radiotherapy is also of value in treating the coin lesion suspected of being carcinoma, if surgery is contraindicated because of the general condition of the patient or advanced age. If tuberculosis cannot be ruled out, radiotherapy should be given under cover of antituberculosis chemotherapy. When the lesion shows signs of shrinking after radiotherapy, the chemotherapy may be withdrawn. Some advise that elderly patients with such an opacity should have a single 'test' dose of radiotherapy sufficient to produce shrinkage of a carcinoma but insufficient to upset the patient. Only if the lesion remains the same size or enlarges after radiotherapy should antituberculosis therapy be commenced. Cytotoxic drugs have a very limited use in the elderly patient. They are of particular value in large malignant pleural effusions when they are introduced into the pleural space after the fluid has been aspirated.

Pain is a distressing symptom in bronchial carcinoma and the amount of analgesic required may be reduced if the patient is given chlorpromazine or thioridazine in doses of 75–300 mg/day. Analgesics of value include the milder paracetamol, codeine, dihydrocodeine, methadone and later morphine or diamorphine. The amount of analgesic necessary is that required to prevent pain, and the nurse's attention should be drawn to the necessity of giving such analgesics the moment the patient complains of distress or worry in the endeavour to avoid pain as much as possible. It is not enough to leave instructions that these preparations should be given when the pain is severe. The whole therapy of the patient and the patient's morale is ruined if pain becomes a pattern of daily life. Nerve root pain produced by a peripheral carcinoma eroding bones at the apex of the lung is relieved by radiotherapy.

If the patient is troubled by a useless unproductive cough then linctus methadone hydrochloride (Physeptone) 5 ml may be of use.

The prognosis of bronchogenic carcinoma in the elderly is extremely variable. The progression of the tumour may be remarkably slow.

Spontaneous pneumothorax

This condition commonly occurs in healthy young males, but it may present in the elderly. The most common cause of a spontaneous pneumothorax is the rupture of a subpleural bulla allowing air into the pleural space. It can complicate a variety of diseases involving lung tissue notably chronic pulmonary emphysema, pulmonary tuberculosis, bronchial carcinoma and lung abscess.

Treatment

Once the diagnosis has been made emergency treatment is required if there is evidence of increasing intrapleural tension; marked dyspnoea especially if accompanied by cyanosis is a suggestive sign. Relief is given by inserting a small venous catheter through a thoracentesis needle and aspirating the intrapleural collection of air through a water seal drain. Such a case demands hospital admission and the patient should be given morphine sulphate 10 mg subcutaneously to prevent coughing and to relieve pain during the journey to hospital except, of course, in chronic bronchitis.

Where the pneumothorax is small and the degree of dyspnoea is slight, the only treatment required is a short period of rest in bed. Cough if present should be treated by codeine linctus in a 5 ml dose. The patient should have a chest x-ray at weekly intervals until re-expansion of the lung is complete. If there is a large pneumothorax and dyspnoea is moderately severe then after admission to hospital air can be taken off the pleural space. In old people with chronic bronchitis and emphysema recurrent pneumothorax may require poudrage with iodized talc. This operation can easily be done under a local anaesthetic. It is important to remember that the aetiology of this spontaneous pneumothorax must be sought and appropriate treatment given for it.

Bronchiectasis

The term bronchiectasis denotes chronically dilated bronchi as demonstrated by bronchography or by pathological examination. It is only of clinical importance if it produces symptoms. The aetiology of bronchiectasis is not clear in every case and at one time congenital malformation of the bronchus was considered an important cause. However, in the great majority of patients bronchiectasis is acquired, usually due to pneumonia complicating measles or whooping cough in childhood. A suppurative bronchopneumonia in the adult may cause bronchiectasis. Post-primary pulmonary tuberculosis commonly results in bronchiectasis which is rarely symptomatic because it is usually in the well-drained upper lobes. Obstruction of a bronchus by a carcinoma is another cause but the importance of the bronchiectasis in the situation is over-shadowed by the gravity of the primary diagnosis.

The symptoms that bronchiectasis may produce include chronic cough productive of large amounts of sputum, recurrent chest infection and episodes of haemoptysis. It may be difficult to distinguish this condition from chronic bronchitis and the two may co-exist, but there is no evidence that one leads to the other. The symptoms of bronchiestasis commonly start in childhood or after a severe pneumonia while those of chronic bronchitis appear later in life.

Treatment

The principles of medical treatment remain the same as in younger people; every effort should be made to improve the patient's general health, for example if anaemia is present it should be corrected. Respiratory infection should be treated by antibiotics; sputum is sent for culture and sensitivity testing and when the results are available, the appropriate antibiotic is prescribed; this treatment is given until the sputum is mucoid. Antibiotic therapy needs to be repeated when an exacerbation of infection occurs. Postural drainage is employed to prevent pus from accumulating in the dilated bronchi, but caution should be taken to make sure that the patient is fit to undergo this manoeuvre. Immediately before the postural drainage some patients benefit from the use of bronchodilators, or from the inhalation of steam, and this can be medicated with 1 teaspoonful of compound tincture of benzoin to 1 pint of hot water. Upper respiratory infection, e.g. sinusitis, should be dealt with as thoroughly as possible. Haemoptysis can be a very troublesome symptom and in old age surgery is not usually a suitable remedy. The haemoptysis should be treated with a mild sedative or, depending on the patient's age, prognosis and general condition, morphine, 15 mg subcutaneously. Urgent blood transfusion may be necessary. The place of surgery in the treatment of the elderly patient with bronchiectasis is extremely limited and rarely has to be considered.

Pulmonary tuberculosis

The incidence of all forms of tuberculosis has reduced during this century but the incidence and death rate from pulmonary tuberculosis increase with age in adult males. Elderly people, especially single or widowed men, with chronic bronchitis are found quite unexpectedly to have pulmonary tuberculosis. The disease may mimic or co-exist with carcinoma of the bronchus. Patients who have a history of diabetes mellitus, long-term steroid therapy, previous gastric surgery, alcoholism, self-neglect or chronic mental illness are particularly at risk of tuberculosis. Respiratory symptoms are the usual presentation but cases of cryptic miliary tuberculosis may present with pyrexia of undetermined origin, unexplained anaemia and weight loss without the usual clinical and radiographic features of the disease. Occasionally acute bronchopneumonia is discovered, at postmortem, to have been tuberculosis.

Unnecessary deaths are likely to occur in elderly patients due to a failure or delay in making the correct diagnosis and failure to institute appropriate treatment for tuberculosis (British Thoracic and Tuberculosis Association 1971).

Treatment

Old people with pulmonary tuberculosis are usually best treated initially in hospital and if the sputum is positive they should remain there until conversion has been achieved. With modern drug treatment strict bed rest is indicated only for febrile or toxic patients. A high-protein diet should be given and vitamin supplements may be indicated. It is often extremely difficult to teach elderly men hygienic habits and time in hospital can be profitably used in social education. The importance of drug compliance should also be emphasized. Before treatment is started sputum should be cultured for the tubercle bacillus and sensitivity tests carried out if organisms are grown. If the patient cannot produce sputum repeated laryngeal swabs should be taken. Sputum or laryngeal swabs should also be taken at monthly intervals.

Two drug regimens can be used. The 9-month regimen comprises an initial 2-month phase of isoniazid and rifampicin supplemented with either ethambutol or streptomycin, followed by a continuation phase of 7 months treatment with isoniazid and rifampicin. The 6-month regimen comprises an initial 2-month phase of isoniazid, rifampicin and pyrazinamide supplemented with either ethambutol or streptomycin followed by a continuation phase of 4 months treatment with isoniazid and rifampicin. Throughout the treatment periods drugs may be given daily or intermittently two or three times a week. Intermittent supervised therapy may be advisable in patients who are unrealiable or non-compliant.

Isoniazid is given orally in a single daily dose of 300 mg. It is highly effective, easy to take, and very cheap. Adverse effects are few, although rarely peripheral neuritis may occur; to avoid this possibility some give pyridoxine, 10 mg daily, as a supplement.

Rifampicin is given orally in a daily dose of 600 mg (450 mg if patient weighs less than 50 kg). It is largely excreted in the bile and in the first 2 months of treatment liver function may be disturbed as evidence by a rise of serum transaminases, occasionally accompanied by a rise of serum bilirubin. Patients, even although jaundiced, rarely feel much upset, and if rifampicin treatment is continued liver function usually returns to normal. If liver function deteriorates rather than improves, rifampicin should be stopped until liver function tests return to normal, and then the drug restarted. In patients with initially deranged liver function, rifampicin should obviously be used with caution and liver function monitored. With daily treatment, hypersensitivity reactions are very rare. Skin rashes and nausea may occasionally occur.

Ethambutol is given orally in a dose of 15 mg/kg body weight per day. The dosage is carefully regulated because the drug may cause optic neuritis in certain individuals and the tendency is dose related. It is best to test the patient's visual acuity initially, and warn him to stop the drug if he notices anything wrong with his eyes. A test of visual acuity may show that in fact there has been no deterioration; if there has been, withdrawal of the drug is followed by recovery in almost all cases. At the dosage suggested visual impairment is rare and the drug is remarkably free from other adverse effects.

Pyrazinamide is given orally in a dose of 20–30 mg/kg body weight per day. This drug may cause arthralgia associated with hyperuricaemia in the first few weeks of treatment and it is contraindicated in patients who are known to have gout. Hepatitis is a rare side effect of treatment.

Streptomycin is given intramuscularly in a dose of 500–750 mg daily. The dose should be adjusted in relation to measurements of plasma streptomycin concentrations in patients over 60 years of age. Important side effects include ototoxicity and nephrotoxicity particularly in the elderly or in patients with renal failure.

Antituberculosis drugs should be taken in a single dose before food. Preparations are available in which isoniazid is combined with rifampicin or with ethambutol to ensure that two drugs are always taken together in the appropriate dosage.

When a patient is so ill that he may die before antituberculosis drugs have had time to take effect, prednisolone may be given in a dose of 100 mg daily for a few days to buy time. Prednisolone in addition to antituberculosis drugs is also of value in the treatment of tuberculous pleural effusions since it tends to prevent the re-accumulation of fluid after aspiration. It should be given in an initial daily dose of 20 mg and reduced over a period of weeks.

There are four important stages in the management of pulmonary tuberculosis (Cole 1985). In the first or pre-treatment phase, hepatic and renal function should be assessed and a suitable drug regimen chosen. The second stage comprises the initial 2-week phase of intensive drug therapy when the patient becomes accustomed to regular drug treatment. The third stage is after 2 months of treatment when the bacteriological sensitivities of the infecting organism become available and the original drug choice can be confirmed or changed and the patient then enters the continuation phase of treatment wih isoniazid and rifampicin. The final stage is reached at 6 months or 9 months when all drugs are discontinued unless a longer course is indicated because of suspected poor compliance or known drug resistance. Relapses are unusual in patients who have complied with a full course of treatment. Antituberculous drug treatment is so effective that thoracic surgery is no longer required.

The doctor who makes a diagnosis of tuberculosis must notify the case to the appropriate public health authorities. All individuals including relatives, carers or health professionals who have had close personal contact with the infected patient should have a chest radiograph and tuberculin testing performed. Treatment of active cases may be complex because of drug resistance, drug side effects and compliance difficulties and should be carried out in collaboration with a thoracic medicine specialist.

REFERENCES

Austrian R. (1981) Pneumonia in the later years. *Journal of the American Geriatric Society* **29**, 481.

Bates M. (1970) Results of surgery for bronchial carcinoma in patients aged 70 and over. *Thorax* **25**, 77.

British Thoracic and Tuberculosis Association (1971) A survey of tuberculosis mortality in England and Wales in 1968. *Tubercle* **52**, 1.

Cole R.B. (1985) Modern management of pulmonary tuberculosis. *Prescriber's Journal* **25**, 110.

Howell T.H. (1965) Problems of respiratory disease in old age. *Journal of the Indian Medical Profession* **11**, 5206.

Rudd R. (1984) Corticosteroids in chronic bronchitis. *British Medical Journal* **288**, 1553.

Scottish Health Service CSA Information Services Division (1981) *Scottish Health Statistics 1979*, Vol. 2, p. 11. Edinburgh, HMSO.

Thomson N.C. (1987) Management of chronic bronchitis and chronic airflow obstruction. *Prescriber's Journal* **27**, 15.

9
Blood Diseases

Age-associated changes have been observed in some of the constituents of blood but none are probably of any clinical significance (Hale *et al.* 1983). Values outwith the accepted normal laboratory ranges require appropriate investigation.

Anaemia

Anaemia is a common clinical problem in the elderly and the diagnosis should be based on the estimation of the haemoglobin content of the blood. Signs and symptoms of anaemia may be present, but they may be absent, and the diagnosis may be missed if the doctor depends only on his clinical judgement. A full blood count investigation and blood film detects the presence of anaemia, its severity, and it may indicate the type of anaemia.

Anaemia is present when the haemoglobin level is below 12 g/100 ml, and it is recommended that every case of anaemia thought to be of macrocytic variety should be referred to a hospital for investigation. Many cases of macrocytic anaemia require considerable elucidation by elaborate diagnostic methods; for treatment initiated before complete diagnosis can make the finding of the appropriate deficiency very difficult. If iron-deficiency anaemia is found this too may well require further investigation unless there is some obvious source of bleeding, e.g. haemorrhoids. In such a case rectal examination would require to be performed and if the bleeding had stopped a prompt response, i.e. an increase in haemoglobin level of 1.5 g in 3 weeks, would be expected to iron. If this does not occur reappraisal of the diagnosis is necessary and such a case should be admitted to hospital for further investigation. Particular attention should be directed to a possibility of occult bleeding from the gastrointestinal tract and nutritional studies may be valuable.

Anaemia in the elderly is frequently due to multiple factors including inadequate dietary intake, chronic infection, renal insufficiency, poor absorption of iron or self-medication with drugs like aspirin. In an elderly patient with unexplained anaemia occult malignancy must be excluded.

There is no evidence that anaemia is ever due to the ageing process, although there appears to be a gradual decrease in the haemoglobin, red blood cell count and packed cell volume within the normal range in the elderly. Most surveys have confirmed that the prevalence of anaemia increases with age and it appears to be more common in females.

The symptoms of anaemia in the elderly are the same as would be expected at any age, but it is more common for patients as they grow old to present with breathlessness and ankle oedema, while angina pectoris and even mental confusion may occur due to severe anaemia. Some old people suffer from very severe degrees of anaemia and make very little complaint. This usually means that the anaemia has come on very slowly and is just one more reason why estimation of haemoglobin level is the only possible way of diagnosing an anaemic state.

The anaemias in old age are:

1   Normochromic normocytic anaemia. Conditions associated with this type of anaemia are:
   (a) Acute blood loss.
   (b) Depression of bone-marrow function (with probable increased destruction of red blood cells) caused by:
      (i)   Infection.
      (ii)   Chronic renal failure.
      (iii) Rheumatoid disease.
      (iv)   Malignant disease.
      (v)   Scurvy.
      (vi)   Protein deficiency.
2   Hypochromic anaemia. The common causes are:
   (a) Iron deficiency.
   (b) Chronic gastrointestinal bleeding.
   (c) Sideroblastic states.
3   Macrocytic anaemias. These may be due to:
   (a) Vitamin B_{12} deficiency.
   (b) Folic acid depletion.
   (c) Scurvy.
   (d) Myxoedema.
4   Haemolytic anaemia.
5   Aplastic anaemia.
6   Myelosclerosis or myelofibrosis.
7   Polycythaemia vera.

Normochromic normocytic anaemia

Acute blood loss

Anaemia of acute blood loss is usually normochromic and normocytic and the aetiology is usually apparent. The patient gives a story of haematemesis, severe epistaxis, haemoptysis, haematuria or melaena. On occasion, no such history is obtainable due either to confusion or forgetfulness and a severely anaemic patient is discovered in whom the diagnosis is made by a process of exclusion. In the treatment of this condition it should be kept in mind that old people do not tolerate readily a sudden state of severe anaemia and have not the homeostatic mechanisms in reserve that young people have. It is thus important to transfuse early and in small amounts rather than wait until massive transfusion is required. The use of packed red cells is to be preferred.

Depression of bone-marrow function

(with probable increased destruction of red blood cells) caused by:

Infection. Anaemia is more commonly due to a chronic source of infection, but it can occur with acute infection and there is no doubt that toxaemia from bedsores can produce a rapid fall in haemoglobin. The finding then of a moderate degree of normocytic normochromic anaemia should make the physician look for a source of infection, such as, infection of the urinary tract, bronchiectasis, tuberculosis, or an abscess either at an injection site or as part of a deep infected bedsore. The patient may make no complaint of this localized infection. Treatment here would comprise eradicating the source of infection using the appropriate antibiotic and it should not be forgotten that small repeated transfusions may be of great value in improving the ability of the patient to overcome the infection.

Chronic renal failure. Normochromic normocytic anaemia due to chronic renal failure is not uncommon. This can be expected with a blood urea which is persistently above 50 mg% (8.3 mmol/l) and this type of anaemia is found where there is chronic pyelonephritis, chronic nephritis or prostatic disease of some standing. The treatment is essentially that of the lesion in the renal tract, the treatment of chronic infection or of prostatic obstruction. If the disease is one of the kidney itself and there is not any great possibility of direct therapy, and as such patients become adjusted to a lower level of haemoglobin it is commonly stated that transfusion is best avoided if the haemoglobin level does not fall below 8 g/100 ml. When this occurs, or in other circumstances when it is desired to improve the haemoglobin level during, for example, the treatment of the prostatic obstruction, it is necessary to give a blood transfusion. However, in chronic uraemia the effects of the transfusion are transient. This type of anaemia does not respond to iron, folic acid or cyanocobalamin.

Rheumatoid disease. The anaemia of rheumatoid disease is usually normochromic, but can be hypochromic or macrocytic. Oral iron is seldom effective in this condition but a slow response is sometimes found with iron given intramuscularly and in those patients who have a hypochromic anaemia a course of parenteral iron is worth trying. Another possible cause of hypochromic anaemia could be blood loss due to aspirin therapy. The anaemia, if macrocytic, requires investigation as it may be associated with vitamin B_{12} deficiency. It can be seen, therefore, that when anaemia does occur in rheumatoid arthritis the haematological investigation should be complete as there is a prospect of treating this anaemia if the correct factor is provided.

Malignant disease. The anaemia associated with malignancy occurs in more than 50% of affected patients, and this occurrence cannot be correlated with the presence or absence of metastases. There may be an increased haemolysis although the Coombs test is only rarely positive. In a proportion of cases there are secondary metastases in the bone marrow, and the tumours most likely to spread to marrow are primary growth of prostate, breast, lung and thyroid. The anaemia is usually leucoerythroblastic, but there may be evidence of normochromic and normocytic anaemia. The treatment is the treatment of the tumour. Anaemia also occurs in malignant blood disorders in the elderly, and if it is leucoerythroblastic a diagnosis of myelosclerosis must also be considered, whereas in leukaemia the anaemia is usually normochromic and normocytic.

Scurvy. Treatment of this is considered under the sections on macrocytic anaemia and vitamin deficiency.

Protein deficiency. There remains some doubt as to whether there is in fact an anaemia due to pure protein deficiency. It must be extremely rare in the United Kingdom and its treatment would be ensured by the treatment of the malnutrition.

Hypochromic anaemia

Iron deficiency

A common cause in old age is iron-deficiency anaemia, possibly aggravated by achlorhydria. There is no doubt that the iron intake of elderly people is sometimes inadequate. Dietary iron deficiency should not be assumed, however, to be the cause and another factor in producing this type of anaemia is chronic blood loss, which exhausts the iron stores within the body. Frequent causes of this condition in the older patient are hiatus hernia, gastric and duodenal ulceration, carcinoma of the gastrointestinal tract, ulcerative colitis, diverticulitis, haemorrhoids, and following operation on the gastrointestinal tract.

The treatment of this iron-deficiency anaemia is concerned first of all with correcting the cause. If the diet is defective advice should be given to modify iron intake and absorption. Iron absorption may be up to 25% from meat, but it may be below 10% from vegetable foods and in some cases less than 1%. Foods that may inhibit iron absorption include wheatbran, eggs, milk and tea. Appropriate supplements may be required if malabsorption is present and blood loss should if possible be checked by treatment of the underlying condition.

The fundamental requirement in these conditions, however, is iron; this is given in order to raise the haemoglobin and to replenish the stores of iron. The usual method is to administer the iron by mouth and to continue for 1–2 months after the haemoglobin is normal but to keep the iron treatment going indefinitely if blood loss, for example from haemorrhoids, is continuing. Iron should not be given at random for anaemia. This can delay diagnosis if the patient is not iron deficient, e.g. in conditions where haemolysis is occurring. Iron deficiency without anaemia is common in the elderly and if it persists, anaemia appears within a few months. Assessment of the patient and investigations should be performed as for iron-deficiency anaemia.

Oral preparations of iron include tablets of ferrous sulphate BP 200 mg, ferrous gluconate 300 mg, ferrous succinate 100 mg, or ferrous fumarate 200 mg. The first preparation is the cheapest and possibly the best. It is reported to cause gastrointestinal upsets, but if the tablet of ferrous sulphate is taken with meals and a small dose given to begin with and increased gradually, e.g. one tablet daily for 1 week, one tablet twice a day for a second week, and one tablet three times a day for the third week, then there is unlikely to be much in the way of adverse effects. This is, however, a slow method of giving iron, and it is possibly easier if a patient is upset by ferrous sulphate to switch to another preparation, e.g. ferrous gluconate or one of the other tablets mentioned above. It is usually possible to find one that does agree with each individual. The use of ferrous fumarate has much to commend it as the substance is dispensed as a dull brownish tablet not likely to be confused with a sweet by children. Some old people prefer liquid preparations and among those available is the ferric ammonium citrate mixture, BPC, with a dose of 10 ml three times per day and there are also liquid preparations of ferrous fumarate and ferrous succinate.

Oral iron therapy is indicated in all cases of iron-deficiency anaemia unless there is a failure to respond to oral medication which may be due to a lack of patient compliance, gastrointestinal adverse effects, continuing severe blood loss or resistant malabsorption. Parenteral iron therapy does not increase the haemoglobin concentration any faster than oral therapy.

Parenteral iron can be given by a course of deep intramuscular injections over a period of 10 days. Iron-dextran injection (Imferon) or iron-sorbitol injection (Jectofer) may be used by intramuscular injection. Each preparation contains 50 mg of iron/ml. Imferon may be given intramuscularly in elderly patients, but it must be injected deeply to avoid troublesome skin staining. Local tenderness may occur. The total dose is calculated from a formula based on the weight of the patient and the degree of anaemia and this is provided in the manufacturers' literature. A test dose of 1 ml is followed by 2 ml doses on alternate days increasing up to 5 ml doses if the preparation is tolerated. Jectofer can be given intramuscularly but must not be given intravenously. It is injected deeply into the buttock and the usual daily dose is 1.5 mg/kg of body weight. The total number of injections in a course is usually 10–20.

Total dose iron infusions are time saving and reasonably safe if applied with care in the elderly. Imferon may be given in saline at a rate of 1 litre of fluid over 4–6 hours. The initial rate of flow is kept at 10 drops/min for 10–30 minutes as a test dose and then increased to 45–60 drops/min. The patient is monitored for at least 1 hour after the end of the infusion and the procedure can be carried out at a day hospital. Local reactions may include venous spasm or phlebitis and general reactions may give rise to symptoms such as nausea and vomiting, fever, tachycardia and headache and abdominal pain.

Chronic gastrointestinal bleeding

Chronic gastrointestinal bleeding is often the cause of iron-deficiency anaemia in older patients. The source of blood loss is most commonly haemorrhoids or hiatus hernia associated with oesophagitis. Other important sources include peptic ulceration, alimentary malignancies, oesophageal varices, diverticular disease of the colon or the ingestion of non-steroidal anti-inflammatory drugs. An important but less common cause of bleeding is from small vascular mucosal lesions in the right side of the colon viz angiodysplasia. Colonic assessment to exclude occult malignancy is essential in elderly patients with iron deficiency anaemia who have demonstrable benign lesions on upper gastrointestinal endoscopy (Cook *et al.* 1986). The treatment is that of the cause of blood loss and the administration of iron therapy (p.132).

Sideroblastic states

A hypochromic anaemia without iron deficiency may be due to a sideroblastic state characterized by an impaired marrow utilization of iron.

In the primary acquired form, a full or partial response to oral pyridoxine (100–1000 mg daily) may occur. Therapy may be required for several weeks. Folic acid deficiency may co-exist with sideroblastic anaemia and marrow examination may show evidence of megaloblastosis which does not always respond to folate replacement therapy. Secondary acquired sideroblastic anaemia may occur in association with diseases with impaired nutrition, e.g. malabsorption, malignancy, alcoholism or post-gastrectomy. Secondary sideroblastic anaemia may occur in myeloproliferative disorders or as a manifestation of drug toxicity, e.g. antituberculous therapy, paracetamol or cytotoxic agents. Secondary states may respond to treatment of the primary cause, and folic acid and/or pyridoxine is often more effective than in the primary form of the anaemia.

Macrocytic anaemias

Vitamin B_{12} deficiency

The most important of this group is Addisonian pernicious anaemia; essentially this is an anaemia affecting older people. Females are probably affected more commonly than males, and it is unusual for patients to be referred to hospital as suffering from anaemia. People come for advice because of swollen ankles or of heart failure that has failed to respond to routine measures, or intermittent diarrhoea. Occasionally the doctor is called in because of difficulty in walking or of mental symptoms. The anaemia is frequently of great severity because it has developed slowly and the patient has learned to adapt to it. It has been repeatedly noted that there is a rapid improvement in cardiac function with vitamin B_{12} therapy long before any significant change has been noted in the haemoglobin level. Mental symptoms are found not infrequently and depression, apathy, paranoid manifestations and confusion may be encountered. It must always be remembered that subacute combined degeneration may be present without anaemia.

The diagnostic criteria for pernicious anaemia are a macrocytic blood picture, a megaloblastic bone marrow, a reduced serum level of vitamin B_{12}, and demonstration of a deficiency of intrinsic factor. The serum B_{12} level falls with age but most would accept 160 pg/ml to be the lower limit of normal. It should be noted that patients receiving chlorpromazine or promazine can have false low serum vitamin B_{12} results. There are many more refined techniques for establishing the diagnosis in doubtful cases, but if the above criteria are satisfied and a reticulocyte response proportional to the severity of the anaemia occurs following treatment with vitamin B_{12}, the diagnosis can be taken as established. The certain diagnosis of pernicious anaemia depends on the absence of intrinsic factor which prevents absorption of vitamin B_{12} in the ileum. If it is considered necessary to separate pernicious anaemia from other types of vitamin B_{12} deficiency, proof of intrinsic factor deficiency can be shown by using radioactive vitamin B_{12}. A serious complication of pernicious anaemia in 4% of cases is gastric carcinoma and for this reason faecal occult blood examination should be performed regularly. If there is any doubt about the diagnosis a barium meal is essential.

Other causes of vitamin B_{12} deficiency include malabsorption of vitamin B_{12} due to the postgastrectomy syndrome, other types of the malabsorption syndrome and in severe dietary deficiency states.

A suggested course of treatment of pernicious anaemia is an intramuscular injection of 1000 µg of hydroxocobalamin daily for 5 days, then an injection of 250 µg is given weekly until the red cell count is normal. Maintenance dose of hydroxocobalamin 1000 µg every 2 or 3 months should be satisfactory. Some physicans recommend that after the initial reticulocyte response has been observed in a fresh case of pernicious anaemia, a course of iron therapy should be given for 2 months to avoid any possibility of iron shortage owing to the rapid production of erythrocytes.

There is still some doubt about the correct treatment of a critically ill collapsed patient who may have a blood count of under one million red cells and a haemoglobin content of around 3 g/100 ml. Packed red cells from 1 litre of blood given very slowly in not less than 6 hours intravenously frequently tide the patient over the critical 4 days until the vitamin B_{12} has time to act. This quantity of packed cells contains a very small amount of vitamin B_{12} and should not upset subsequent vitamin B_{12} estimation. This procedure should be reserved for patients whom it is anticipated will have a poor prognosis in the initial period of hospitalization. Transfusion is seldom necessary in treating patients with megaloblastic anaemia. Nevertheless, when the haemoglobin is less than 5 g/100 ml or haematocrit less than 15% the chance of cardiac failure is probably lessened by transfusion. It must be emphasized that once vitamin B_{12} therapy has been commenced it must be continued for the rest of the patient's life.

Lawson *et al.* (1972) drew attention to the high mortality of megaloblastic anaemias and the danger of sudden death during treatment; deaths were mainly due to cardiovascular causes and pulmonary oedema. During folic acid or vitamin B_{12} treatment the plasma potassium concentration fell sharply by almost 1.0 mEq/l on average and in some cases values below 2.5 mEq/l were recorded. Estimates of red blood cell potassium concentration before treatment showed some subnormal values in many cases, suggesting that these patients often had pre-existing potassium deficiency. There were good theoretical grounds for expecting plasma potassium to fall during treatment since supplying the missing haemopoietic factor was likely to result in the rapid production of new cells and the incorporation of normal intracellular constituents. Diarrhoea or polyuria might be contributing to this hypokalaemia as 50% of pernicious anaemia patients have episodes of diarrhoea and evidence of poor renal function is often found. A sharp fall in plasma potassium might cause cardiac arrest and also precipitate digitalis toxicity. These patients should have their serum potassium levels examined before and during treatment.

In megaloblastic anaemias due to disorders of the gastrointestinal tract it may be necessary to give more than one factor: for example, in steatorrhoea a gluten-free diet, folic acid and vitamin B_{12} may be necessary. In megaloblastic anaemia associated with partial or total gastrectomy the treatment is similar to that for pernicious anaemia, namely, adequate therapy with vitamin B_{12}. This applies also when this type of anaemia is seen following a gastroenterostomy or where there has been extensive resection or disease of the terminal ileum where vitamin B_{12} is normally absorbed.

In conditions of intestinal stricture or fistulae involving the small intestine or where there are blind or stagnant loops of small intestine, bacterial overgrowth may occur. The oral administration of an antibiotic such as tetracycline or chlortetracycline, 250 mg four times daily, may produce a haematological response, but this is best combined with the intramuscular injections of hydroxocobalamin just as for pernicious anaemia. As soon as possible surgical correction of the intestinal abnormality should be undertaken, but if this cannot be performed then short courses of chlortetracycline given intermittently are of value in improving the diarrhoea. The vitamin B_{12} injections will require to be continued permanently in such instances.

Folic acid depletion

Megaloblastic anaemia due to folic acid deficiency may be of nutritional origin in elderly people with inadequate diets lacking in liver, fruit and fresh vegetables. The effects of a poor diet may be aggravated by the presence of tuberculosis, rheumatoid disease or after partial gastrectomy. Scurvy is usually associated with severe folate deficiency.

Folic acid deficiency and megaloblastic anaemia may be associated with malabsorption, hepatic cirrhosis, malignancy, chronic haemolytic anaemia, chronic inflammatory diseases, alcohol abuse and it may occur in patients on long-term anticonvulsant therapy, e.g. phenobarbitone, phenytoin or primidone. Other drugs that may cause megaloblastic anaemia due to folate deficiency include antimitotic agents, sulphasalazine and nitrofurantoin. Neurological features of folic acid deficiency may include a mild peripheral neuropathy and psychiatric manifestations. Confusional states may be presenting features in elderly patients.

Scurvy

Anaemia is usual in scurvy. This may be normocytic or macrocytic. The normocytic anaemia may be due to blood loss into the skin and deeper tissues and there may also be an element of haemolysis. The macrocytic anaemia may be associated with megaloblastic erythropoiesis due to vitamin C deficiency or folic acid deficiency. If the anaemia does not respond to saturation with vitamin C it may be necessary to add iron on the principle that this is an iron deficiency anaemia, provided the anaemia is not megaloblastic. If the anaemia is megaloblastic it may respond to folic acid and a few cases may respond to vitamin C as the sole therapeutic agent.

Scurvy is not now a very common disorder and it is not always associated with anaemia. The order of treatment should always be to correct the scorbutic condition by giving adequate vitamin C and also to ensure that the patient in future takes a diet which contains sufficient ascorbic acid. Vitamin C is present in green vegetables, fruit, tomatoes, potatoes, liver and kidney. If the anaemia did not respond to vitamin C further investigation would be necessary.

Myxoedema

Mild or moderate anaemia occurs in two-thirds of patients with myxoedema. The anaemia is usually normocytic or slightly hypochromic but it may be macrocytic. The macrocytosis may be due to reticulocytosis from recent blood loss or to a possible association with megaloblastic anaemia, particularly pernicious anaemia. Thyroxine replacement therapy generally improves the anaemia of hypothyroidism, but concurrent iron-deficiency anaemia or megaloblastic anaemia must be fully investigated and managed separately.

Haemolytic anaemia

Acute acquired haemolytic anaemia is rare in the aged but chronic acquired haemolytic anaemia is more common in the over 50s. The haemolytic anaemias are rare, however, and have certain essential features, such as persistent anaemia, constant reticulocytosis, hyperbilirubinaemia and excess urobilinogen in the urine and faeces.

Haemolytic anaemias can be caused by certain drugs and chemicals and haemolysis is seen in a number of other disorders, e.g. collagen disorders, malignant lymphomas and myeloproliferative disorders.

Idiopathic auto-immume haemolytic anaemia is usually associated with warm antibodies, but a variety associated with cold antibodies affects predominantly the elderly and is known as cold haemagglutinin disease. In warm and cold antibody auto-immune haemolytic anaemia the direct Coomb test is usually positive.

The main line of treatment for the auto-immune haemolytic anaemias of the warm antibody variety is by corticosteroids and prednisolone is the preparation commonly used in an initial dose of 10–15 mg every 6 hours. As haemolysis subsides the dose of corticosteroids is reduced, in most cases to 40 mg of prednisolone or less per day and this can often be discontinued after 6–8 weeks. If patients fail to respond to steroids isotope studies may show that splenectomy should be performed. If splenectomy is not indicated or not successful, immunosuppressive agents such as azathioprine may be tried. Very careful control is necessary.

The benefits of blood transfusion are usually transient in the management of haemolytic anaemias. There is often great difficulty in cross-matching blood. Fresh blood should be used if possible and transfusion should be kept to a minimum.

Aplastic anaemia

This rare type of anaemia is sometimes divided into two main groups:
1   idiopathic aplastic anaemia
2   secondary aplastic anaemia

The idiopathic form is not uncommon in elderly people and in this disorder the bone marrow is difficult to obtain, with a great reduction in all elements and the sample may show only a few scattered cells in a gelatinous and fatty matrix. Clinically the patient presents with a steadily progressive anaemia, fever, associated with haemorrhage into the skin or from the mucous membranes and, on occasion, ulcers in mouth and throat. The blood picture reveals a normocytic normochromic anaemia with a persistently low reticulocyte count and leucopenia. The platelet count usually falls to figures less than $100\,000/mm^3$.

In secondary aplastic anaemia the same symptoms and blood findings occur. There may have been an idiosyncratic reaction to a drug or a viral infection, e.g. hepatitis. Certain agents can produce aplastic anaemia if a sufficient dose is given and these include cytotoxic drugs and radiation. A long list of drugs is known to have an association with this form of anaemia. Aplastic anaemia is more likely to occur after a second exposure to a drug. Drugs most often implicated include the antibiotics chloramphenicol and sulphonamides, anti-inflammatory agents such as phenylbutazone, penicillamine and gold salts, antithyroid preparations, anticonvulsants, phenothiazines, chlorpropamide and less commonly antihistamines and thiazide diuretics.

Treatment

The first principle is to try to find if the patient has a primary idiopathic aplastic anaemia and if there is a cause for it. This usually means that all drug therapy is stopped, while extensive inquiry is made as to the different medications that have been taken in the possibility that one of them might be producing this illness. In the meantime it is essential to keep the patient adequately supplied with haemoglobin until the marrow functions again and to achieve this steroids and blood transfusion are given. Potential sources of infection should be kept to a minimum and the patient should be nursed in a clean and preferably sterile area. If infection occurs, antibiotics are recommended, in view of the neutropenia that is present, and it is wise to give the patient ample amounts of all known haemopoietic factors such as vitamin B_{12}, folic acid, iron and vitamin C. Not all agree that the effect of haematinics should be tried but often the precise diagnosis is doubtful and while it is being confirmed the patient's life is in danger.

Oxymetholone by mouth in a dose of 4 mg/kg of body weight daily sometimes gives a good response and can be continued for several months. The dosage should be halved when there is evidence of a remission. This drug is not so hepatotoxic as testosterone but liver function tests should be done.

If a transfusion is required more frequently than once every 10 days, an increased rate of haemolysis can be assumed. This, of course, is not a very accurate method of diagnosis but does suggest that blood transfusion is failing to hold the patient's condition. It would be essential, therefore, to think of splenectomy at this stage, especially if the marrow was found to be active although all blood elements were reduced. In cases that bleed because of thrombocytopenia, blood transfusion with fresh blood should be tried and a course of steriods given. Platelets may be given before red cell transfusions and this may reduce the risk of the development of severe thrombocytopenia and resultant catastrophic haemorrhage. When a heavy metal has been implicated in the causation of aplastic anaemia dimercaprol should be administered.

It can be seen that the treatment of aplastic anaemia is a difficult and complicated one and where possible the advice of a haematologist should be obtained.

Myelosclerosis or myelofibrosis

This is a disease of the older age group and is insidious in origin, running a chronic course. It is usually idiopathic and on occasion has been found to pass into a stage of chronic myeloid leukaemia after an interval of many years. There is anaemia, malaise, gross splenomegaly and hepatomegaly; the anaemia is commonly of the leucoerythroblastic type and thrombocythaemia may occur. The marrow is increasingly replaced by fibrous tissue or osseous connective tissue.

Treatment

Blood transfusion at intervals is necessary to keep the haemoglobin at a reasonable level and this may be all that is required for years. However, gastrointestinal haemorrhage may occur necessitating immediate transfusion. If haemolysis becomes a prominent feature, then steriods in the form of prednisolone, 40–60 mg a day for 2–3 weeks, and then on a lower dose may be essential. Splenectomy or splenic irradiation should be considered if hypersplenism occurs or if massive splenomegaly becomes intolerable for the patient.

Some patients with myelofibrosis are helped by oxymetholone. This can be combined with busulphan in cases where white cell and platelet counts are moderately elevated, and a single daily dose of 4 mg of this agent is given before breakfast, a watch being kept on the leucocyte count. If such treatments are being considered, it would be essential of course to consult an expert in haematology in the use of such antimitotic agents.

Polycythaemia vera

This is a disease of middle and old age and the over-production of erythrocytes in this illness results in an increase of the volume and viscosity of the blood. This may be accompanied by leucocytosis and thrombocythaemia and in many instances the illness terminates as acute or chronic myeloid leukaemia.

In the elderly this disease may present as an acute stroke due to cerebral infarction or haemorrhage or with less dramatic symptoms which may include dizziness, headache, visual disturbances, intermittent claudication, rest pain or gangrene of the legs or Raynaud phenomenon in the hands. There may be an increased tendency to bruising or more severe bleeding, e.g. expistaxis or gastrointestinal haemorrhage. Pruritus is often a commanding symptom. The typical blood picture shows a haemoglobin level of over 18 g/100 ml with a packed cell volume of 60–70%. The spleen is enlarged and firm in about 75% of cases.

Secondary polycythaemia may occur when there has been diminution of plasma volume, e.g. after vomiting, diarrhoea or sweating, and is also seen as a compensatory mechanism when there is incomplete oxygenation of the blood, as in chronic cardiac and pulmonary disease or due to the toxic effects of poison, e.g. carbon monoxide. Polycythaemia may also be present in Cushing syndrome and may occur in association with tumours especially of the kidney.

Treatment

When these other causes have been excluded the treatment of polycythaemia vera is directed towards a reduction of the number of red blood cells in the circulation. Three main types of treatment are available:
1   venesection
2   radioactive phosphorus
3   administration of drugs

Venesection. This is regarded as unsatisfactory as the only method of treatment. Its effect is only temporary and even when repeated frequently the red cell count may remain high with persistence of the increased blood viscosity. In addition, venesection does not lessen the thrombocythaemia, which is one of the important factors leading to increased susceptibility to thrombosis in this disease. It is especially efficacious, however, in producing rapid relief of symptoms particularly cerebral symptoms. It is usually possible to remove 200–500 ml of blood on alternate days until the packed cell volume is returned to the normal range. Thereafter it would be desirable to maintain the packed cell volume below 45%. In severe cases the blood may be very viscous and venesection is difficult as the blood flow is very slow and clots readily. This problem can be ameliorated by the intravenous administration of 5000 i.u. of heparin immediately before venesection which is then performed using a standard taking set.

Radioactive phosphorus. The myelosuppressant treatment of choice in the elderly is ^{32}P. This substance can be given orally or possibly better intravenously as a solution of sodium acid phosphate following venesection to a normal packed cell volume. A common intravenous dose for a man is 5 mCi and for a woman 4 mCi, but this is usually calculated by the radiotherapist and varies between 4 and 7 mCi according to the mode of administration, the weight of the patient and the severity of the disease. If the response is satisfactory the platelet count falls first and the degree and rapidity of this fall indicate the likely subsequent reduction of the red cell count. After a month the patient feels some improvement and the red cell count falls during the succeeding 2 months. If the response is inadequate, another smaller dose of radioactive phosphorus can be given and if treatment is satisfactory a remission lasts for 1–3 years. This treatment is not accepted universally as being safe as it has been stated that it is a possible cause of the transformation of the polycythaemia to acute leukaemia. This may take over 10 years to develop and is a less significant consideration in the elderly.

Drug therapy. Busulphan should be administered in a dose of 4 mg/day for a period of 4–6 weeks alternative with 4 weeks off therapy and a total of 6–12 weeks drug administration should produce remission. With this regimen maintenance therapy is not required. This drug has a particular effect on the platelet count and is therefore of special value in patients with marked thrombocytosis.

Hydroxyurea is a useful alternative myelosuppressive agent. This drug should be given orally in an initial daily dose of 20–30 mg/kg of body weight with titration of the dose to maintain the desired effect. Distressing pruritus may respond to myelosuppressive therapy alone and additional relief may be obtained with the use of cimetidine in an oral dose of 300 mg three times a day.

THE LEUKAEMIAS

Acute leukaemia

Over the age of 50 years an abrupt rise in the death rate from all forms of leukaemia occurs and it has been recorded that there is a natural increase in leukaemia above that age and that the more acute forms are largely responsible for that increase. In the elderly, acute leukaemia is usually myeloblastic or myelomonocytic. Males are predominantly affected. Frank haemorrhage is rare and fatigue, anorexia, dyspnoea and infection are the most common symptoms. The peripheral blood often shows a mainly monocytic picture and a mainly myelocytic pattern in the marrow.

There is as yet no clear understanding of the natural history of acute leukaemia in the elderly. Advanced age at the time of diagnosis is usually associated with shortening of the expected survival time for the patient. Low white cell counts and high platelet counts and high haematocrit values are associated with a longer survival. Females have a longer survival time and conservative treatment does prolong the survival time and improve the quality of life. The elderly have as good a remission rate and survival time as younger patients with acute myelogenous leukaemia if they are managed with optimal intensive chemotherapy (Foon & Zighelboim 1981).

The aims of conservative treatment in the elderly are to keep the patient as symptom-free as possible, to avoid and to remedy complications as they occur and to provide for the patient the maximum amount of comfort. Decisions as to further treatment are complicated and difficult and depend on many factors, such as the physical and mental condition of the patient, ignoring the present state of leukaemia. On occasion it is considered necessary to give transfusion of whole blood and this preferably should be fresh. Platelet transfusion may be needed and certainly oral antibiotics to control infection, while analgesics also may be required to keep the patient free from discomfort. The general principles of specific therapy are to induce and maintain a remission and to re-induce the remission if relapse occurs on maintenance therapy. In acute myeloblastic leukaemia remission may be induced with a combination regimen which may include cytosine arabinoside, daunorubicin, thioguanine, vincristine and prednisolone. The management of acute leukaemia in elderly patients should be supervised carefully by an expert haematologist.

Chronic leukaemia

In the elderly the common form of chronic leukaemia is lymphatic. This is often mild and asymptomatic, the abnormality being found in blood and bone marrow. On many occasions this condition does not require treatment but observation.

Treatment then should not be undertaken as soon as the diagnosis is established but should be postponed until the following situations demand it, either alone or in combination (Table 9.1).

Table 9.1 Indications for treatment in chronic lymphatic leukaemia.

1   Lymphadenopathy or splenomegaly producing discomfort
2   Marrow failure
3   Systemic symptoms
4   Marked skin infiltration
5   Auto-immune complications, e.g. haemolytic anaemia

When anaemia occurs there is quite frequently haemolysis, and it is justifiable to use prednisolone. This sometimes has an excellent effect. If obvious or occult haemolysis is not present, iron and blood transfusions may be given. In this condition careful thought is necessary before transfusions are used, but this is so commonly a chronic illness and the patient may feel so much better after a transfusion that it is frequently justifiable, particularly when the marrow becomes hypoplastic. Specific therapy is usually best avoided but here again it is impossible to lay down definite rules. If a patient is otherwise well, chlorambucil may be used in a dose of 0.15 mg/kg. If symptoms are relieved in 6 weeks and white cell count and platelet count are satisfactory, the drug can be discontinued or given in half the recommended dose for another 6 weeks. Cyclophosphamide may be helpful but it is rarely justifiable to use the powerful mustard antimitotic drugs. Radiotherapy may be given for large gland masses if the masses are causing discomfort or embarrassment. Infection is common in this condition and this is due in part to the reduced γ-globulinaemia, so that oral penicillin can be given as a prophylactic measure and the appropriate antibiotic prescribed when an infection occurs. When repeated infections occur the use of γ-globulin may be considered although generally this form of prophylaxis has not proved to be very effective. It must be stressed once more that the whole patient must be treated bearing in mind his mental and physical state, his social conditions and his own wishes, and to proceed recklessly with powerful antimitotic drugs thus rendering the patient's last days troublesome and unhappy is not sound policy.

Chronic myeloid leukaemia

This is not a numerically important disease in geriatric practice. If it does occur and treatment is recommended, then busulphan is the drug of choice given by mouth in a dose of 0.06 mg/kg body weight daily. At first, white cell and platelet counts require frequent checks and dosage should be reduced to a maintenance level of 1–2 mg daily when the white cell count has reached 10 000–20 000/mm^3. This maintenance dose varies according to individual sensitivity. In this condition there may also be an iron-deficiency anaemia which may require therapy.

Multiple myelomatosis

Multiple myelomatosis is predominantly a disease of middle and old age. It is more common in males than females and the patients present with bone pain, frequently in the back, or because of symptoms of anaemia. Pain round the chest can occur from spinal nerve root compression and paraplegia may be seen from compression of the cord. Macroglossia and pain upon percussion of bones may be noted, while spontaneous bleeding or fractures, tumours in bones or collapse of vertebrae, or renal insufficiency may be found. The diagnosis is based upon the radiological findings and the result of marrow examination. Determination of the electrophoretic pattern of the serum proteins helps but Bence-Jones proteinuria is not a constant finding.

Treatment

In the rare case of the solitary myeloma this is best treated by local excision if it is in an accessible situation. Radiotherapy is the most effective means of relieving pain and this would be used in patients with localized areas of bone destruction or pressure on nerve roots. Cyclophosphamide, as 15 mg/kg body weight intravenously once weekly, or 3 mg/kg body weight per day orally, is a useful preparation in producing amelioration of bone pain. As agranulocytosis occurs quite frequently following the administration of this substance, twice weekly white cell counts are necessary. The adverse effects of cyclophosphamide are mainly gastrointestinal but marrow depression and haematuria have been described. The drug is reputed to be platelet sparing but alopecia is a common distressing adverse effect. If there is no improvement in the patient's condition after 6 weeks, it can be taken that the drug is not going to be useful. If, however, improvement has occurred, the drug should be continued. Melphalan is a more powerful drug, usually given orally, in a dose of 0.05–0.1 mg/kg body weight per day in divided doses for 7–10 days, but whenever there is any sign of marrow depression the dose should be dropped to a small maintenance dose. Prednisolone is used where there is thrombocytopenia or hypercalcaemia and is often given with melphalan. Great care must be exercised with any of these drugs if there is uraemia, low initial dose being the rule, but the renal failure is not a contraindication to treatment since it may be due to the disease itself. The decision about treatment in multiple myeloma is a difficult one, but if the patient's general health is good and his chronological age not a true index of his physical state, specific therapy is almost certainly worth-while especially in the presence of pain. Allopurinol may be required for hyperuricaemia.

   The prognosis in myelomatosis is related to the degree of anaemia, blood urea and level of clinical disability. In the absence of anaemia and with a normal blood urea the probability of surviving for 2 years is 76%. If however the haemoglobin is less than 7.5 g% or the blood urea is above 10 mmol/l in a patient with restricted activity, then the likelihood of surviving for 2 years is only 9% (MRC 1980).

Lymphadenopathy

Local lymph gland enlargement may be found in association with regional sepsis or spreading carcinoma but generalized lymphadenopathy is likely to indicate leukaemia or a malignant lymphoma. The diagnosis of the cause of lymphadenopathy rests with the histological examination of biopsy specimens.

Malignant lymphomas include Hodgkin disease and the non-Hodgkin lymphomas, the latter being subdivided into low and high grade malignancy. These disorders are not uncommon in old age and they usually present with local or generalized lymphadenopathy and hepatosplenomegaly with systemic symptoms including weight loss and fever. In elderly patients the disease is often widely disseminated by the time of presentation. Older patients have a higher incidence of infradiaphragmatic involvement associated with a more aggressive clinical course of the illness.

Management of the lymphomas should be supervised by specialist oncologists and radiotherapists. Treatment is determined according to the clinical features and the staging of the disease. Intensive radiotherapy for localized Hodgkin disease can result in a high cure rate. In recurrences, or if the disease is generalized, chemotherapy is indicated.

The prognosis of a non-Hodgkin lymphoma of high grade malignancy is usually poor in elderly patients particularly if the illness is associated with bone marrow or gastrointestinal involvement. Long-term disease-free survival is however possible in appropriately staged and intensively treated patients (Mead *et al.* 1984). Standard treatment includes chemotherapy combined with radiotherapy.

Use of anticoagulants in the elderly

Warfarin requirements vary widely between individuals and there is a greater sensitivity to the effects of warfarin with age (O'Malley *et al.* 1977). Heparin requirements are generally less variable than for warfarin and there is no difference in heparin requirements in the elderly compared with younger patients. However the elderly (especially women) appear to be particularly susceptible to the bleeding complications of heparin (Jick *et al.* 1968).

The risk of bleeding is related to the duration of anticoagulation and it is therefore important to reduce the period of anticoagulation to a minimum but still gain the benefit of the drug therapy.

Oral warfarin therapy should be started with a flexible induction regimen allowing for titration of the initial loading dose and maintenance dose depending on the British Comparative Ratio (BCR) of the blood measured daily during the first 4 days of treatment (Fennerty *et al.* 1984). During maintenance therapy the optimum range of BCR is the lowest degree of anticoagulation consistent with the benefit in any particular condition. For venous thromboembolism a BCR between 2 and 3 is adequate while for intra-arterial or intracardiac thrombosis the BCR should be maintained between 3 and 4.5 for adequate protection (Routledge 1985). Heparin should be commenced with a loading dose of 5000 international units (i.u.) followed by 1400 i.u. per hour by intravenous injection. Infusions of heparin may be safer than intermittent injections because they are associated with a lower risk of bleeding (Routledge 1985). Maintenance therapy is tailored in accordance with the kaolin/cephalin clotting time (KCCT) of whole blood samples. The desirable therapeutic KCCT lies within the range of 1.5 to 2.5 times control time.

There are various regimens advised to start and maintain anticoagulation in patients with the risk of thromboembolism. One practical approach includes a total period of 5 days of heparin and warfarin is introduced in the third, fourth and fifth days.

It is convenient to describe the use of anticoagulants as follows:

1   advisable
2   doubtful
3   contraindicated

Advisable

1   These substances are used in the prevention and treatment of a leg vein thrombosis (phlebothrombosis). They are not usually given in thrombophlebitis where there is inflammation in the superficial veins. Thrombosis in the paralysed leg of a hemiplegic predisposes to pulmonary embolism and the risk is greatest in the acute phase 6–10 days after the episode. Fibrinogen half-life values combined with leg scanning can give early warning of thrombosis. This can show when anticoagulant therapy should be commenced. There is less risk of aggravating or provoking a cerebral haemorrhage if treatment with anticoagulants can be withheld for a week.
2   Anticoagulants are also of value in pulmonary embolism mainly in order to prevent the recurrences which are so frequent.
3   In cerebral embolism it is now agreed that these drugs are of value. Many clinicians wait for 3–5 days so that any tendency for the initial ischaemic infarct to bleed may pass and the infarct be allowed to stabilize. The anticoagulants are given in order to prevent the further dissemination of emboli from the original clot. In such cases heparin is not used but oral anticoagulants only. Anticoagulants should not be given in cerebral

embolism associated with infective endocarditis. Mycotic aneurysms are common and haemorrhage is an ever-present danger. Anticoagulants should be continued for at least 6 months and tapered off at the end of 1 year.

4   In patients who have had myocardial infarction with evidence of thromboembolic phenomena. The usual length of treatment is 1 year.

5   Patients who have cerebral embolism due to atrial fibrillation with mitral stenosis or a mixed mitral valve lesion should have anticoagulants continued for life unless the source of embolism can be removed by mitral valve surgery.

6   Hyperthyroid patients with atrial fibrillation have a risk of systemic embolization and long-term oral anticoagulation should be considered if the dysrhythmia persists in the euthyroid state or if an embolism has occurred.

7   Patients with heart valve prostheses.

Doubtful

1   Routine anticoagulant therapy does not influence early mortality in myocardial infarction but it may protect against thromboembolism. Short-term parenteral heparin therapy should be given to high-risk elderly patients after severe infarction in prolonged bed rest, with obesity or where a previous history of venous disease is elicited. Anticoagulant regimens can be stopped when the patient is fully ambulant.

2   Perioperative low dose subcutaneous heparin has been widely advocated to prevent postoperative deep vein thrombosis and pulmonary embolism in high-risk elderly patients undergoing abdominal or lower limb surgery.

Contraindicated

1   Anticoagulants are of no proven value in completed strokes. If there is any possibility of a stroke being due to cerebral haemorrhage their use is dangerous.

2   Anticoagulants are probably of no value in the treatment of patients with transient ischaemic attacks and prolonged anticoagulant therapy could precipitate stroke in this group.

3   Anticoagulants should not be prescribed in a patient with a stroke in evolution, i.e. a stroke that advances slowly over several hours. The risk of precipitating cerebral haemorrhage makes this course of action inadvisable.

4   Anticoagulant therapy is contraindicated if the patient has active

ulceration of the gastrointestinal tract, severe renal or hepatic disease, anaemia, pericarditis or significant systemic hypertension.

REFERENCES

Cook I.J., Pavli P., Riley J.W., Goulston K.J. & Dent O.F. (1986) Gastrointestinal investigation of iron deficiency anaemia. *British Medical Journal* **292**, 1380.

Fennerty A. *et al.* (1984) Flexible induction dose regimen for warfarin and prediction of maintenance dose. *British Medical Journal* **288**, 1268.

Foon K.A. & Zighelboim J. (1981) Treatment of acute myelogenous leukaemia in older patients. *New England Journal of Medicine* **305**, 1470.

Hale H.E., Stewart R.B. & Marks R.G. (1983) Haematological and biochemical laboratory values in an ambulatory elderly population: an analysis of the effects of age, sex and drugs. *Age and Ageing* **12**, 275.

Jick H., Slone D., Borda I.T. & Shapiro S. (1968) Efficacy and toxicity of heparin in relation to age and sex. *New England Journal of Medicine* **279**, 284.

Lawson D.H., Murray R.M. & Parker J.L.W. (1972) Early mortality in the megaloblastic anaemias. *Quarterly Journal of Medicine* **41**, 1.

in the Elderly (Ed. Swift C.G.) Oxford, Medical Education Services Ltd.

(1984) Poor prognosis in non-Hodgkins lymphoma in the elderly: clinical presentation and management. *Quarterly Journal of Medicine NS* **211**, 381.

Medical Research Council Working Party on Leukaemia in Adults (1980) Prognostic features in the third MRC myelomatosis trial. *British Journal of Cancer* **42**, 831.

O'Malley K., Stevenson I.H., Ward C.A., Wood A.J.J. & Crooks J. (1977) Determinants of anti-coagulant control in patients receiving warfarin. *British Journal of Clinical Pharmacology* **4**, 309.

Routledge P.A. (1985) Anticoagulants in the elderly. In *Cardiovascular Therapeutic Problems in the Elderly* (Ed. Swift C.G.) Oxford, Medical Education Services Ltd.

10
Endocrine Diseases

Thyroid disease

Thyroid function is well preserved in most elderly people but thyroid disorders are not uncommon and mental confusion, anaemia, constipation, and ischaemic heart disease may be caused by hypothyroidism or co-exist with it. Thyrotoxicosis may present with diarrhoea, congestive heart failure or confusion. Many a thyrotoxic patient has been initially suspected to have myxoedema. The useful tests are the tri-iodothyronine (T_3) resin uptake, serum T_3, thyroxine (T_4), and TSH (thyroid-stimulating hormone), free thyroxine index (FTI) or effective thyroxine ratio (ETR) and radioactive iodine uptake tests.

In a review of the prevalence of thyroid disease in the elderly in the community Campbell et al. (1981) suggested that it was not justifiable to screen elderly populations for thyroid disease using laboratory tests. A knowledge of the ways in which thyroid disease may present in the elderly and a willingness to perform appropriate investigations if there is any clinical feature suggesting thryoid abnormality should ensure that most patients with thyroid disease are diagnosed.

Hypothyroidism

Bahemuka & Hodkinson (1975) found a prevalence of hypothyroidism of 2.3% in 2000 consecutive admissions to a geriatric unit and community studies have shown a varying prevalence rate of hypothyroidism in the elderly. Tunbridge et al. (1977) showed a prevalence rate of 0.5% of overt hypothyroidism in women over the age of 65 years. Hypothyroidism is more common in women and the symptoms depend on its degree. It is most often due to auto-immune thyroiditis (Hashimoto disease), but radio-iodine therapy and thyroidectomy produce a proportion of cases, as do drugs, e.g. resorcinol applied to varicose ulcers, and hypopituitarism. Diagnosis may be difficult because of the very slow progression of the disease and the resemblance of many of its manifestations to those of ageing. The classical symptoms are lethargy, constipation, intolerance to cold, vague rheumatic pains, paraesthesiae in the hands and deafness.

151

Occasionally depression or hallucinations may lead to admission to a mental hospital. The appearance of the patient shows dry, coarse and thickened skin, enlargement of the lips and nostrils, obscuration of the prominence of the malar bones and malar flush. The body hair is sparse, the head hair coarse, and the eyelashes tangled. The voice is croaky and cerebration slow; the reflexes are slow to relax; a normal contraction is followed by delay before the muscle relaxes. The occasional patient may show striking cerebellar signs, e.g. ataxia. Body temperature is low, and hypothermia is an important and often lethal hazard. The cardiac silhouette is enlarged, often because of pericardial effusion. Anaemia may be present and is usually moderate in degree due to deficiency of thyroxine or iron, while true pernicious anaemia can occur.

Hypothyroidism due to pituitary disease is rare in the elderly. Diagnosis is assisted by the history, especially of a premature menopause or severe postpartum haemorrhage, by evidence of failure of other endocrine glands (e.g. absence of pubic hair, low blood pressure), by the finding of dry fine rather than coarse skin, and, in those cases due to pituitary tumour by expansion of the sella turcia or suprasellar calcification on x-ray of the skull.

The diagnosis of primary hypothyroidism is confirmed by evidence of a low serum thyroxine and a raised TSH level, the serum T_3 levels are of no diagnostic value. Low serum thyroxine levels may occur in euthyroid patients with hypoproteinaemic states and in these cases the free thyroxine index is a helpful diagnostic test. Asymptomatic patients with a raised serum TSH and the presence of thyroid antibodies but with a normal serum thyroxine progress to a hypothyroid state at a rate of approximately 10% per annum (Tunbridge *et al.* 1981). The decision to treat such patients before they have overt hypothyroidism is a difficult one. Thyroid function tests should be repeated at 6-monthly intervals and treatment should be commenced when a hypothyroid state is confirmed.

Treatment

In elderly patients the initial dose of thyroxine should be 25 µg daily increasing to 50 µg after 1 week and then by 50 µg daily every 2 weeks to a maintenance single daily dose of 100–200 µg. Treatment should be life-long. Elderly people often do not take maintenance thyroxine in the recommended dosage and sometimes they stop taking it altogether. Appropriate follow-up should include re-examination of thyroid status at 12 or 18-monthly intervals. Maintenance thyroxine requirements may reduce with age in some individuals (Young *et al.* 1984). In practice, enough thyroxine should be given to maintain a normal concentration of serum T_4 with a detectable but normal serum TSH (Toft 1985).

In many cases a balance may need to be struck between undertreatment of hypothyroidism and precipitation or aggravation of angina or heart failure. It may be wiser in such patients to keep the maintenance dose of thyroxine at 50 μg daily. If angina becomes a problem during the initial stages of thyroid replacement a β-adrenergic blocking agent may be useful. Care must be taken to prevent the development of hypotension.

Hyperthyroidism

This condition is less common than hypothyroidism in old age, but it is even more likely to present atypically. When it presents with typical symptoms and signs, diagnosis is not difficult. The old person who is thin, alert, active and agitated and has a goitre and atrial fibrillation, must be investigated with this diagnosis in view; on occasion a retrosternal thyroid may be enlarged. Heart failure is not infrequent and weakness and wasting of muscles, especially of the shoulder and hip girdles, may be severe. A few patients show apathy and lethargy rather than overactivity. Refractory heart failure may be due to hyperthyroidism. All patients who present with isolated atrial fibrillation should have thyroid function tests performed.

A raised serum thyroxine confirms the diagnosis, but if the patient is clinically hyperthyroid and has a normal serum thyroxine then the serum T_3 should be measured as a raised T_3 may be the earliest biochemical indicator of developing hyperthyroidism. A high serum thyroxine may be detected in patients on oestrogen therapy but measurement of the free thyroxine index clarifies the diagnosis. A raised serum thyroxine may be associated with a low serum T_3 due to reduced conversion of thyroxine to T_3 which may occur in non-thyroidal illnesses. The serum levels of T_4 and T_3 normally return to the normal range when the patient recovers from his illness.

Treatment

Radio-iodine treatment is the method of choice in the elderly unless the thyroid is very large and surgical relief of mediastinal obstruction necessary. The maximum effect of radio-iodine is not apparent until at least 3 months, and indeed more than one dose is often needed. If there is rapid atrial fibrillation or heart failure, carbimazole should be given (10–15 mg three times daily) together with digitalis and diuretics, until hyperthyroidism is controlled. It should then be stopped for a few days, radio-iodine given, and carbimazole resumed for a further 6–8 weeks. β-Adrenergic blockers are often useful in patients with tachycardia.

As radio-iodine therapy is followed after 10 years by an incidence of hypothyroidism of 35% or more the treated thyrotoxic patient should be followed up for life.

Diabetes mellitus

Carbohydrate intolerance is known to increase with age. The definition of diabetes presents particular problems in old age. In diabetes surveys less than 1% of people over 70 have been found to have previously unrecognized diabetes, but glucose tolerance tests on elderly people without glycosuria have shown abnormalities of diabetic type in a further 1–2%, or even up to 30%. Diabetes mellitus is diagnosed when the fasting blood glucose concentration equals or exceeds 7 mmol/l (126 mg/dl) on more than one occasion, or when the blood glucose concentration 2 hours after a 75 g oral glucose load equals or exceeds 10 mmol/l (180 mg/dl) irrespective of the fasting concentration. A state of impaired glucose tolerance (IGT) exists when the 2-hour blood glucose concentration falls between 7 and 10 mmol/l. The management of IGT depends upon individual circumstances, but many patients may benefit from treatment since this is likely to reduce the frequency of arterial disease and the specific complications of diabetes such as retinopathy (Keen & Fuller 1980).

The practical problem of diagnosis is complicated by the fact that although the renal threshold for glucose may be as low in the elderly as in the young, so that renal glycosuria is not rare, it is often considerably raised; thus blood sugar levels of 13.9 mmol/l (250 mg/dl) may not be accompanied by glycosuria. The diagnosis of diabetes must thus always rest on the blood sugar, never solely on the presence of glycosuria. The use of glucose tolerance tests for the diagnosis of diabetes in the elderly is often impracticable and the plasma glycosylated haemoglobin (GHb) estimation offers a useful screening test to detect the presence of diabetes. The elderly person is not required to fast, only a small sample of blood is required and urine collection is unnecessary (Martin *et al.* 1984).

Diabetes is usually discovered in old age as a result of symptoms such as thirst, weight loss, polyuria, and pruritus vulvae, any of which should lead to testing of the urine and estimation of the blood sugar. Many present with evidence of complications, such as sepsis in the feet due to neuropathy or peripheral vascular disease, or failing vision due to cataract or retinopathy, and many are found, and many more should be found, as a result of routine urine testing during the course of an unrelated illness or at an out-patient or consultative clinic. Presentation in coma is rare.

When the diagnosis of diabetes is established the patient should be examined with particular emphasis on peripheral vascular disease, neuropathy, cataract and retinopathy, and the exclusion of urinary infection and pulmonary tuberculosis.

Complications

All the complications of diabetes may occur in the elderly and evidence of them is frequently found when the diagnosis is made.

Neuropathy. The definition and diagnosis of neuropathy in elderly diabetics may be difficult, since its manifestations, e.g. sensory loss, especially of vibration sense in the legs, loss of the ankle jerks and later the knee jerks, can occur in old age. However, loss of pain and touch sense and nocturnal pain in the legs should be regarded as due to diabetic neuropathy.

Neuropathic pain can be distinguished from pain due to ischaemic changes: there is usually relief from movement but not from hanging the legs over the side of the bed. The diabetic state should be controlled and carbamazepine 200–400 mg at night may relieve nocturnal pain. In time the pain may disappear spontaneously.

Trophic ulceration and sepsis in the feet, which sometimes lead to septic arthritis and osteomyelitis of the metatarsals, may result from the sensory loss. These septic lesions must be carefully distinguished from those of peripheral vascular disease, since their treatment is quite different. The septic lesions respond to local surgery, e.g. drainage of abscesses, removal of destroyed bone, combined with antibiotic therapy and proper control of diabetes; gangrene due to peripheral vascular disease, i.e. occlusion of major arteries, usually requires amputation at a level compatible with healing.

In addition to the symmetrical mainly sensory neuropathy already discussed, the condition of diabetic amyotrophy occurs in the elderly. In this there is weakness and wasting of the muscles of the hip and thigh, usually painful, and often initially asymmetrical. The knee jerk is lost, but there is no sensory loss. This condition may come on soon after the diagnosis of diabetes or may be its first manifestation. It is important not to confuse it with sciatica or 'femoral neuritis'. It tends to progress for a few months, then to remain stationary, and then to improve with control of diabetes, with restoration of muscle power to normal in 12–18 months. In this it is unlike the sensory neuropathy, which rarely shows any marked change for the better no matter how careful the treatment of diabetes.

Diabetic autonomic neuropathy is a further group of conditions not infrequently encountered in the elderly. Three syndromes are of importance. Postural hypotension may occur and syncopal attacks on standing must be distinguished from hypoglycaemic effects. Diabetic diarrhoea may be episodic or continuous and may be accompanied by nocturnal faecal incontinence. Many patients with this disorder respond to antibiotic treatment with tetracycline and the addition of metronidazole may well be helpful. The third syndrome of bladder disorder is probably under-diagnosed and it is due to a dilated atonic bladder with the eventual development of overflow retention. Temporary catheterization and treatment of any urinary tract infection often result in functional improvement, but surgical treatment of the bladder neck may be necessary and is usually highly effective.

The eyes. Visual failure in elderly diabetics may be due to cataract, retinopathy, or any other non-diabetic cause. Cataract is probably no more common in elderly diabetics than in non-diabetics, but cataract severe enough to require surgical treatment is about five times more common. The presence of diabetes should never deter or delay the decision to seek specialized advice about the question of cataract extraction.

Retinopathy is as frequent in elderly as in young diabetics. So-called 'malignant' retinopathy, with new vessel formation, preretinal haemor-rhage and proliferation of fibrous tissue is uncommon, and visual symptoms are usually due to destruction of the macula by massive exudate. There is little evidence that meticulous control of diabetes greatly improves the prognosis of established retinopathy in the elderly diabetic, but photocoagulation has been shown to benefit macular disease. Clofi-brate may increase the rate of disappearance of hard exudates, but often with little improvement in vision.

The arteries. Atherosclerosis of cerebral, coronary, mesenteric, or per-ipheral leg arteries is common in diabetes mellitus.

The kidney. Proteinuria may be due to specific diabetic renal disease (nephropathy) or may accompany urinary tract infection. Massive protein-uria and the nephrotic syndrome are rare, but slowly progressive chronic renal failure sometimes occurs.

Ketoacidosis. This condition is characterized by hyperglycaemia, glyco-suria, dehydration, ketosis and acidosis. It is unusual in elderly diabetics and occurs in insulin-dependent patients. This complication is usually precipitated by a failure to take insulin or due to the stress of infection or surgical procedures. It may occasionally be the presentation of diabetes mellitus in a previously undiagnosed patient. Patients with ketoacidosis require intensive medical care. The principles of management include correction of acidosis, fluid and electrolyte replacement, insulin therapy and treatment of any underlying cause. Low dose insulin should be administered by continuous infusion or by intermittent intramuscular injections.

Hyperosmolar non-ketotic coma. This occurs mainly in elderly patients with mild non-insulin dependent diabetes and may be the initial presentation of the disease. It is often precipitated by infection or drugs, e.g. steroids or diuretics. Stupor or coma usually develops slowly over several days in a patient who has had a preceding period of thirst, polyuria and weight loss. Dehydration is a major feature and the blood glucose usually exceeds 35 mmol/l with a plasma osmolality in excess of 330 mosmol/l. The serum sodium and chloride may be markedly elevated. Acidosis and severe ketosis are absent. Circulatory shock is a common complication of this condition. Treatment includes intravenous hypotonic fluids, routine parenteral broad spectrum antibiotics and some benefit may be obtained by the use of subcutaneous low dose heparin to prevent thromboembolic complications. Insulin requirements are usually low and often less than half the dosage necessary to treat the hyperglycaemia of diabetic keto-acidosis. Despite appropriate management the mortality rate of hyperosmolar non-ketotic coma may be as high as 50%. Death is most often due to overwhelming infection or a vascular event.

Treatment

The keynote of the treatment of diabetes in the elderly should be simplicity. Old people have great difficulty in understanding complicated regimens and in remembering to carry them out. The objective should be as good control of blood sugar levels as is compatible with an enjoyment of life.

All diabetics should be given dietary advice, preferably initially by a dietician and thereafter the advice should be reinforced by a health visitor or a nurse specializing in the care of diabetic patients. Calorie restriction and weight reduction are usually required. The patient should be encouraged to take a high carbohydrate, high fibre diet with a reduced intake of simple sugars, cholesterol and high saturated fats. The elderly diabetic is much more likely to comply with a modified diet if it is not too restricted or complex. Urine testing is important in assessing progress and should also be taught. Once glycosuria has been controlled, it is usually only necessary to test after the largest meal of the day and not more often than once or twice weekly. An initial watch must be kept on blood sugar levels.

Many elderly diabetics can be controlled by diet alone, especially those who are overweight, have few symptoms, and blood sugar levels when first seen which are not very high, e.g. under 16.6 mmol/l (300 mg/dl). Many more can be controlled by the addition of an oral antidiabetic agent. The sulphonylureas, glibenclamide and tolbutamide have a short to intermediate duration of action and are indicated for use in elderly diabetics. Chlorpropamide (Diabinese) has a prolonged action and is best avoided in the elderly because of the risk of severe hypoglycaemia. Tolbutamide (Rastinon) should be given in oral doses of 500 mg twice or thrice daily and glibenclamide (Daonil) can be given once daily with breakfast in doses of 2.5–15 mg. The sulphonylureas are usually well tolerated but care should be taken in the very elderly or if the patient has renal failure.

A proportion of diabetics who cannot be controlled by sulphonylureas alone, either initially or because of failure of action after months or years, can be controlled by the addition of a biguanide. Metformin (Glucophage, 0.5–1.5 g daily) may be given, but gastrointestinal adverse effects (nausea and anorexia) are frequent and may compel discontinuance.

Perhaps 20% of elderly diabetics require insulin. A single daily subcutaneous injection of a long-acting preparation such as insulin zinc suspension is appropriate. It is best to begin with small doses, such as 16 units, and to increase by small amounts, e.g. 4 units every three days, until only slight glycosuria is present. Hypoglycaemia must be avoided almost at all costs, since at best it discourages the patient and those who care for him, and at worst may lead to serious mental impairment, particularly if repeated. If insulin is required, it is therefore better not to insist on optimum control, but to regard blood sugars of 8–11 mmol/l as satisfactory.

Proper control of diabetics is essential during intercurrent illness, e.g. pneumonia, cardiac infarction, congestive heart failure, etc. In general, the diet should be that appropriate to the illness, rather than specifically to diabetics, oral hypoglycaemic agents should not be given, and insulin should be given to control the blood sugar. Repeated small doses of soluble insulin every 8–12 hours with frequent urine tests are most satisfactory. If the illness is at all severe or likely to last more than a day or two the patient should be in hospital.

Hypoglycaemia may be difficult to diagnose and may present as diffuse brain upset, i.e. mental confusion, or focal cerebral disorder, for example hemiplegia, or cause headache, vasoconstriction, or sweating. Any acutely developing neurological or psychiatric symptoms in a diabetic on insulin or an oral hypoglycaemic agent must be treated as hypoglycaemia until proved otherwise. Glucagon because it can be given parenterally in a dose of, for example, 0.5 mg may be more suitable for administration in the patient's home than intravenous glucose.

Follow-up of the elderly diabetic is essential to ensure that the regimen is as simple as can be, that doses of oral agents or insulin are correct and that proper care is being given for any complications that may be present. Regular chiropody should be arranged for a patient with any foot lesion. Since treatment is life-long good rapport between patient and doctor is vital and much patience and tolerance may be needed by both. This is perhaps especially true when the patient has lived into old age with his diabetes; here the rule for the doctor must be to make only such alterations as are essential. No regimen which has worked well for many years should be altered simply because it does not conform to the doctor's prejudices.

Other endocrine disorders

Endocrine diseases, other than those affecting the thyroid and diabetes, are rare at any age. The occasional case of hypopituitarism, Cushing syndrome and hyperparathyroidism occurs in old age. When Cushing syndrome is diagnosed in the elderly an underlying neoplasm, usually a bronchogenic carcinoma, should always be suspected.

Hypercalcaemia is more common in the elderly than in younger age groups. The most common group of causes of hypercalcaemia in old age includes malignancy with or without metastatic bone disease. Elderly females are at special risk of developing primary hyperparathyroidism (Mundy *et al.* 1980). They usually present with asymptomatic hypercalcaemia or with an acute hypercalcaemic syndrome manifest by confusion and dehydration. Other clinical features may include tiredness, dysphagia, nausea and vomiting, constipation, cardiac dysrhythmias and muscle hypotonia. Most patients have no evidence of bone or renal disease. One-third of affected patients will however have classical bone disease including skeletal pain, radiographic evidence of loss of bone tissue and spontaneous fractures.

The diagnosis of primary hyperparathyroidism is confirmed by estimation of the serum parathyroid hormone (PTH) level by the technique of radio-immunoassay. Mild, asymptomatic elderly patients without evidence of hyperparathyroid bone disease may require no specific treatment and can be kept under medical surveillance. The most effective treatment for the condition is surgical removal of the parathyroid adenoma. Parathyroidectomy is well tolerated by elderly patients irrespective of their age (Heath *et al.* 1980). Prolonged medical treatment has not yet proved generally to be satisfactory, but in some patients, who may be unfit for surgery, short-term biochemical and symptomatic benefit may be obtained with the use of oral phosphate or diphosphonates, for example sodium etidronate.

Hypocalcaemia may be associated with severe renal impairment, steatorrhoea, osteomalacia, chronic diarrhoea, iron-storage disease, malignant disease and a history of neck surgery or irradiation. Idiopathic hypoparathyroidism may present for the first time in old age and manifestations may include confusion or late onset epilepsy (Graham *et al.* 1979).

Phaeochromocytoma is uncommon in old age but it may present with severe labile hypertension. Surgical removal of the tumour can be successfully achieved and this may render the patient normotensive (Cooper *et al.* 1986).

REFERENCES

Bahemuka M. & Hodkinson H.M. (1975) Screening for hypothyroidism in elderly inpatients. *British Medical Journal* **2,** 601.

Campbell A.J., Reinken J. & Allan B.C. (1981) Thyroid disease in the elderly in the community. *Age and Ageing* **10,** 47.

Cooper M.E., Goodman D.G., Frauman A., Jerums G. & Louis W.J. (1986) Phaeochromocytoma in the elderly: a poorly recognized entity? *British Medical Journal* **293,** 1474.

Graham K., Williams B.O. & Rowe M.J. (1979) Idiopathic hypoparathyroidism: a cause of fits in the elderly. *British Medical Journal* **1,** 1460.

Heath D.A., Wright A.D., Barnes A.D., Oates G.D. & Dorricott N.J. (1980) Surgical treatment of primary hyperparathyroidism in the elderly. *British Medical Journal* **280,** 1406.

Keen H. & Fuller J.M. (1980). The epidemiology of diabetes. In *Metabolic and Nutritional Disorders in the Elderly* (Ed. Exton-Smith A.N. & Caird F.I.) Bristol, John Wright.

Martin B.J., Knight P.V., Kesson C.M., O'Donnell J.R. & Young R.E. (1984) Glycosylated haemoglobin: its value in screening for diabetes mellitus in the elderly. *Journal of Clinical and Experimental Gerontology* **6,** 87.

Mundy G.R., Cove D.H. & Fisken R. (1980) Primary hyperparathyroidism: changes in the pattern of clinical presentation. *Lancet* **1,** 1317.

Toft A.D. (1985) Thyroxine replacement treatment: clinical judgement or biochemical control? *British Medical Journal* **291,** 233.

Tunbridge W.M.G. *et al.* (1977) The spectrum of thyroid disease in a community: the Whickham survey. *Clinical Endocrinology* **7,** 481.

Tunbridge W.M.G. *et al.* (1981) Natural history of autoimmune thyroiditis. *British Medical Journal* **282,** 258.

Young R.E., Jones S.J., Bewsher P.D. & Hedley A.J. (1984) Age and the daily dose of thyroxine replacement therapy for hypothyroidism. *Age and Ageing* **13,** 299.

11
Diseases of the Kidney and Prostate

With increasing age the resting renal blood flow and glomerular filtration rate diminish and both the excretory and reabsorption capacities of the renal tubules decrease. Thus as people grow older renal efficiency gradually deteriorates and as all functions of the kidney decline at about the same rate, it can be concluded that nephrons are lost in their entirety. The remaining units are adequate to maintain renal function under resting conditions but reserve capacities are substantially reduced in the ageing individual. Reduction in renal mass with age has been documented and it has been shown that compensatory hypertrophy decreases with age, for example after removal of one kidney. The total renal function in the elderly may be only 50% of that of the young adult even in the absence of a rise in blood-urea level. The usual measure of renal function, the glomerular filtration rate, decreases 46% from 20 to 90 years of age. At the same time renal blood flow decreases 53% (Shock 1968). Within a narrowed range of adaptability the kidney of the older individual appears capable of maintaining a normal acid base balance. The kidneys of older people are less well able to respond to fluctuations in hydration, solute load, and renal perfusion. Diminished total cell mass is associated with a decreased content of body water, a reflection of the decreased water content of the intracellular space. The total body potassium decreases with the diminished cell mass. The body desiccates with age. Hyponatraemia may result from injudicious use of diuretics, some of which can cause uninterrupted sodium loss, which may on occasion result in acute renal failure. Prolonged use of laxatives and diuretics may result in significant loss of potassium and tablets that combine potassium with a diuretic may not be sufficient to compensate for this.

RENAL DISEASE

Renal lesions are not a major cause of death in old people. In 1969, Black & Moore surveyed urinary infection in the elderly stating that renal disease following urinary infection was the most common single cause of death from kidney disease, the death rate from re-infection after infancy was higher in women than in men until the age of 65 but in the elderly the death rate was higher in men.

Acute renal failure

1   Intrinsic acute renal failure.
2   Prerenal or extrarenal failure.
3   Postrenal failure.

Intrinsic acute renal failure

Kumar *et al.* (1973) analysed the development of acute renal failure in 122 patients over the age of 70 years. Patients with a past history of renal disease and those with acute-on-chronic renal failure were excluded. The diagnosis of acute renal failure was based on the presence of oliguria and rising blood urea levels. In 84 patients the renal failure was attributed to ischaemic renal damage. Dehydration and electrolyte imbalance was an important factor in 59 patients and 38 had undergone major surgery. Profound hypotension was recorded in 33 patients after various catastrophes, e.g. myocardial infarction, gastrointestinal haemorrhage, leaking aortic aneurysm, acute pancreatitis, respiratory failure and drug-induced anaphylaxis. Thirteen patients had bronchopneumonia and renal failure developed secondary to dehydration and toxaemia. The use of antibiotics, especially tetracycline, was thought to have caused acute renal failure in nine patients, while in two, the only preceding event was the use of intravenous contrast media. In summary the causes were ischaemia, toxaemia with dehydration and drugs. Drugs of particular danger in the elderly are the non-steroidal anti-inflammatory agents and the aminoglycoside antibiotics. The clinical features are gastrointestinal, e.g. anorexia, nausea, vomiting, diarrhoea and respiratory dyspnoea with other symptoms depending on the causative factors.

Treatment

In addition to routine care of the bladder, prevention of infection and dietary control, correction of electrolyte and fluid balance is of prime importance. Prophylactic use of antibiotics is usually avoided, but when indicated by proven infection, antibiotics are used under bacteriological control and with serum assays when the drugs are nephrotoxic. Tetracyclines are best avoided because of the risk of deterioration in renal function. Levy (1981) advises for acute established renal failure careful monitoring of fluid balance with fluid intake restricted to 500 ml/day with the previous 24 hours losses from urine, vomiting or diarrhoea added. Diet, oral if possible, should provide over 2000 calories of carbohydrate and should cover requirements of essential carbohydrates. Correction of electrolyte imbalance and dialysis where indicated are other recommendations. Deteriorating clinical condition, urea above 30 mmol/l, severe acidosis and hyperkalaemia are indications for dialysis, usually of the peritoneal type. Episodes of hypotension are treated with the liberal use of hydrocortisone, intravenous fluids, blood transfusion and antibiotics if bacteraemia is considered to be present. The most important cause of death is infection: bronchopneumonia or septicaemia; myocardial infarction is the second most common cause.

Dehydration and electrolyte imbalance are the major precipitating factors of acute renal failure with major surgery the second most important cause. Infection is both a causative factor and a complication. The use of nephrotoxic antibiotics must be avoided in the elderly since they may cause renal failure, especially if other factors are present.

In elderly patients with acute renal failure the prognosis should not be regarded as being hopeless by reason of the patient's age alone, and every effort should be made to offer all available forms of treatment.

Prerenal or extrarenal failure

As detailed above, dehydration may complicate the clinical picture and introduce an extrarenal element which in other cases may be anaemia or a myocardial infarct. The kidneys of old people already depleted in total number of nephrons are very liable to fail because of extrarenal uraemia. Simple dehydration caused by weakness or other illness such as a cerebral infarction or salt and water deprivation must be considered. Cardiac infarction or congestive heart failure may be producing a poor renal blood flow precipitating this condition. Other causes such as loss of fluid from gastrointestinal haemorrhage, or from shock after trauma or burns may cause uraemia. These are the types of uraemia to be stressed in the elderly as the simple measures of treatment for the appropriate condition remedy the disease, and the diagnosis can be made by clinical observation with haemoglobin estimation and biochemical help. This extrarenal or prerenal uraemia is more likely to occur in patients with existing renal damage.

Postrenal failure

Postrenal uraemia is associated with obstruction at any point in the urinary tract. The most common cause is prostatic obstruction, and because it tends to be intermittent and insidious in onset it is usually a factor in producing damage to the renal parenchyma either from hydronephrosis or infection or both. Prompt surgical treatment of prostatic obstruction is essential. Carcinoma of the prostate or obstruction to the ureter or bladder outflow by calculi produces the same syndrome.

Chronic renal failure

This is due to progressive organic renal disease and in the elderly this is most likely due to chronic or recurrent pyelonephritis with hydronephrosis from intermittent obstruction to the urinary outflow, while pyonephrosis as a complicating factor is occasionally found. Amyloid disease of the kidney is sometimes seen and kidney disorders due to collagen disease, diabetes, gout, myelomatosis and renal vein thrombosis may be discovered. Uraemia associated with hypertension is not common but such a kidney would be liable to be affected by the extrarenal causes of uraemia.

Clinical findings

The symptoms of weakness, apathy, drowsiness by day, with not infrequently confusion at night, progress to those of headache, loss of appetite and vomiting; muscular weakness develops and a foul breath is sometimes noted with a dry brown tongue. The skin lacks moisture and is of yellowish colour; there is often a complaint of pruritus. Troublesome diarrhoea may occur and involuntary twitching may be noted, while a normocytic anaemia may be found. Respiration becomes deep and is often Cheyne–Stokes in type, and because of associated left ventricular failure paroxysmal nocturnal dyspnoea may occur. Pericarditis, bronchopneumonia and spontaneous bleeding, e.g. from stomach or into the skin, can develop suddenly and the latter especially is often seen as a terminal event. The diagnosis may be very difficult and requires full biochemical help and in the absence of a reliable history is often one of exclusion. In geriatric practice such a diagnosis is impossible to make without the full facilities of a general hospital.

Treatment

Fluid and electrolyte balance must be restored. The factors precipitating the condition, e.g. myocardial infarction, congestive cardiac failure or blood loss, must be treated promptly. A low circulating blood volume should be corrected and surgical opinion sought early if an obstructive element in the urinary tract is suspected. When uraemia is due to chronic renal failure treatment becomes complex and is often of little avail. If the blood urea level is running above 17 mmol/l the protein content of the diet should be restricted to the essential amino-acids. An adequate fluid intake, 3 l/day is prescribed in the endeavour to obtain 2 litres of urine. Salt restriction is likewise not indicated unless oedema or congestive cardiac failure is present. Oedema in chronic renal failure may be relieved by frusemide or bumetanide in large doses. Acidosis, if present, should be corrected initially by sodium bicarbonate 2–10 g/day orally and then if long-term administration is necessary changed to sodium citrate to prevent the development of skeletal demineralization. Occasionally excessive loss of salt occurs in the urine and this may happen if chronic pyelonephritis is the cause of the renal failure. This is revealed by a persistently low value for serum sodium and on clinical examination a weak, confused patient is found who is almost certainly hypotensive. Clinical improvement follows the administration of 5–10 g of salt by mouth per day. Anaemia in chronic renal failure (p. 131) is usually unresponsive to iron, folic acid or hydroxocobalamin. The patients are often well adjusted to their low haemoglobin level and unless the haemoglobin falls below 8 g/100 ml blood transfusion is not advisable, and unfortunately when it becomes necessary the effect of the blood transfusion is usually transient. Nausea, vomiting and itch may be relieved by chlorpromazine 25 mg intramuscularly which may also help the restless. Chloral hydrate derivatives or temazepam are the recommended hypnotics in such cases, but if these are unsuccessful morphine may be required. Thioridazine 25 mg three times per day may allay the worry and distress of these patients and sometimes lessens the hiccough. Mainten-ance haemodialysis should be considered bearing in mind the importance of the quality of life and that the younger old survive longer on dialysis than the very old. Ambulatory peritoneal dialysis is also effective in the elderly. Renal transplants are not usually advised but can be carried out; the dangers of adverse effects due to high doses of prednisone therapy is a possible contraindication. Towards the end of their life these patients require peace and symptomatic relief and every effort should be made to provide this rather than meticulous correction of the biochemical abnor-mality.

Metabolic bone disease due to chronic renal failure may be overlooked in elderly people. This manifests itself by spontaneous bone pain and inability to walk and responds to treatment with vitamin D. Calcium blood levels must be watched carefully during this therapy.

Acute glomerulonephritis

Arieff, Anderson & Massry (1973) reported five cases each with a different presenting clinical picture and postulated that acute glomerulonephritis is not a single disease but rather represents a pattern of reaction of the kid-ney for many different reasons. While streptococcal infection is probably the main underlying cause, immune responses of the kidneys to antibodies and other generalized diseases such as systemic lupus erythematosus, polyarteritis, Goodpasture syndrome, Henoch–Schonlein purpura, thrombotic thromboctytopenic purpura, haemolytic uraemic syndrome, and bacterial endocarditis may lead to a clinical picture of acute glomerulonephritis.

While the classical case of acute glomerulonephritis presents no diagnostic difficulty in elderly patients, the initial diagnosis may be that of congestive heart failure or infection and renal disease is not considered. The most common manifestations are those of oedema, dyspnoea, circulatory congestion, infection and non-specific symptoms such as anorexia, nausea, vomiting, diarrhoea and muscle pain. Hypertension is less common. While protein, blood cells and red blood cell casts are usually present in the urine, the absence of any of these findings does not rule out the diagnosis and the laboratory findings may be singularly unhelpful.

Anaemia, elevated erythrocyte sedimentation rate and hypoalbuminaemia are variable. While in most individuals renal biopsy is not recommended, it may occasionally be necessary for diagnosis. Elderly patients with acute glomerulonephritis are prone to oliguria.

In undiagnosed uraemia in the elderly, acute glomerulonephritis should be excluded and moderate or marked renal failure should be treated as potentially reversible. In such cases there is the usual history of pharyngeal infection with a change in volume and colour of urine. Breathlessness, especially on exertion, is common in patients over 40 years of age, while haematuria is noted in nearly every patient; treatment is similar to that for acute renal failure.

Nephrotic syndrome

Fawcett *et al.* (1971) found that patients aged 60 years and over accounted for 25 out of 100 consecutive adult cases of the nephrotic syndrome. Amyloidosis did not have a higher incidence in the higher age group and five of the elderly patients with minimal-change lesions were treated with prednisolone. In four, a complete remission from the nephrotic syndrome followed, while the fifth patient's course was unknown. These results suggested that when the patient's other circumstances allowed, the nephrotic syndrome in an elderly patient should be investigated and managed as in younger age groups.

Pyelonephritis

This is the most common type of renal disease with its greatest incidence in the ninth decade (McKeown 1965). Prostatic disease, calculi, neurological disease, prolonged recumbency and diabetes are among the predisposing causes of acute pyelonephritis. This illness usually shows itself by loin pain, frequency of micturition and pyrexia. Some cases of pyelonephritis are due to abnormalities or obstruction of the urinary tract and the bulk of the evidence suggests that the infection travels up the ureter from below, but transient bacteriaemia is the cause in other cases.

This illness is more difficult to diagnose in the elderly in its chronic form and the symptoms may include one or more of the following: tiredness, backache, anaemia or weight loss, renal failure or hypertension. A urinary infection may be discovered during the routine investigation of some other illness; the first indication may be proteinuria, hypertension or both, or even advanced renal failure in a previously symptomless patient. A significant number of elderly persons who are apparently normal have occult renal disease mainly chronic interstitial pyelonephritis. An elderly person with unexplained fever or with vomiting without obvious cause or with depression might have this illness and symptoms may be absent or unheeded. It is said that about half the chronic cases have a normal blood pressure.

The diagnosis of pyelonephritis depends largely on bacteriological and radiological investigation. A specimen of midstream urine in men or a clean voided midstream specimen in women is sent to the laboratory. If this is not possible, as for example in incontinent patients, a sterile plastic bag can be attached to the penis or a sterile tinfoil tray placed under the thighs of a female patient after washing the genitalia with saline. The urine obtained can be transferred to a sterile container. In mentally confused or obese women it may be necessary to catheterize the patient to obtain a suitable specimen of urine. If this has to be done it is recommended that 60 ml of a one in 5 000 solution of chlorhexidine diacetate be instilled into the bladder at the end of the catheterization. The presence or absence of proteinuria is an unreliable index of urinary infection. The diagnosis of urinary infection is made by culturing the urine and performing a bacterial count. More than 100 000 organisms/ml denote infection while counts between 10 000 and 100 000 are doubtful and a repeat examination is necessary. The presence of pus cells in the urine is suggestive of infection which must be confirmed by culture. Urine from the renal pelvis and blood may also be cultured. Serum antibodies may be present against the infecting organism and are indicative of renal involvement. Other tests employed include straight x-ray of abdomen, abdominal ultrasound and intravenous pyelography. If renal function is impaired and the blood urea is of the order of 17 mmol/l or more there is usually insufficient concentration of the dye to give a shadow.

Treatment

Immediately the disease is suspected a culture of urine should be sent for bacteriological examination; the aim of therapy is to eradicate infection from the urinary tract quickly and completely. Before this result is known treatment should be started at once with co-trimoxazole, two tablets per day, although Asscher (1981) considers that trimethoprim on its own is more effective especially for out-patients. The dose is 200 mg every 12 hours or once daily if renal impairment is present. Alternative anti-biotics are sulphadimidine or ampicillin.

Cephalexin (Ceporex) orally or gentamicin parenterally are useful preparations when bacteriological results indicate that they are likely to be effective.

The correct antibiotic treatment depends on the sensitivity of the organism and while the antibiotics mentioned above may be started, if there is no clinical response the antibiotics should be changed at once to the one indicated by the bacteriologist's report.

It is essential to continue the chemotherapy for at least 7 days. For recurrent infection long-term therapy can be undertaken with appropriate doses of co-trimoxazole. If infection persists an alternative antibiotic to which the organism is sensitive should be used.

Tests of cure by urine culture must be undertaken; in any recurring infection the possibility of renal or bladder calculus or other form of obstruction to urinary outflow should be considered.

Hydronephrosis and pyonephrosis

In older people these conditions are not uncommon and the cause is likely to be intermittent obstruction to urinary flow coupled with ascending infection. Unsuspected bilateral hydronephrosis with severe secondary renal damage is often found at necropsy in patients who die in chronic renal failure. On occasion, individuals who are severely wasted with gross signs of toxaemia and a terminally rising blood urea are found at autopsy to have gross pyonephrosis when no infection could be demonstrated.

PROSTATE GLAND

As the individual ages the prostate changes and the resulting obstruction if it occurs bears little relationship to the size of the gland. Large adenomata can occur with no residual urine while severe obstruction may take place with a small fibrous contracted prostate.

Benign prostatic hypertrophy

Disease of the prostate gland is a common condition in elderly men and is associated with some degree of discomfort or difficulty in passing urine. Older patients do not report their symptoms usually until a late stage and direct enquiry about the function of micturition is an essential part of history taking. The size of the gland on rectal examination is frequently unrelated to the symptoms and when the history and observation of the patient suggests prostatic hypertrophy the urological surgeon should be contacted promptly. An unexpected finding of uraemia requires the exclusion of prostatic obstruction as a cause. A complete knowledge of the patient's medical and surgical status is essential before operation and necessary investigations include flow studies, urine culture, blood levels of urea, creatinine, acid phosphatase and haemoglobin. Every effort should be made to prepare the patient for operation as adequately as possible.

Treatment is by transurethral resection of the prostate or prostatectomy. It is not reasonable to deny surgery of the prostate to men on grounds of age alone, if they are otherwise healthy. Ninety-five per cent of prostatectomies are performed transurethrally and mortality is less than 3%. If the patient is admitted as an emergency the mortality is trebled due to the increased incidence of infection and impairment of renal function. Contraindications to operation are cardiac pain at rest, intractable cardiac failure, respiratory disease so advanced as to limit mobility and a recent cerebrovascular accident. If the patient has had a myocardial infarction it is usually advisable to wait 3 months from the incident. A patient with a pacemaker can be operated on provided the pacemaker is in the pectoral region as diathermy will destroy one in the lower abdomen. Most patients retain sexual potency after prostatectomy if sexual activity existed before the operation.

In patients unsuitable for operation gestronol hexanoate (Depostat) by intramuscular injection once per week for 6–8 weeks has been tried. Phenoxybenzamine (Dibenyline) in a dose of 10 mg/day increasing to 10 mg twice per day if there are no adverse effects has been used when there is a particular reason to delay operation. Contraindications are hypotension or angina and common adverse effects are hypotension with giddiness, tachycardia and stuffiness of the nose (Chisholm 1981).

Carcinoma of the prostate

This is a common disease of old men and it is rare before 50 but the disease increases rapidly in occurrence to 80 years. Among those aged 80 years,

80% will have histological evidence of carcinoma of the prostate. Thus its incidence is later than benign prostatic hypertrophy, and it said to remain localized initially up to 3 years and then it may spread to bladder and metastasize to bones, especially the pelvis, vertebrae, or proximal femur; the next most frequent sites are lungs, liver and aortic nodes. Thus, carcinoma of the prostate is frequently present in very old men without causing symptoms. Prostatic cancers are divided into clinical, latent and occult. Clinical is when the disease is producing symptoms and is diagnosed by history. Latent cancers are those foci, morphologically resembling prostate cancer that do not themselves produce symptoms. They are usually found incidentally at prostatectomy or necropsy and have not at that time disseminated. Occult cancers are those producing metastases while the primary remains insignificant in size or hidden.

Symptoms are frequently due either to obstruction to bladder outflow or to the metastases, for example pain in the back or legs or weight loss and weakness and persistent anaemia; oedema of the lower limbs with lymphadenopathy may be discovered. Haematuria is usually a late symptom. It can be seen, therefore, that this illness is very difficult to detect clinically at an early stage.

The diagnosis depends eventually on rectal examination and if the prostate feels hard, an x-ray of pelvis is essential to exclude prostatic calculi. In carcinoma of the prostate the gland is hard, fixed and has ill-defined margins; the swelling may be nodular. With focal disease acid phosphatase is likely to be normal; once disease spreads beyond the confines of the gland both total and prostatic fraction of acid phosphatase will be raised. Radio-immunoassay of acid phosphatase is very sensitive and may be raised in focal disease. Estimation of blood levels of urea and electrolytes are useful as overflow obstruction can cause renal impairment. The frequency of bone involvement indicates the need to check levels of calcium, inorganic phosphate and alkaline phosphatase. Hypercalcaemia is commonly due to bone invasion but can also be caused by non-metastatic hormonal effects. These estimations are important in the investigation of illness in elderly men as the treatment of prostatic carcinoma in its early stages is effective. If the diagnosis is doubtful, examination of the prostatic fluid obtained after massage of the prostate may reveal carcinoma cells or needle biopsy may be positive and cysto-scopy may show appearances that are suggestive of carcinoma of the prostate. Once the diagnosis is established a bone scan should be performed to detect metastatic disease and in most cases immediate consultation with an urologist is essential; when there are complications a team approach with radiotherapist and physician specializing in diseases of the elderly is indicated as well.

Radical prostatectomy is in practice performed in a relatively small group of cases but carries a high survival rate, 90% 10-year survival with lesions less than 1 cm in diameter; unfortunately the risk of urinary incontinence is high. For the bulk of cases transurethral resection may be needed to overcome obstruction of the urinary tract, while obstruction in extreme old age or the presence of advanced local disease or metastases indicates the need for stilboestrol. The use of oestrogen in every patient with carcinoma of the prostate is unnecessary and may be harmful. It is probably not required in the presence of focal disease with well differentiated cells. If the histology reveals undifferentiated cells early treatment is justified. Stilboestrol is given orally in a dose of 1 mg three times per day and should be continued for the rest of the patient's life. If fluid retention is a problem a diuretic should be given. A fall in serum acid phosphatase, if this was initially raised, would usually be indicative of satisfactory progress. When a rapid therapeutic response is essential the use of intravenous fosfestrol tetrasodium (Honvan) over a period of 7–10 days in a dose of 1000 mg/day is advised. This substance may also be used if the initial clinical response to stilboestrol is unsatisfactory or if symptoms recur after remission in a dose of 100 mg three times daily by mouth. The development of venous thrombosis, pulmonary embolism, heart failure or a stroke are indications for stopping the oestrogens and recurrence of local symptoms would then be treated where possible by transurethral resection and when applicable painful metastases by radiotherapy. The complications of stilboestrol therapy are gynaecomastia and fluid retention with dependent oedema; diuretics control the oedema. Polyestradiol phosphate (Estradurin) has the advantage of being effective when given as a single injection once monthly. Where tumour staging of disease is used one extending beyond the capsule or into the seminal vesicles or tumour fixed or invading neighbouring structures respond to external beam radiotherapy.

Bilateral orchidectomy is the treatment of choice where there are cardiovascular contraindictions to oestrogen administration. Advantages are that feminization does not occur, the breasts do not become painful, impotence is not inevitable and there is no need to remember to take tablets. When there is bone pain this may be relieved by radiotherapy and if this fails hypophysectomy may be of value. The place of cytotoxic drugs requires further elucidation but a combination of oestrogen and a cytotoxic agent estramustine phosphate (Estracyt) may be considered when primary treatment has failed. The recommended dose is 140 mg four times daily and this requires adjustment according to the presence of adverse effects such as nausea and vomiting. Prognosis (Chisholm 1981) for overall survival for 5 years is about 60%; for patients who present with metastases at the time of diagnosis, the interval between diagnosis and death averages less than 3 years. The average 15-year survival for early localized tumour is about 30%.

Prostatitis

Acute inflammation of the duct and acini is commonly due to infection with *Escherichia coli, Streptococcus faecalis* or *Staphylococci.*

Initially symptoms are fever, rigors and a feeling of weakness. Frequency of micturition, pain on passing urine or in the perineum or groin may be noted. Rectal pain and painful defaecation may occur while haematuria at the end of micturition is often present. Severe perineal pain may indicate that a prostatic abscess has formed and this condition is sometimes associated with retention of urine. On rectal examination the prostate gland is tender, swollen and may feel nodular. Direct examination of the expressed prostatic secretion can provide evidence of the infection and confirmation rests on the culture of the causative organism.

Treatment consists of rest in bed while co-trimoxazole and erythromycin are the drugs of choice but bacteriological culture will give accurate information on this. The main problem of therapy is that antibiotics have difficulty in reaching the prostatic fluid.

REFERENCES

Arieff A.I., Anderson R.J. & Massry S.G. (1973) Acute glomerulonephritis. *Modern Geriatrics* **3,** 77.
Asscher A.W. (1981) Urinary tract infection. *Journal of the Royal College of Physicians of London* **16,** 232.
Black D.A.K. & Moore T. (1969) Urinary infection in the elderly. *Geriatrics* **24,** 126.
Chisholm G.D. (1981) Benign prostatic hypertrophy and carcinoma of the prostate. *Prescriber's Journal* **21,** 278.
Fawcett I.W., Hilton P.J., Jones N.F. & Wing A.T. (1971) Nephrotic syndrome in the elderly. *British Medical Journal* **2,** 387.
Kumar R., Hill C.M. & McGeown M.G. (1973) Acute renal failure in the elderly. *Lancet* **1,** 90.
Levy D.W. (1981) Acute renal problems in old age. In *Acute Geriatric Medicine* (Ed. Coakley D.) London, Croom Helm.
McKeown I. (1965) *Pathology of the Aged.* London, Butterworth.
Shock N.W. (1968) The physiology of ageing. In *Surgery of the Aged and Debilitated Patient* (Ed. Powers J.H.) Philadelphia, W.B. Saunders.

12
Diseases of the Bladder and Urinary Incontinence

BLADDER

The urinary bladder accommodates approximately 500 ml urine and fills slowly without much increase in intravesical pressure. It is capable of emptying itself completely and can hold as much as 2000 ml urine but when filled to this capacity there is usually pain except in some very old people or if this volume has been reached over a long period of time. Awareness of distension reaches consciousness at about 250 ml but no intrinsic contractions of the bladder occur then unless they are consciously allowed by the individual in order to empty the bladder. When the bladder is full to capacity there is an urge to micturate with a rapid rise in intravesical pressure, but this desire can be suppressed if socially inconvenient by cortical inhibition of the spinal reflex arc. If bladder filling continues a pressure is reached where further cortical inhibitory control is impossible and voiding occurs. When micturition is desired contraction of the detrusor muscle and funnelling of the bladder outlet occurs. The bladder neck and the urethra are opened and the pelvic muscles relax and voiding takes place. The rising intravesical pressure is conveyed by afferent impulses by the parasympathetic nerves and the detrusor muscle continues to contract smoothly and urine is expelled at a steady rate until the bladder is empty. Detrusor muscle contraction that cannot be suppressed is called unstable or an unhibited contraction.

Closure of the urethra takes place initially in the male at the external sphincter and in the female about the midurethra. The external sphincter in males and in females the proximal urethra maintain continence when intra-abdominal pressure is raised in coughing or straining. In normal people, straining during micturition increases the rate of urine flow but in some males with enlargement of the prostate such action decreases the urine flow. Voluntary interruption of micturition is achieved by contraction of the striated muscle of the pelvic floor and the distal sphincter. Detrusor relaxation is a slower process but is usually completed as striated muscle activity declines. Any urine proximal to the region of the external sphincter empties back into the bladder.

173

With advancing age there is a gradual decline in the tone of voluntary muscle with diminished strength of the pelvic floor and the external sphincter. Diverticula and trabeculation in the bladder are found with increasing frequency in old age.

In women declining levels of oestrogen result in atrophic changes which cause not only senile vaginitis but also marked thinning of the tissues of the external genitalia and of the lower urinary epithelium.

Symptoms associated with bladder dysfunction

Nocturnal frequency (nocturia) is usually the first symptom of increased frequency of micturition. It may be caused by irritation or inflammation of the bladder wall which makes the stretch receptors more sensitive. Frequency is a symptom of bacterial cystitis, bladder stone, tumour or a neurological lesion. When retention of urine with a large residual volume of urine in the bladder at the end of micturition is present, frequency may occur.

Urgency of micturition is a common symptom in the elderly and the signal denoting the sensation of fullness of the bladder probably declines over a lengthy period so that the individual is unaware of the usual rise of tension denoting bladder fullness. The desire to micturate then arises only when the stimulation from the bladder is greatly increased by the actual bladder contraction just before the onset of micturition. With increasing age the higher centre control weakens so that instead of being able to post-pone micturition for an hour or more after the sensation of fullness has been experienced the older person may be able to delay micturition only for a matter of minutes. Frequency and urgency in the absence of infection, mechanical or neurological abnormalities may be due to overactivity of the detrusor muscle and this is called detrusor instability resulting in the unstable bladder. This shows uninhibited contractions which occur at any capacity and may take place during normal filling or following any rise in intra-abdominal pressure such as coughing or change of posture. This is common in men with an enlarged prostate showing obstruction; such patients will often be incontinent and this fact should be known before operation or surgical intervention may fail to cure the incontinence.

Painful micturition (dysuria) is characteristic of lower urinary infection while hesitancy, i.e. a delay between voluntary initiation of micturition and the occurence, if associated with diminution in the urinary stream, is usual in patients with prostatic obstruction. Dysuria may also be used to describe difficulty in passing urine.

The most common symptom is nocturnal frequency which is noted more frequently as age increases and is generally associated with loss of cortical inhibition over the sacral bladder centre. Urinary incontinence is commoner in women and is found more often as age advances. When it is severe it is frequently associated with dementia. Precipitancy of micturition and scalding on micturition are also common while difficulty in passing urine is noted more often in men while urinary tract infection occurs more frequently in women.

Special diagnostic methods

Cystometrogram

A cystometer is a manometer attached to a catheter in the bladder which reveals pressure changes within the bladder as the bladder fills. The pressure in the rectum is also measured and thus the intravesical and the intra-abdominal pressures are recorded simultaneously. Cystometry is performed with the patient awake to obtain information regarding the sensory aspects. By this type of investigation the types of neurogenic bladder can be identified and the unstable bladder discovered.

Peak flow rate

Peak flow rate is a useful measurement to record, however the volume voided must be known as flow rates are related to bladder volume.

High voiding pressures with low flow rates suggest outflow obstruction. High voiding pressures with normal flow rates are probably due to detrusor hypertrophy in response to increased resistance while low flow rates with low detrusor pressure indicate a deficient detrusor.

Micturating cystogram

The micturating cystogram is of value and the pressure recordings of the cystometrogram can be taken simultaneously with x-ray screening of the bladder filled with a radio-opaque fluid. By this method differentiation can be made between neurogenic and non-neurogenic causes of incontinence. Bladder neck obstruction will be revealed by the presence of trabeculation and eventually by diverticula.

Cystoscopy

Cystoscopy will show the presence of inflammation, hypertrophy and other abnormalities such as stone, papilloma and carcinoma of the bladder.

Haematuria

The history of the incident should be taken, but in elderly people the account given is often unreliable and certain methods of investigation are now standard procedure. The urine stick test is very sensitive and can detect as few as 5×10^6 red cells per litre of urine. A red cell count of more than 100×10^6 per litre of urine in centrifuged specimen is regarded as abnormal and in older people must be taken seriously.

Concomitant treatment with anticoagulants should not be blamed for microscopical haematuria as some people who develop haematuria while taking warfarin have urological disease.

After exclusion of a local genital cause for the bleeding by examination straight x-ray of bladder and kidneys, urine culture and cytology, intravenous urography and cystoscopy are necessary. If no cause can be found a follow-up should be arranged for repeat analysis of urine and cytology every 6 months and if bleeding continues cystoscopy and urography undertaken at intervals of 1 year. About 50% of older patients with haematuria have carcinoma of the bladder (Bullock 1986).

Common causes of haematuria in the elderly are as follows:

Cystitis

Haematuria can occur in haemorrhagic cystitis. This condition tends to relapse frequently, and while occasionally it is painless it is often associated with painful, frequent micturition. The finding of evidence of an infected urine together with haematuria is not sufficient to establish this diagnosis, which is essentially one of exclusion.

Papilloma of the bladder

Not all papillomas are malignant, but they must be considered as potentially so and repeatedly subjected to cytoscopic observation. Most papillomas can be treated effectively by diathermy through a cystoscope, and in the malignant forms of bladder growth there is usually an associated infection and the patient may complain of dysuria and frequency as well as haematuria. The diagnosis is made by cystoscopic examination and by biopsy.

Tumours of the kidney

These usually present as cases of haematuria often with pain on the affected side and the diagnosis is made by pyelography. Surgical removal is the only effective treatment.

Urinary stones

Stones in the upper urinary tract are said to be uncommon over 60 years and are not always painful. Non-obstructive stones may be found lying in the renal pelvis, often of great size and frequently without pain, but usually associated with renal infection. If the patient is very elderly the associated infection should be treated but surgical removal of the kidney is not, as a rule, advised.

Bladder stone is a relatively common disease of old age and is often found where urinary tract infection is recurrent and does not yield properly to treatment. A stone of moderate size can be crushed without difficulty and the fragments removed. If associated with prostatic enlargement the prostate may have to be dealt with and both conditions can then be treated by perurethral methods. The recently developed technique of extracorporeal shockwave lithotripsy appears to be a safe, effective and economical method of treating renal and ureteric calculi with a low incidence of side effects in expert hands (Das *et al.* 1987).

Disease of the prostate

It is said that benign enlargement of the prostate is more liable to cause bleeding than malignant disease and that the bleeding is due to the highly vascular state of the enlarged prostate.

Other conditions

Acute glomerulonephritis, tuberculosis of the kidney, blood disorders and treatment with anticoagulants are other causes of haematuria. Tuberculosis of the kidney is an eminently treatable cause of haematuria and the diagnosis is made by pyelography and urine culture and the treatment is by antituberculosis drugs and steroids. In patients with leukaemia, haematuria can occur; and it is essential to note whether the patient has been receiving anticoagulant therapy as this is a relatively common cause of haematuria.

Cystitis

This is a common illness in elderly people, and in men is usually associated with urinary stasis following urethral stricture or prostatic disease. In women it is sometimes impossible to find a cause for stasis but cystitis is frequently associated with a cystocele. In both sexes where cystitis does not yield rapidly to appropriate therapy the complications of bladder stone and bladder tumours should be considered. Cystitis is also liable to occur where the patient has been in bed for some considerable time or is suffering from disease of the nervous system associated with bladder dysfunction, and occasionally the infection is introduced into the bladder by catheterization. The symptoms of acute cystitis are frequency, a burning feeling on passing urine, and sometimes quite severe pain in the lower abdomen. On occasion, haematuria may be found in cystitis among the elderly. The diagnosis depends on examination of the urine and a midstream urine in both sexes should be obtained where possible and submitted to bacteriological examination. Cystitis must be distinguished from the urethral syndrome that may cause similar symptoms but without detectable bacterial infection of the urine; in elderly women this is commonly associated with senile vaginitis but may also be found after gynaecological surgery. In cystitis there are usually many white blood cells in the urine. It is customary to commence treatment before the results of the sensitivity to antibiotics are available, and it is common practice also to start treatment without cystoscopic and radiological investigation in a first attack. In the very elderly the more elaborate searches for an underlying cause are only performed if the cystitis fails to clear promptly or recurs. Carcinoma of the bladder may present as a cystitis that has occurred for the first time in an elderly person and some recommend cystoscopy in cases of recent onset in older people. While haematuria is common in uncomplicated cystitis, the sudden onset of this in a previously fit elderly individual would render cystoscopy advisable. The patients are advised to drink plenty of fluid and in severe infection, co-trimoxazole, two tablets twice per day may be given orally provided that the renal function is satisfactory. Trimethoprim or amoxycillin are alternative drugs. In this condition therapy should last 7–10 days. Choice of antibiotic may have to be altered as a result of the bacteriologist's report or failure of clinical response to therapy. After an interval of 10 days a midstream specimen of urine should be repeated for test of bacteriological cure.

Cancer of the bladder

This occurs most commonly in the seventh decade and more frequently in women; the presenting symptom is usually painless haematuria. Frequency with painful micturition may also be noted while a urinary infection occurring for the first time in old age should be regarded as suspicious especially in women.

Clinical examination is in most cases unhelpful and a cystoscopy is essential. An x-ray of chest and an intravenous pyelogram are also necessary. Treatment is planned in consultation with the urological surgeon and help may be necessary from the radiotherapist; radical cystectomy is being undertaken in some centres while for metastatic or unresectable tumours chemotherapy has been used. Due to the toxicity of this regimen it is wise to recommend specialist chemotherapy units (Hargreave 1985).

Retention of urine

The main problem with elderly people is an accurate diagnosis, and one difficulty is that there may be no complaint by the patient of retention of urine. A distended bladder is recognized as one of the most common causes of restlessness, and uraemia from prostatic obstruction with a dry tongue and full bladder can occur without the patient complaining of urinary disturbance. Faecal impaction must be excluded as an underlying cause, and in all cases of retention of urine rectal examination must be performed. The diagnosis is even more difficult in those who are mentally confused. In men, a frequent cause is prostatic disease and here there may be a history of increasing frequency of micturition over a number of months. The attack of acute retention in such a condition may be precipitated by the patient becoming cold or ill or being unable to empty an over-distended bladder at an inconvenient movement. On occasion, the condition may be precipitated by drunkenness, and retention may be produced by the use of a diuretic drug. Retention of urine in women is not so common and may be due to a gynaecological condition, bladder neck obstruction, or occur after major pelvic or hip surgery, or associated with a cerebrovascular accident, especially one of recent origin. Some patients are psychologically incapable of voiding urine while lying down and thus may develop retention.

Treatment

The treatment of retention of urine depends on the cause of the condition and no attempt at diagnosis should be regarded as complete without a rectal examination; another factor is the availability of immediate skilled aid and if the retention is acute and the patient is near a hospital emergency admission is the best policy. If the cause is thought to be prostatic enlargement a urologist should be consulted at once. As a rule most patients with acute retention require admission to hospital and subsequent operation. If the elderly patient has developed painful retention and lives far from a hospital he should be given an effective dose of morphine and placed in a warm bath; if urine is passed the emergency is over. Even the successfully relieved patient almost certainly requires further diagnostic assessment in hospital in the immediate future. If drug therapy fails unless catheterization is possible in the patient's house hospital admission becomes essential. In such cases infection is the greater danger and every care must be taken to avoid introducing this to the bladder. For patients who can be sent immediately to hospital direct admission to a surgical ward should be arranged as a casualty department, because of the risk of infection, is not a suitable place to pass a catheter. Catheterization is as essentially an aseptic procedure as lumbar puncture. Any attack of acute retention with a history of prostatism is an absolute indication for a prostatectomy. The patient requiring a prostatectomy may benefit from the insertion of a Foley catheter. In a rational patient a Gibbon flexible catheter is easy to insert and comfortable for the patient. If it is impossible to pass a catheter skilled assistance is required and it may be necessary to use a suprapubic catheter. If the patient is being considered for a prostatectomy a careful history must be obtained and a full clinical examination performed with a check on cardiac status, haemoglobin, urea and electrolytes, bacteriology of the urine and ideally a pyelogram; there is no need to postpone operation for this as the pyelogram can be done later. Some patients require long-term catheterization in the management of chronic retention and incontinence when they are unfit for surgery. In women, when no mechanical obstruction to outflow is suspected, the use of carbachol 0.25 mg subcutaneously may be tried. This substance should not be used if the patient is very ill. When the individual responds it may be possible to continue treatment with oral carbachol and so especially in cases of recent cerebrovascular accident achieve control over the bladder. Catheterization with the modern small plastic self-retaining catheter and cover with antibiotics is not so dangerous as in former years, but it is still an undertaking which should only be contemplated if there is no other remedy. If no cause for the retention of urine has been discovered then the urologist should be consulted at an early date and further activity should be the result of a joint plan. Postoperative bladder problems are discussed by Watkins & Vowles (1979) and among other relevant points made it is noted that most men find it difficult to micturate satisfactorily until they are able to stand, and they slip easily into a state of retention with overflow which presents as incontinence.

Incontinence of urine

Incontinence of urine is present when urine is passed repeatedly otherwise than into suitable containers and when this occurrence is outwith the patient's control. The International Continence Society (1976) defined it as a condition in which involuntary loss of urine is a social or hygienic problem and is objectively demonstrable. A more clinical definition is – incontinence is involuntary excretion or leakage of urine in inappropriate places or at inappropriate times twice or more often a month regardless of the quantity of urine lost (Thomas *et al.* 1980). Incontinence is a symptom and not a disease and the causes are numerous. Urinary incontinence occurs in 16% of women 75 and over and in 15% of men 85 and over; these figures increase greatly if residential homes with 32% incontinent people and geriatric units with 50% are considered (Brocklehurst 1986).

Treatment depends on the aetiology and has to be flexible and purposeful to obtain results. Incontinence is a justifiable reason for seeking hospital admission as once this symptom has developed its cause should be looked for as quickly as possible in order to make a correct diagnosis and start treatment.

Incontinence of urine is often the symptom that renders elderly people unable to be kept in their own homes and to the individual is a catastrophe. The act of voluntary micturition is complicated: as the bladder fills a rise in internal pressure occurs and information about this is sent to the spinal cord and brain stimulating the desire to micturate. As a result of social training, if it is inconvenient to micturate, impulses from the cerebral cortex inhibit contractions of the bladder and the desire to pass water is postponed. If the bladder volume exceeds 600 ml the pressure within it can no longer be lowered and as the volume increases there is an uncontrollable act of micturition.

Centres for control and co-ordination of micturition exist in the lower end of the spinal cord, the hypothalamic region and in the cerebral cortex. This latter site provides conscious control mainly of an inhibitory nature. With increasing age the tone in the bladder increases and the capacity decreases and if cortical control is affected by cerebrovascular disease these changes become exaggerated and voluntary control lessened.

The healthy older person tends to pass urine more frequently and has a degree of urgency of micturition. In extreme old age as the need to hurry to the lavatory increases by a strange irony of fate the gait becomes slower.

Local causes of urinary incontinence

Block of outflow of urine. This is seen most commonly in elderly men due to prostatic hypertrophy. The incontinence is of the overflow variety and examination often shows an enlarged bladder to be present, and rectal examination discloses an enlarged prostate. These cases are eminently curable; the patient is often alert and co-operative and the urine may be sterile. The advice of a urologist should be sought at once and when possible catheterization postponed until he has examined the patient. This also applies to other forms of obstruction such as those due to stricture, bladder neck hypertrophy and stones. Faecal impaction of the rectum is another common cause. Sometimes there is no organic obstruction and the bladder is atonic and apparently unable to contract adequately. This is often the cause of urinary retention in the female. In such cases the bladder wall may become very thin and be very difficult to palpate. If the patient is asked to stand the floor may be flooded. A similar type of incontinence may be caused by drugs with anticholinergic actions such as the antidepressants. Straight x-ray of abdomen is valuable to disclose the presence of stones, and intravenous pyelography is helpful in estimating kidney function and showing any structural abnormalities of the renal tract. Phimosis with balanitis may be the cause of difficulty in micturition and yields to surgery. Inspection of the genitalia is essential in all cases of incontinence. Symptoms of outflow obstruction are hesitancy, loss of stream, feeling of incomplete micturition, increased frequency, nocturia, urgency of micturition and possibly urge incontinence. Post-prostatectomy incontinence is most commonly the result of bladder instability which presents after relief of the obstruction. A post-micturition dribble in the male may be due to failure of the bulbocavernous muscle to expel urine remaining in the bulb of the urethra at the end of voiding.

Gynaecological conditions. Urethral caruncle, vaginitis and uterine prolapse are some of the causes of incontinence while stress incontinence brought on by coughing, laughing, or walking, is often due to weakness of the bladder sphincter and the pelvic floor. Vaginal examination should be performed and inspection made for cystocele and procidentia and gynaecological opinion should be sought. Stress incontinence can occur in men following sphincter destruction at prostatectomy.

Urinary infection. While chronic urinary infection does not exert a major influence in the production of incontinence, acute urinary infection may be related to incontinence. It is generally agreed that old people who are confined to bed are more likely to be incontinent. Dysuria and frequency without bacterial infection in the aged female is called the urethral syndrome. This may be due to changes in the hormone-sensitive squamous epithelium of the distal urethra resulting in an atrophic urethritis.

General causes of urinary incontinence

The common cause of urinary incontinence in the elderly with stroke or other type of organic cerebral disease is due to uninhibited detrusor activity – the unstable bladder. The uninhibited detrusor activity renders the bladder neck incompetent. There is loss of the normal warning period between the first desire to micturate and micturition itself and spontaneous contractions of the bladder take place early in filling. When this loss of control is associated with mental confusion the patients are often quite unaware of being incontinent and seem little upset by it. Detrusor instability affects both sexes and the symptoms are frequency, urgency and urge incontinence and trigger incontinence, i.e. at the sound of running water; the bladder is usually hypertonic. Causes of this condition are stroke, dementia, Parkinsonism, normal pressure hydrocephalus and focal frontal lesions.

Spinal cord lesions above the sacral centre may result in an uninhibited bladder. The development of residual urine in these cases depends on the degree of detrusor/sphincter dyssynergia present.

Lesions such as tumour or vascular incidents involving the sacral centre result in an atonic bladder with overflow incontinence while loss of bladder sensation as in diabetes produces progressive distension of the bladder with increased bladder capacity. Typical symptoms are recurrent urinary tract infections and dribbling incontinence or precipitant incontinence.

In severe illness, especially of a terminal nature, incontinence often occurs, especially when accompanied by delirium. Physical disability causing difficulty in walking or in handling a urinal or bedpan can result in incontinence. Emotional disturbance caused by bereavement, being transferred to hospital, resentment or anger may produce incontinence. The older person may feel rejected by relatives, friends and society. Psychological handling of patients is important and no feeling of guilt must be instilled if incontinence occurs.

Incontinence may be caused by drugs such as sedatives, tranquillisers or any substance that produces drowsiness or confusion. Diuretics in some patients may produce incontinence.

Transient incontinence. This may be due to an acute confusional state, an acute cerebrovascular accident, faecal impaction, drugs such as anticholinergic preparations and psychological causes.

Incontinence in stroke patients

If the brain damage is severe or if mental impairment was present before the stroke, the incontinence is likely to be frequent and persistent, and the patient has no knowledge of his bladder function. With lesser degrees of brain injury and if the patient is mentally alert, control is likely to be quickly regained. The most valuable prognostic sign is the mental state, and if confusion is present the incontinence is likely to persist. Patients who are only incontinent at night usually have less severe mental damage and a better prognosis. Other factors that adversely influence the prognosis are poor general health of the patient and local abnormalities of the urinary tract such as obstruction to the outflow of urine, muscular weakness, or bacterial infection. The cystometric findings are usually of detrusor instability.

Many individuals have difficulty in making their wants known because of aphasia and incontinence may be due to this alone. Patients may be shy about asking for attention, especially female patients, and severe bladder distension may occur, followed by an overflow type of incontinence. While in men following a stroke, the patient may only have one good hand and movements may be clumsy, causing difficulty in handling the urinal or with fly buttons and incontinence may be accidental in nature. The cause for the incontinence should be sought and faecal impaction, urinary retention and urinary infection should be excluded. Such patients require regular toileting, charting of the incontinence and active encouragement and reassurance.

Investigation

A detailed history of the illness is essential, with particular reference to the type and duration of the incontinence and the patient's sensation and attitude to it. Thorough medical examination including an accurate assessment of mental state should be performed; special watch should be kept for depression. Inspection of the genitalia and a rectal examination are routine procedures. Thereafter, if the patient is admitted to hospital the incontinence should be recorded on a special chart which provides information as to the amount, whether the incontinence is during the day or night and the response to treatment. A clean specimen of urine is cultured to discover any infection present and serum urea and electrolytes to assess the kidney function. Special investigations are performed in selected cases such as cystoscopy and pyelography. More elaborate urodynamic studies are becoming increasingly available and are of help in difficult cases. Cystometry is the most useful and will demonstrate detrusor instability or outlet obstruction often with secondary detrusor instability – a most important finding to make before prostatectomy is performed. Other conditions revealed by cystometry are stress incontinence, atonic and hypotonic bladders.

Diagnosis is absolutely essential in planning treatment.

Treatment

If a patient is said to be incontinent, the nature of the disability must first be ascertained, and this includes finding out if in fact incontinence is present or if, for example, an elderly gentlemen is unable to avoid spilling the urinal when he tries to take it out of the bed. An incontinence chart is used to record the frequency of the loss of urine and the time at which it is worse, e.g. during the day or night. Is there also incontinence of faeces? This makes the diagnosis of chronic brain failure more likely. The incontinence record is invaluable in determining the progress or otherwise of the individual and of great help when the time comes for discharging the patient, e.g. to an old person's home, as evidence of the complete continence. Knowledge of the frequency of incontinence and the duration of the disability are essential in making a correct diagnosis.

Incontinence of urine is rarely due to one single cause, but some of the factors involved may well be amenable to treatment. It must be emphasized that the whole patient must be dealt with, while local causes must be attended to, and faecal impaction must be kept in mind as a contributory factor. Acute urinary infection should certainly be treated, and oestrogen therapy may help senile vaginitis, which has been incriminated as a cause of incontinence. The general health should be reviewed, anaemia, toxaemia, cerebral anoxia, or over-sedation with drugs may impair cortical control. When a block to urinary outflow is present or a gynaecological condition exists, specialist advice should be sought from a urologist or a gynaeocologist.

The term 'designing towards continence' (Hood 1976) implies a complete reorientation of planning of accommodation at home or in hospital in dealing with incontinent patients. Many old people are unable to walk more than 10 metres before becoming incontinent once they have the desire to micturate so there must always be a toilet or a commode a short distance from the patient. Beds must be low enough for the old person to rise at night. Mandelstam (1977) has demonstrated the advantages for incontinent patients of clothes that can be removed quickly. The garments must be chosen to suit the individual (Malone-Lee *et al.* 1983). In modern hospitals where incontinent patients are being cared for it is essential to provide labour-saving equipment for bathing, handling and lifting overweight disabled elderly people and modern methods of foul linen disposal and an abundant supply of disposable pads, pants and suitable clothing must be available.

Nursing measures. The patient should be kept as active as possible and encouraged to be out of bed for as long as the physical condition allows. The very fact of being upright, and not lying flat, means that gravity helps to make micturition easier and acts as a preventive measure against incontinence. Regular supervised visits to the lavatory are necessary if the patient is able to walk, or regular bedpan or urinal rounds, for people unable to get to the toilet, should be a routine of geriatric wards, or where old people are nursed at home. In looking after incontinent patients the value of the bedside commode should not be overlooked. During the night, for incontinent male patients, a urinal bottle may be left in position supported and underlaid with incontinence pads, and for females, plastic bedpans of small size and flat triangular shape may be placed under the thighs. Scrupulous care of the genital and buttock areas is necessary consisting of frequent washing and drying followed by an emollient ointment of zinc oxide, kaolin and cod liver oil such as Thovaline, or a silicone barrier cream like Siopel. A plastic unspillable male urinal is available and prevents accidental wetting of the bed by clumsy handling of the urinal (Spil Pruf, Rusch).

Restriction of fluids after 6 p.m. sometimes helps patients whose incontinence is mainly nocturnal, and of course, watch must be kept so that impaction of the rectum with faeces is not overlooked.

Encouragement by nursing and medical staff is necessary, and the patient must be made to feel that it is important to remain dry. Kindness is essential in the treatment of incontinence; difficulties common to most elderly patients are sometimes not understood especially by untrained staff, such as lack of awareness of those with clouded perception or problems in communication with deaf or aphasic patients and realization of the postural difficulties of those with arthritis or stroke when using a bedpan. The part played by depression in incontinence is important and an adequate number of nurses is essential in the geriatric unit if cure of urinary incontinence is to be obtained.

Transmarginal inhibition is a situation where a patient fails to use a bedpan or a urinal, gets into bed or clean clothes, and promptly soils them. Such an event could be induced by emotional trauma caused by admission to hospital, nursing or residential home. In treating incontinence there is a need for allowing the patient ample time to pass urine and of ensuring privacy.

When an elderly individual is admitted to hospital, it must be kept in mind that for years this person may have herself got out of bed to go to the toilet during the night, and the administration of a hypnotic or failure to show the old person where the toilet is may result in an incontinent patient in the morning. The bed in hospital may be too high for the patient to get out, and common sense regarding reorientation must be applied when the old person comes into hospital.

Medical aspects

Prostatic enlargement is a significant cause of urinary incontinence in elderly males and must be dealt with if this is the cause of the trouble. The presence of detrusor instability should, if possible, be ascertained before any operation is undertaken. In the male electronic devices have a special part to play in the control of post-prostatectomy incontinence. Expert advice should be obtained (Rosen 1981). Simple ideas like improving the mobility of the patient can transform the situation, e.g. from the use of levodopa in parkinsonism, or by helping to relieve depression with drug therapy. Bladder retraining programmes aiming to increase gradually the interval between acts of micturition until a near normal pattern is established may be of use in detrusor instability.

Stress incontinence in women is often amenable to gynaecological plastic repair, and age is no barrier. Any active woman is usually fit for surgery. Many gynaecologists stress the value of local oestrogen therapy where the vaginal skin is thin before surgery. Depending on the gynaecological condition, varying surgical procedures are available, and in good hands the great majority of patients can be cured of stress incontinence by surgery. Good results following electrical stimulation of the pelvic musculature have been reported and it is possible in many cases to retrain these muscles and thus physiotherapy may be of value. Exercises can diminish frequency of micturition and nocturia (Shepherd 1980). Electrical control of incontinence is sometimes of value in the female who is waiting for gynaecological repair, or in women who refuse any form of surgery. Electrical devices are worn either intravaginally or intra-anally but are rarely of use in elderly patients. They are of little use if the patient is confused. It is worth recalling that any woman with incontinence must have an examination of the vulva as well as of the rectum.

Drug treatment

In general the use of drugs in the treatment of urinary incontinence has been disappointing. Anticholinergic drugs are of value in the control of unstable bladder contractions, uninhibited neurogenic and irritable bladders; the aim is to increase the volume of the bladder at which the first desire to micturate is experienced and to reduce the force of the uninhibited detrusor contraction. All of these drugs may cause dry mouth and blurred vision. Contraindications to their use include achalasia or obstructive oesophageal lesions, glaucoma or prostatic obstruction. Flavoxate hydrochloride (Urispas) can be given in doses of 200 mg three times a day. Terodiline hydrochloride (Terolin) has anticholinergic and calcium antagonist properties. This drug should be prescribed in doses of 12.5 mg twice daily. Side effects can include, in addition to anticholinergic effects, weight gain, tremor and leg oedema. Propantheline bromide (Pro-Banthine) can be given orally in a dose of 15 mg three times per day. Imipramine (Tofranil) is sometimes effective especially in nocturnal incontinence and is also an anticholinergic drug. It is given orally in a dose of 25 mg in the evening or, for daytime use, of 10 mg three times per day up to 25 mg at similar time intervals. The main adverse effect is postural hypotension.

Cholinergic drugs have been used with caution to re-establish voiding after surgery or in selected patients with the atonic type of neurogenic bladder, e.g. bethanecol. Cholinergic drugs can cause severe adverse effects such as sweating and abdominal colic. The anticholinesterase preparation, distigmine bromide is an alternative choice and can be used orally. Finally oestrogen preparations must be kept in mind where atrophic (senile) vaginitis is a component in causing urinary incontinence. Judge (1969) used 1 mg of quinoestradol (Pentovis) daily in the dose of 0.25 mg four times a day in patients in whom the presence of urinary infection had been ruled out. He found the optimum effect took over 4 weeks to develop and the drug should only be given in courses of around 6 weeks.

Success in treating incontinence of urine depends on an accurate physical and mental assessment of the patient, and the use in combination of the therapies available. An overall success rate of 50% can be expected with the best management. The major factor governing success is the mental state. The best results can be expected where there is local disease with no disturbance of mental health. In demented patients with incontinence the outlook is bleak and they often require long-term hospital care.

Newman (1969) felt that incontinence that followed change in environment might be prevented. In some cases the condition might be functional, and an understanding of the needs of the old person might help greatly. Urinary incontinence occasionally seems to be used by the elderly as the only protest mechanism left to them.

There are emotional aspects of incontinence in the elderly, and Sutherland (1971) while admitting that the large majority of cases of incontinence was caused by physical or organic factors, stated that there were certain psychological aspects demanding attention; the emotional reaction of the patient to incontinence and the emotional reaction of those who care for the incontinent patient, and the management of the problem in the light of these factors. For satisfactory treatment, awareness of our own attitudes must be accompanied by the reassurance that they need not promote guilt on our part. We must not translate them into our handling of the patient. All the sensitivity, insight, patience and understanding that could be mustered must be used and our approach must be on a very personal level. There seems no doubt that when depression is present it is worth trying a course of antidepressant drugs.

Appliances

Appliances are of use only in a minority of patients, as the co-operation of the patient is required, and this is difficult to obtain if any mental disturbance is present. For intractable incontinence, incontinence pads with elastic pants for females, marsupial or Kanga pants, may be tried. For men various attachments to the penis have been described and the Maguire urinal or the Bard penile sheath may be of use. Useful information is given in the booklet by Mandelstam (1980) and in a review by Smith (1988). An indwelling catheter may have to be used when the patient is very incontinent and confused, or when bedsores are a problem. The introduction of plastic disposable catheters has made management easier, but catheters require proper attention, regular changing, and a watch kept for infection.

In conclusion, no treatment will be satisfactory for urinary incontinence unless a correct diagnosis has been made, and this means among other things, a careful inspection of the urogenital system, for example any woman reporting incontinence must have an examination of the vulva as well as the rectum. Thought must also be given to the planning of housing for the elderly, sheltered housing for older people and hospital geriatric units. The elderly must have easy and rapid access to a toilet which must be large enough to take a wheelchair. The facilities of mirror, wash-hand-basin and WC must be suitable for old people with adequate hand grip provision and easy to use apparatus. No flimsy fitting should be installed which might be used in error as a help in standing.

In designing day accommodation there should be a WC close by, and any waiting area should be so equipped. In most hospital wards there is inadequate signposting with no directions to the toilets and the lighting in lavatories at night is often poor. Simple remedies may often be surprisingly successful and the long tried commode may on occasion solve the problem of urinary incontinence.

REFERENCES

Brocklehurst J. (1986) The ageing bladder. *British Journal of Hospital Medicine* **35**, 8.

Bullock N. (1986) Asymptomatic microscopical haematuria. *British Medical Journal* **292**, 645.

Das G. *et al.* (1987) Extracorporeal shockwave lithotripsy: first 1000 cases at the London Stone Clinic. *British Medical Journal* **295**, 891.

Hargreave T.B. (1985) Radical cystectomy. *British Medical Journal* **290**, 338.

Hood N.A. (1976) Urinary incontinence. *Health Bulletin* **34**, 354.

International Continence Society (1976) First report on the standardisation of terminology of lower urinary tract function. *British Journal of Urology* **43**, 39.

Judge J.G. (1969) The use of quinestradol in elderly incontinent women. A preliminary report. *Gerontologia clinica* **11**, 159.

Malone-Lee J.G., McCreery M. & Exton-Smith A.N. (1983) *A Community Study of Incontinence Garments*. Department of Health and Social Security Report. London, HMSO.

Mandelstam D. (1977) *Incontinence*. London, Heinemann Medical.

Mandelstam D. (1980) *Incontinence and its Management*. London, Croom Helm.

Newman J.L. (1969) The prevention of incontinence. *8th International Congress of Gerontology Proceedings* Vol. 2, p. 75. Federation of American Societies for Experimental Biology.

Rosen M. (1981) Male urinary incontinence. *British Journal of Hospital Medicine* **25**, 215.

Shepherd A.M. (1980) Re-education of the muscles of the pelvic floor. In *Incontinence and its Management* (Ed. Mandelstam D.) London, Croom Helm.

Smith N. (1988) Aids for urinary incontinence. *British Medical Journal* **296**, 772.

Sutherland S.S. (1971) The emotional aspects of incontinence in the elderly. *Modern Geriatrics* **1**, 270.

Thomas T.M., Flymat K.R., Banner J. & Meade T.W. (1980) Prevalence of urinary incontinence. *British Medical Journal* **281**, 1234.

Watkins J.S. & Vowles K.D.G. (1979) Postoperative problems in the aged. In *Surgical Problems in the Aged* (Ed. Vowles K.D.G.) Bristol, John Wright.

13
Stroke

Epidemiological evidence indicates that the frequency and severity of cerebrovascular disease have reduced in the past 20 years (Wolf *et al.* 1986). Cerebrovascular disease is however still a major cause of morbidity and mortality in the elderly. The major forms of the disease are stroke, transient ischaemic attack (TIA) and the multi-infarct state. The risk of cerebrovascular disease rises steeply within increasing age and approximately 75% of all strokes occur in patients over 65 years of age.

Treatment of a stroke

Once the diagnosis of stroke has been made, the immediate treatment is concerned with adopting life-saving methods in this initial phase of catastrophe. In many cases the patient is unconscious and then the aim is to prevent death from asphyxia, from dehydration or from infection. Asphyxia must be avoided by clearing the airway which can be blocked by dentures, by secretion or by food debris. The head should be slightly elevated on one pillow and turned to the side and care taken that the patient does not inhale any vomited food material. An airway should be inserted if necessary and suction may be employed to clear obstructing material. Respiratory difficulty may arise during transport of the patient. Before travel the mouth should be cleaned, artificial dentures removed and a clear airway established, and the patient should be placed in the pronelateral position and accompanied by a trained person. The patient may be deeply unconscious, but many people who appear semi-conscious can hear and respond. Efforts should be made to communicate with the patient and encouragement given. If the patient responds, a drink of water should be given by the physician to see if the patient can swallow; this particular observation is most important and is one that must be undertaken by a doctor. The ability to swallow should return in many cases in 24–48 hours, but if this does not happen it may be necessary to insert a nasogastric tube or to give fluids intravenously.

The major determinant of whether a stroke patient should be admitted to hospital is his residual functional capacity and ability to carry out activities of daily living rather than the degree of neurological deficit

(Table 13.1). Patients with TIAs or minor strokes can be readily managed at home in satisfactory social circumstances but attention should still be given to excluding a treatable underlying cause with appropriate history, examination and limited investigations.

Table 13.1 Indications for hospital admission.

Immobility
Reduced conscious level
Dysphagia
Severe hypertension
Cardiac dysrhythmias
Diabetes mellitus
Atypical onset

In the disabled stroke patient complications such as dehydration, bedsores, chest infection and stiff shoulder can be prevented by adequate nursing care at an early stage. Well-established routines of professional nursing care have been developed to treat the stroke patient in the acute phase in hospital. Bedsores can occur very rapidly and the time immediately following hospital admission is a time of high risk. These sores may not all occur on the sacral area; they can develop on heels or elbows or at any point where constant unremitting pressure is not relieved. An alternating pressure mattress is useful but nothing can take the place of highly skilled nursing. Adequate support of the major joints prevents subluxation deformities and preserves functional ability of the joints. In patients with altered conscious levels or dysphagia, the airway must be protected and adequate fluid and electrolyte balance and nutrition maintained. A helpless and unconscious patient very readily develops hypostatic pneumonia and if a pyrexia and chest signs occur a broad spectrum antibiotic, e.g. amoxycillin should be given orally or if necessary by injection.

A paralysed arm or leg may feel cold to the touch and carers may attempt to warm the limb. An unguarded hot water bottle may be placed against a paralysed limb and if the patient cannot move the limb and has no sensation in it, a burn may result.

If the patient from the onset of his illness has been conscious he may not realize he is paralysed and is liable to fall out of bed in the attempt to get up and walk. He may instinctively try to get to the bathroom and so fall. He may not be able to say what he wants, so every restless patient should be offered a urinal, bedpan or commode.

A close watch must be kept on the bladder as retention of urine is common initially and incontinence may simply be due to overflow. Usually as the patient regains consciousness the bladder control recovers over the next 48 hours but if retention is noted it should be relieved by a modern small plastic self-retaining catheter. If there is no sign of spontaneous recovery of bladder function, a subcutaneous injection of carbachol, 0.5 ml (0.125 mg) can be given with the catheter left in position to ascertain if this substance is effective and also if there is any untoward reaction. If no adverse effects are noted, such as pallor or sweating, the dose may be increased to 1 ml (0.25 mg). This is contraindicated if the patient's general condition is poor and prognosis bad. If the bladder responds to the carbachol then an injection of 1 ml (0.25 mg) may be tried in 6–8 hours with the catheter removed. If this is successful and further treatment is required, twice daily injections of carbachol may be used initially and then oral dosage of 1 mg of carbachol tried once a day increasing slowly to 2 mg twice a day for a few days. It is on occasion not possible to feel the distended bladder especially in females and, if an overflow incontinence is suspected, standing the patient up with assistance may result in a flooding of the floor thus revealing that a distended bladder has been present. In such cases oral carbachol is usually successful. Urinary incontinence is common and catherization should not be used for reasons of nursing expediency. The patient should be given the chance of becoming continent, and permanent catherization should be considered only if it is clear that the incontinence is unlikely to improve and is damaging the skin. It is wise to wait for at least 8 weeks after the stroke. An exception to this rule would be to allow a patient with severe incontinence to return home (Akhtar & Garraway 1982).

Faecal impaction in the early stages of illness is a common cause of restlessness, and a rectal examination is essential to exclude this condition and prostatic enlargement. If a constant search for the cause of restlessness is not made and strong sedatives are used to keep the patient in bed he may well be rendered so drowsy and immobile that he dies from the very things endeavour has been made to prevent, namely, dehydration, pneumonia and large sloughing bedsores. Restlessness may be due to faecal impaction as mentioned above or retention of urine, or lying in a wet bed or being in strange surroundings. The appropriate therapy must be applied. Thioridazine is a useful preparation even at this stage in a dose of 12.5–50 mg three times a day. If pain is the cause of restlessness this must be relieved (p. 216). For a hypnotic, temazepam 10–30 mg or triclofos syrup in a dose of 1–2 g (10–20 ml) may be useful.

The initial management is to prevent the patient from dying, and at the same time to make sure that his general positioning in bed is such that deformities do not occur. Care must be taken to treat footdrop by a pillow or covered board at the end of the bed and to avoid making it worse by having the bedclothes too firmly stretched across the lower part of the bed.

Investigation

Stroke patients should have basic medical investigations performed (Table 13.2).

Table 13.2 Basic investigations in stroke.

Urea and electrolytes
Liver function tests
Syphilis serology
Blood sugar
Urinalysis
Full blood count
ESR
Chest radiograph
12 lead ECG

Dehydration may be difficult to detect clinically; an elevated blood urea and serum sodium may be the only manifestations. Dehydration can extend the area of neuronal damage and should therefore be treated actively if necessary with intravenous fluids. Blood sugar estimation will help exclude hyper- or hypoglycaemia which can present with focal neurological signs which usually resolve completely on correction of the metabolic upset. Polycythaemia and thrombocythaemia are rare causes of stroke but they should be excluded as the risk of further strokes can be reduced by specific treatment. Raised serum levels of γ-glutamyl transferase or mean cell volume may indicate a background of alcohol abuse. An ESR of more than 100 mm in 1 hour should be further investigated to exclude cranial arteritis or infective endocarditis. The ECG may show evidence of myocardial infarction, dysrhythmias or conduction defects which may be amenable to specific drug treatment or implantation of a cardiac pacemaker. Echocardiography is indicated if valvular heart disease is thought to be the source of embolic cerebrovascular disease. Chest radiography will detect unsuspected pulmonary disease or cardiac enlargement. More specialized neurological investigations are indicated if the pathological diagnosis underlying stroke is in doubt. Of those patients with a clinical first stroke, approximately 80–90% have a cerebral infarct and 10–20% have haemorrhage. Infarct and haemorrhage cannot be reliably distinguished on clinical grounds alone. An isotope brain scan can exclude subdural haematoma but this investigation has been generally superseded by computerized tomography (CT). A CT scan will exclude intracranial tumour or abscess and will differentiate infarct from haemorrhage within 2 or 3 weeks of the onset of the stroke illness. Electroencephalography is not usually indicated. Lumbar puncture and examination of the CSF is indicated if meningeal irritation is present and if subarachnoid bleeding is suspected. Cerebral angiography is rarely indicated during the acute stages of stroke illness in elderly patients.

Drug treatment in acute stroke

As yet no specific drug treatment, during the first few days of a stroke, has been shown convincingly to affect overall mortality or resultant neurological disability. Various methods have been promoted to reduce the incidence of cerebral oedema and limit infarct size but they have not been validated. Treatment with vasodilators, anticoagulants, thrombolytic agents and haemodiluting agents, e.g. low molecular weight dextran are as yet of no proven benefit in acute stroke disease.

Surgical treatment of acute stroke

Subdural haematoma is the most important indication for surgical intervention in cerebrovascular disease. The diagnosis may be suggested by the presence of classical symptoms, e.g. headache, fluctuating drowsiness and mild hemiparesis but this condition may also present with dysphasia, epilepsy, hemianopia or dense hemiplegia. In intracerebral haematoma the surgical indications for clot evacuation are still unclear. Surgery is generally not indicated unless there is raised intracranial pressure and the best results are likely to be obtained in lobar or cerebellar haematoma.

Continuing management

Whenever the patient becomes alert, and even remotely capable of understanding what is happening, continued reassurance is given. It has been well said that the patient who has had a stroke suffers from the effect of his stroke, depression following its occurrence, and fear. This fear especially of the future must be kept in mind constantly.

Rehabilitation in a more active way is now starting, bearing in mind the four aspects of the illness:
1   The physical illness.
2   The disability that may result from this.
3   The mental changes that occur.
4   The social conditions of the patient.

The patient is allowed out of bed when he is conscious, afebrile, has no tachycardia and looks as if he could get up. The feeling of well-being is rather indefinite but is sensed both by the patient and those who are constantly with him.

The assessment of hemiplegia

There are six areas to be covered by assessment (Adams 1974) (Table 13.3).

It is worth noting that a hemiplegic patient cannot be expected to be in better condition physically or mentally after a stroke than before it. A relative or friend who knew the patient before the illness should be asked about the patient's previous state of health.

Table 13.3 Assessment of hemiplegia.

Exercise tolerance
Motivation
Sensory impairment
Mental capacity
Motor deficit
Postural control

Exercise tolerance is defined as the strength or endurance required by the hemiplegic to make the most of recovery, and cardiac complications are the most important hinderances to power and effort in elderly people. Stroke victims have often co-existing ischaemic heart disease and they are also at special risk of developing symptomatic postural hypotension.

Motivation is obviously a most important factor in the rehabilitation of the hemiplegic. It is greatly helped by regularly repeated reassurance that independence and self-care and return to a normal social life is possible.

Sensory defects are discovered by careful examination while impaired vision and the presence of hearing defect may complicate the issue. Hemianopia is often missed in cerebrovascular disease.

Mental capacity can be assessed using one of a number of available mental test questionnaries.

Motor deficit is checked in three ways:
1. The extent and severity of late spasticity.
2. Postural abnormality and the threat of contracture.
3. The degree and distribution of returning voluntary power.
   In this way progress can be estimated.

Postural problems are complicated because the mechanisms of co-ordination and integration are complex. The patient who cannot stand with confidence cannot walk reliably. Postural problems can be noted early in recovery; patients who have difficulty in supporting themselves upright in bed and who, even when propped up with pillows, have to be watched constantly or they fall sideways. Such patients may not realize when a change of posture is occurring and some individuals are unable to determine when they are in fact in the upright position.

Prognosis following a stroke

The mortality rate in the first 4 weeks after a first stroke ranges from 20 to 60% (Dennis & Warlow 1987). Intracerebral haemorrhage and extensive cerebral infarction are associated with a poorer prognosis than smaller cortical or posterior fossa infarcts. In subsequent years 5–10% of first stroke survivors die usually of vascular disease of the heart or brain. The recurrence rate of stroke is approximately 10% per year.

In the immediate assessment of a stroke the features detailed in Table 13.4 are associated with a grave prognosis.

If the patient survives the first 14 days then useful indices of continuing bad prognosis would be as in Table 13.5.

Table 13.4 Features associated with poor prognosis in acute stroke.

Reduced conscious level
Cheyne–Stokes respiration
Pupillary abnormalities – Fully contracted
                         – Widely dilated
                         – Unequal
Conjugate deviation of eyes
Bilateral extensor plantar responses
Hypothermia
Hyperpyrexia
Signs of meningeal irritation

Table 13.5 Poor prognostic indicators at 14 days after onset of stroke.

Still unconscious
Continued pyrexia
Persistent tachycardia
Massive paralysis with dysphagia
Rapid development of bedsores
Gangrene of limbs
Bronchopneumonia

When the first month is successfully passed then it is necessary to estimate the outlook regarding recovery and successful rehabilitation. The degree of intellectual impairment and the capacity to understand simple instructions are factors of great importance. The time elapsing from the stroke to the first attempts to regain purposeful activity is a guide and of course the extent to which the family can or are prepared to co-operate in the treatment has to be kept in mind.

Intravenous infusion of glycerol may reduce the initial mortality in acute ischaemic stroke but it does not affect the longer term prognosis in terms of mortality or residual neurological deficit (Frithz & Werner 1987). Calcium channel blockers may have a role in the treatment of acute ischaemic stroke. Nimodipine administered orally in doses of 30 mg 6-hourly for 4 weeks and started within 24 hours of the onset of the illness has been shown to improve survival in men and appears to reduce the degree of resultant neurological disability in stroke survivors (Gelmers *et al.* 1988).

High dose steroids should theoretically reduce the intracerebral oedema which may be associated with cerebral haemorrhage or infarction. However, after several promising reports about the use of high dose dexamethasone in acute stroke disease, further studies have not confirmed any clear benefit (Leading Article 1987). Osmotic therapy with mannitol may on occasion be of value in uncontrolled, increasing intracranial pressure.

Hypertension and in particular raised systolic pressure is the most important risk factor for stroke. Great caution must be exerted in commencing or increasing antihypertensive drugs in the first 4 to 6 weeks after a stroke. Cerebral autoregulation is markedly impaired in this early phase and even minor reductions in blood pressure may cause further neuronal damage due to extension of the area of cerebral infarction. Patients with hypotension or postural hypotension may require a reduction or withdrawal of their antihypertensive drugs and this may improve cerebral perfusion. A gradual reduction of blood pressure in severe hypertension with diastolic pressures of more than 130 mm Hg should improve cerebral blood flow. This may be achieved using a β-blocking agent, e.g. atenolol or a calcium channel blocker, e.g. nifedipine.

Prognosis in the stroke patient both as regards life expectancy and ultimate recovery is slowly improving. One year after acute stroke, one-third of patients have died, 45% are independent and 22% have varying degrees of dependency (Dennis & Warlow 1987). One-quarter of hospitalized acute stroke patients require permanent institutionalization. A number of factors will influence the eventual placement of disabled stroke survivors (Hurwitz 1969) (Table 13.6).

The presence of a second disabling condition may adversely affect the level of independence eventually achieved. Pre-existing blindness, amputation of a leg, severe osteoarthritis of hips or knees may lead to the need for continuing hospital care.

Patients with little or no intellectual impairment and not incontinent of urine merit intensive and prolonged rehabilitation even if there is gross physical disability due to motor or sensory loss. Those with serious intellectual deterioration and with gross urinary incontinence which persists for 8 months are unlikely to regain independence and do not justify the prolonged utilization of intensive therapy (Akhtar & Garraway 1982).

Table 13.6 Factors which influence placement of stroke survivors.

Degree of paralysis
Degree of sensory loss
Degree of dementia
Communication disorders
Past attainment, e.g. former occupation
Relatives willingness to help
Availability of rehabilitation facilities
Availability of community services

Rehabilitation of the hemiplegic

This can be taken as an example of the method of trying to make elderly ill people ambulant and independent. In rehabilitating a hemiplegic person it is essential to perform three distinct and separate functions.

1 *Physical rehabilitation*

The effort must be made to make the elderly person use to the maximum the amount of functioning brain tissue that has been left to him. Care must be taken to ensure that if there is any power left in a muscle at all, that the muscle is exploited to the utmost, and the physical rehabilitation of the patient must be pushed as far as is possible. It is worth stating that the elderly, once initiated in the methods of physiotherapy, can stand much more intensive physical treatment than was once thought.

2 *Psychological rehabilitation*

The second essential is to overcome the emotional disturbance that has occurred in the patient's mind, in other words, to rehabilitate him psychologically. The patient may well be depressed and this is a common occurrence rather than a rarity. Encouragement must be given from the start of treatment, and at the same time care must be taken to demonstrate to the patient that something active is being done for him. When the patient is conscious he is asked to lift the weak leg clear of the bedclothes, holding it in a straight line. If the leg can be lifted two clear inches from the bedclothes, then he is told at this stage that there is no question but that he will be able to walk again. Some such test and some such encouragement are essential at the commencement of therapy to make the patient realize that the prospects of recovery are good; the ability to walk again is achievable.

Care must be taken in prescribing antidepressants in the elderly stroke patient. These drugs may cause sedation, confusion or epilepsy in patients with cerebral damage. A tricyclic antidepressant, e.g. dothiepin or amitriptyline may be prescribed in low doses of 25–50 mg daily and gradually increased to 100–150 mg daily in patients with persistent depressive features (House 1987). Electroconvulsive therapy (ECT) should be considered for major depression unresponsive to drug treatment. ECT is usually delayed until 3 months after the onset of acute stroke.

Those individuals with a left hemiplegia and a disorder of spatial appreciation are very difficult to rehabilitate because of lack of insight and denial of disability. Staff require explanation of this especially as these patients are often garrulous, facile and demanding.

3   Social rehabilitation

The last aspect of rehabilitation is the social aspect and while the hemiplegic patient is undergoing treatment in hospital, every effort must be made to fit the social background of the patient to suit the patient's residual disability. This may mean alteration to the house or a new house, or a different way of life from that to which the patient has been accustomed; all this can be planned while the patient is undergoing therapy.

Patient in bed. Physical rehabilitation starts when the patient is unconscious; both arms and legs should be put through a full range of movement as it must always be assumed that a patient suffering from a stroke is going to recover. The nursing is orientated from the start to this attitude of mind. If there is any history of a fall or signs of bruising caution must be used until it is established that there is no fracture. One of the common mistakes made is to misinterpret the inability of a patient to move a limb thinking of this as paralysed, when in fact the patient may have sustained a fracture of, for example, the neck of femur. Lack of pain can be noted on occasion and loss of function may be the principal sign of fracture. Contractures should be prevented and the bedclothes should not be pulled so tightly across the feet that footdrop results. Watch should be kept for deep venous thrombosis of the paralysed leg; early rehabilitation may prevent this. Low dose heparin regimens may be useful in reducing the risk of venous thrombosis and pulmonary embolism.

Criteria for getting a patient up. The stage at which the patient may be sat out of bed can be estimated by the following simple precepts. First, the patient must be conscious; secondly, the patient should be afebrile, and thirdly, have no tachycardia. Finally, and this is the most important criterion, the patient must be judged from his general condition and attitude to be fit enough to stand up to the change of posture. When he starts to sit out of bed he tends to fall to the affected side, and initially he is only allowed out of bed while his bed is being made. This gradual progression of activity should be carefully watched by the doctor.

Rehabilitation to be successful is a team effort, and in hospital the team is composed of the doctor in charge of the case, the nursing staff, the physiotherapist, the occupational therapist, the speech therapist and, not infrequently, the chiropodist. Under the present circumstances in most regions of this country it is difficult, unless the social conditions are exceptional, to rehabilitate a severely paralysed patient in his own home. Milder cases with slight paralysis, however, who have intelligent and interested relatives and friends, can be successfully treated provided the social background is suitable.

Bed-end exercises. Whenever the patient is managing to sit comfortably in his chair bed-end exercises should be used, and these can be modified to suit either the patient's own house or performed in a ward, or in a physiotherapy department. The basis is quite simply that the patient uses the end of the bed or a wall-bar at about the level of his shoulder, and both hands, the weak and the good, are put on this bar. A bed-end board, i.e. a piece of wood that is placed between the legs at the end of a bed to prevent the patient's feet from slipping under the bed, is put in position. The patient pulls himself up from a sitting position to a standing position and initially he may need the help of one or even two physiotherapists. The principle is that the patient is, by active methods, strengthening his own muscles. At first this is extremely difficult for a patient and he must be taught to sit down gracefully and slowly at the end of the exercises. The aim is to teach the patient how to stand up and how to sit down.

Several points are of importance; the patient should be wearing hard shoes, a patient who cannot stand should not be making attempts to walk. If the patient cannot grip with his weak hand the end of the bed or the bar on the wall, the nurse or physiotherapist should place the hand round this bar and hold it on for the patient. Progress is occasionally amazingly rapid even when expectation of recovery is not great.

There are many modifications of this test; for example, once the patient is standing he can lift his weak leg up on top of the bed-end board, or if it is being done in a physiotherapy department, on top of a piece of wood about 2 inches high. He then practises raising the good leg which means standing on the weak leg and is much more difficult, and, for the patient, a hazardous procedure. A further useful exercise is that the patient is asked to take side steps along the bar moving the feet laterally to one side then the other side. These exercises are practised first holding on with two hands to the end of the bed or wall-bar, then with one and finally not holding at all. The patient's sense of balance and posture is restored and eventually he can stand independently. These exercises are in fact designed so that several patients can do them under the supervision of one physiotherapist, or in the absence of physiotherapeutic help a nurse who has been instructed in the routine can supervise the patient's exercises. The time taken to master the bed-end exercises may vary from a day or two to a month, depending on the disability of the patient. The patient is under the psychological handicap of a sudden illness that has deprived him of the power of one side, and he may also have sustained injury to the brain which may have rendered him aphasic and so he may be incapable of understanding more than the simplest of commands. Caution must be exercised at the start of physiotherapy because of the frequent presence of an unsuspected myocardial infarction as a complication, and if the patient is exercised too vigorously cardiac failure may ensue.

This routine of simple, progressive purposeful movements, carried out for short repeated periods, answers the patient's needs at this stage well. He can see the point of these exercises and it can be explained to him quite simply that this is the first step in learning to walk again. It is completely essential to make sure that the patient understands what is going on and also that the physiotherapist is made quite clearly aware of how much exertion the patient can undertake. The idea of a team approach should be constantly preserved, the patient being exercised as much as he can bear, but not more than that.

After the wall-bar work or bed-end exercises, as the patient can now stand, the next stage is walking with a fixed support. The hemiplegic has frequently insufficient grip in the affected hand so a single wall-bar fixed to the wall is used; with the physiotherapist on the affected side he may support himself with the unaffected hand. Some prefer to use parallel bars with a long mirror at the opposite end. Different models are available, but portable, adjustable and collapsible parallel bars are very useful where space is limited. The patient sits at one end, stands up as he has learned to do and walks forward gripping the parallel bars. The physiotherapist is observing this and is all the time instructing him on what to do, taking particular care when he has to turn. The patient should be taught to sit down gracefully and one of the signs of progress noticed is that when he has a little glance backwards to see if there is a seat to sit on, this shows that he is now beginning to realize what it is all about. If the grip of the weak hand results in a dragging progress along the parallel bar, this can be aided by the patient gripping a piece of leather which slides along the bar. The full-length mirror at the end of the parallel bars is helpful, so that the physiotherapist can point out any obvious defects in the mechanism of walking to the patient. When walking exercises start the patient should be wearing comfortable lacing shoes.

The next step is walking on the level with a mobile support, e.g. the Zimmer walk-aid. This is strong, light, well-designed with four feet which have rubber ends to avoid slipping. It has been compared to a mobile pulpit and its best feature is its simplicity; it is so light that the patient has no difficulty in lifting it up, placing it in front of him and then walking up to it. Patients should be leaning forward at this stage of their rehabilitation, so that if they fall they fall forwards on their Zimmer walk-aid and not backwards. The characteristic attitude of people with a stroke, who have rehabilitated themselves, is to lean back as they walk. With this walk-aid the patient can learn to walk on the level and a patient independent at this stage can go home using a Zimmer walk-aid. In many instances the hemiplegic may find a quadruped stick a more useful aid because he can only use one hand. This aid is a strong, light adjustable stick with four feet, each of which has a rubber ferrule. The stance of a patient using one of these devices is to lean heavily on the stick and bring his centre of gravity between it and the good leg; the usual drill in learning to walk is stick, bad leg, good leg, stick, in that order and the patient has to learn to time the movement of legs and stick and gradually to distribute his weight more evenly between his two feet.

Finally, the patient may be able to walk with an ordinary walking stick; this should always have a rubber ferrule and be of a suitable length for the individual. Some hemiplegic patients never graduate to a simple walking stick and can never achieve more than walking on the level.

If progress continues stair work is now carried out on a well-lit staircase with two stout banisters. At first the patient learns to ascend and descend without passing his feet and then he learns to pass his feet in the normal way. It is usual to find that descending steps are more difficult for a hemiplegic than ascending. The affected quadriceps seem to have more difficulty in holding the patient erect while reaching down for the next step than it has when he thrusts his trunk upwards in climbing. Whether the patient leads with the weak or unaffected limb is determined by such concomitant disabilities as abduction or footdrop. Thereafter, similar stairs outside the building, and the comparatively uneven ground outside, are the final stages in physical rehabilitation. A walking aid for use on stairs is of great help: the Zimmer stair climber walking aid. This series of stages is simple, purposeful and progressive, and from the beginning, calculated to impress the patient with the idea of walking again.

More formal and specialized drills must also be considered when a hemiplegic is undergoing physical rehabilitation. Inability to abduct the arm and reach above the head is a serious handicap, for example, in putting on a jacket, or a shirt, or in dressing. One of the advantages of putting both arms and legs through a full range of movement from the time that the patient is unconscious and admitted to hospital is that the frozen shoulder is not found. During the time the patient is learning to walk his arms and hands and fingers are being put through a full range of movements.

Full scapulohumeral movement is the most important adjunct to utility of the upper limb, and a simple exercise is often prescribed for this: the patient sits beneath a single pulley; a cord passing over the pulley is held by the patient at either end and by pulling down on the rope with the good arm the palsied arm can be passively abducted. Where the paralysed hand cannot grasp the rope a leather gauntlet is used which can be hooked on. The flexors, and the quadriceps of the affected lower limb may also need to be built up and this may be carried out by isotonic exercises. By this means the joints as well as the muscles that move them are exercised.

It is occasionally useful, by means of serial splints or malleable plastic, to try and correct deformities and overcome contractures.

In the lower limb it is very common to find the affected foot showing plantar flexion and inversion and this requires correction. The advice of an orthotist should be sought as the use of light plastic back splints, which are simple to apply and not noticeable when suitable garments are worn, has revolutionized the therapy of this condition; the patients no longer need to look like disabled people.

On occasion the patient is left with a flaccid limb and not a spastic one, and this is a grave handicap to rehabilitation. Flaccidity may be helped by a long splint; consultation with a skilled orthotist is always worthwhile. This has many disadvantages as a permanent solution, but as a short-term measure it may allow walking during the time that the affected quadriceps recovers tone and power. The splinted limb sticks out awkwardly when the patient sits and it complicates sitting and standing.

There is a definite place for raising the heel of the affected side in patients handicapped by painful hyperextension of the knees when walking or in the neglected hemiplegic whose knee is left with a residual contracture. This is useful to remember as some degree of residual contracture may resist all attempts at correction. The question of raising one heel may well be worth considering if there are difficulties in rehabilitation and references will be made to this in the treatment of parkinsonism (p. 220).

Other simple exercises that can improve the power of the affected limb in a natural way can be provided by setting the patient the task of piling on top of one another a series of toy building blocks. The patient sits at a table with the blocks in front of him and erects a column of blocks, which may go up to 18 inches, and if he can do this he has regained a useful amount of shoulder abduction, as well as co-ordination of the arm and fingers. Precise exercises such as the transferring of glass marbles from one utensil to another are of great value. Purposeful natural exercises are further exemplified by the use of a button board, which is a device consisting of a series of buttons of various sizes with corresponding buttonholes. The patient is instructed to do and undo these buttonholes, and when he can do this, this is of great value to him in dressing. It must always be borne in mind that as part of the team exercise the patient is also being taught how to dress and how to attend to his everyday personal needs.

On occasion it may be that the patient has no idea of where the upper limb is in space. Such a limb may well be flaccid and falls down to the side and may impede the patient's walking, and in fact throw him off balance. It is worthwhile in such a case placing the affected arm in a sling; there are some elegant methods available for doing this. The purpose of this type of apparatus is simply to prevent the arm from swinging when the patient is walking, thus threatening the patient's balance.

It must be emphasized that during this part of rehabilitation a time may be reached when it is decided that the patient is going to be left with a certain amount of residual disability. It may, for example, be impossible to get the patient beyond the level of a wheelchair existence. There may be too much brain damage; the patient may not be able to cope with the exercises because of his heart condition, and the disability therefore has to be estimated and the life of the patient adjusted to this disability. How long should one continue physiotherapy? Until improvement ceases; even if it takes a year. When should one give up? Not until 2 months have elapsed without progress.

There are now a wide variety of wheelchairs that are attractive, light, and, for example, can be made so that a hemiplegic patient can have both driving wheels on the non-paralysed side, and if he is strong enough he can learn to propel and turn such a chair using one hand.

Surgery in stroke rehabilitation

Surgery in the rehabilitation of the patient following a stroke falls into two main types:
1   destructive
2   reconstructive

1   *Destructive* surgery is reserved for patients with reflex activity, for example flexor spasticity producing pain rendering nursing impossible and causing bedsores and where there is no potential for improvement.

When the lower limbs are in severe flexion and incontinence is present, intrathecal phenol may be used. When the patient is continent then the limbs can be straightened by myotomy and tenotomy with or without neurectomy.

2   *Reconstructive*
   (a) *Lower limbs.* An equinovarus deformity of the ankle is one of the common troublesome disabilities occurring in hemiplegics. This produces difficulty in obtaining toe clearance in the swing phase of gait and results in an unstable base for walking. In the elderly, a fall often occurs, commonly with a resulting fracture. In moderate cases this can be controlled by a suitable short plastic splint. In some cases that are severe, an elongation of the tendo Achillis and transfer of half the tibialis anterior to the outer border of the foot may help. Stuttering gait due to adductor spasticity can be corrected by adductor release or obturator neurectomy or a combination of the two. The painful disabling deformity of clawing of the toes which makes it impossible to wear shoes can be corrected by transferring the long toe flexor to the extensor.
   (b) *Upper limbs.* Reconstructive surgery in the upper limb is seldom necessary in older people. However, where persistent shoulder pain is present and where there is marked spasticity in the subscapularis, the surgical release of the muscle dramatically relieves pain and allows increase in the range of active and passive movements of the shoulder. Severe elbow flexion can be corrected by myectomy of the brachialis muscle and finger flexion can be released by transferring the sublimus to profundus tendons in the forearm.

Speech and speech therapy

Dysarthria is a disorder of articulation and does not involve any disturbance in the proper construction and use of words. Common causes of this condition are a stroke, bilateral corticospinal lesions due to vascular damage of both internal capsules, motor neurone disease and tumour involving both corticospinal tracts in the midbrain. Speech is slurred, production of consonants being severely affected. Much can be done to help the patient except in cases of bilateral paralysis of the tongue with involvement of lips and soft palate where little progress can be expected.

Aphasia means absence of speech, but dysphasia or difficulty in speaking is the more usual symptom found after a stroke episode. The classification commonly adopted is to divide the patients into those suffering from predominantly receptive aphasia and those with predominantly expressive aphasia. There is usually a certain overlap and no absolute and clear-cut separation between these groups. The patient with predominantly receptive aphasia has difficulty in the 'intake' side of this complicated process. He has certain varying amounts of loss of comprehension of the spoken or written word; the words he hears or sees may have no meaning for him. This is an immense emotional shock and understandably his speech and writing performance is poor. In expressive aphasia the patient understands the meaning of words, his full comprehension of the written word may be intact but he may not be able to express himself or read aloud. He may be only able to say 'yes' or 'no', a fact of considerable importance to the doctor taking the history of the illness who may not be aware of this complaint. Such patients can often sing and under severe emotional stress produce familiar words of anger. One of the most difficult problems of management is presented by the deaf patient who has had a stroke and become aphasic. Touch by the stroking of a hand may initially be the only form of contact possible, and with this alone it is possible for the skilled and sympathetic attendant to make rapport with his patient.

Articulatory or verbal dyspraxia is a disorder of articulation that describes the inability voluntarily to produce phonemes to form words in the absence of any paresis of the speech musculature.

The speech therapist working with the elderly requires great patience, much enthusiasm, and the ability to withdraw rapidly when the old person shows signs of fatigue or perseveration. After a stroke it is essential to start speech therapy early whenever the patient has completely recovered consciousness and confusion has gone. It is wise to warn visitors and staff where dysphasia is severe to try to limit the conversation to simple statements or questions. The speech therapist, as a result of her tests, is able to give the doctors and nursing staff clear instructions as to the disability and the correct management of her patient. Nurses in the day-to-day care of patients can be helping all the time with retraining. The demonstration to the patient that he can sing is often a source of encouragement to him. Initially, the patient's confidence must be gained and therapy of too complicated a nature may induce an outburst with loss of emotional control. Encouragement is not enough and thought must be given to the possibility of the stroke being accompanied by a disturbance of affect, e.g. severe depression necessitating specific treatment with antidepressant drugs must be kept in mind. Many of these people are deeply and severely depressed and some of the increased emotional lability can be improved if this is treated energetically. Counting of serial numbers, e.g. one to 20, is a common method of commencing speech therapy or repeating the days of the week consecutively or, as mentioned above, the singing of the first verse of a familiar song and trying to get the patient to sing the second verse. The use of gesture to reinforce words is helpful and, if it is possible, the patient should be encouraged to write. A thick dark pencil which requires light pressure is useful, and if the patient cannot use the right hand the left should be tried. It is essential to try and stimulate interest in what is happening in the ward or at home and books of simple content are often useful; large print books make reading easier. A simple programme as for teaching infants to read is of use and, where applicable, the attempt at building words with alphabet letter bricks is helpful. The nurse should speak to the patient frequently and keep him informed of what is going on.

Speech therapy is directed to returning a patient to his own home and the sooner he can once more be incorporated into society the better.

The speech therapist must remember that social problems, worry about the future and economic uncertainty will serve to retard recovery of her patients.

Dysphasia or dysarthria complicates more than 40% of stroke incidents with resultant difficulty in communication and is a major barrier to rehabilitation in many cases. In dysphasia, spontaneous improvement may be expected in the first 3 months after a stroke but little objective improvement is noted after 3 months. Little is known about the natural recovery of patients with dysarthria but marked improvement has been observed in the first 3 months of speech therapy, after maximum neurological stability post-stroke, with limited further improvement thereafter.

Patients should be seen ideally for short periods daily on 5 days of the week for up to 2 years to obtain maximum benefit. Adverse prognostic factors include the severity of the deficit at the time of initial assessment, the length of time that has elapsed between the onset of the disorder and the first assessment, and the presence of intellectual impairment, emotional lability, anxiety, depression or poor motivation.

Stroke clubs may assist in the language rehabilitation of the dysphasic stroke patient and volunteer schemes involving groups of untrained people have shown some promise in producing an improvement in dysphasic patients in terms of their general attitude, morale and language skills.

Occupational therapy

The part played by the occupational therapist in the treatment of the patient with a hemiplegia is of great importance. She is part of the team and like the other members has a duty to instil a desire to get better in the mind of her patient. She is much concerned with his day-to-day progress working in close collaboration with the doctor, the nursing staff and the physiotherapist. She must make sure that the hemiplegic ultimately makes the full use of the faculties which he has left to him following his organic lesion.

It can be said that over the last few years the function of the occupational therapist in geriatric practice has changed in emphasis. She does, of course continue to work closely with the physiotherapist in restoring muscle function to the level compatible with the patient's age and ability, thus working towards independence particularly in the mobility required for daily living. The main aim is to make the exercises interesting and to ensure that the patient is improving his muscle power by the task he is performing. The patient who operates a loom should be using his shoulder joints to the full or strengthening his quadriceps within the range and power prescribed.

However, it is in collaboration with all members of the treatment team that the occupational therapist's main function lies.

These functions are:

1 To help the patient to retain independence in the general activities of daily living.

2 To retain the ability to enjoy the social aspect of community life which combats the effects of loneliness in old age.

General activities of daily living

Here the ultimate aim is to make the patient live an independent existence in his own home. The patient is trained to dress and undress, to attend to his personal needs, to get in and out of bed and of a bath, and if applicable, to cook. Many gadgets are available to help those who are disabled and in dealing with the elderly patient these have to be of a very simple nature. Activities for daily living are best taught in a model kitchen, bedroom and bathroom, i.e. a daily living flat. In essence the programme starts with self-care, feeding, dressing, bathing, and attending to toilet needs and proceeds to domestic needs, e.g. cooking, laundry and housewifery, and then to outdoor needs, climbing stairs, entering buses, crossing roads and avoiding traffic, and lastly shopping.

The occupational therapist can perform her task better if she visits the patient's home and tries to assess his disability in regard to his return to surroundings she has seen. She may then request the local authorities to make certain alterations and adaptations to the patient's house. She may wish a bath-aid or a bath rail; some form of support may be necessary round the WC. A ramp may be needed to enable the patient confined to a wheelchair to get out of doors. The height of the gas stove may require alteration and appliances like a vegetable spike board may be needed beside the sink. While these alterations are being made the occupational therapist may be training the patient to use these aids. It is easier to rehabilitate an individual who is gaining her balance sitting at the kitchen sink and who realizes full well why the various exercises are being performed and what is the ultimate aim.

The social aspect

Here the main aim is to restore or maintain communication in the form of interpersonal relationships. This is seldom easy for the elderly when sight, hearing, speech, or all three may present difficulties in making contact with others, but it is essential if the lonely isolation of the elderly is to be avoided. Many people are mentally so apathetic and disinterested that this hurdle is a very difficult one to overcome and much encouragement is required.

Group work is indicated and may take the form of simple craft-work, e.g. bold colourful embroidery, soft toys and knitting, in which the patient may achieve quick success thus gaining the satisfaction that brings a return of confidence and combats helplessness and depression. Familiar games are helpful, such as dominoes, draughts, cards; social afternoons which include community singing, or in fact any type of recreational activity that is congenial, are of value here. This is occupational therapy of a supportive nature and should be under the supervision of an occupational therapist but valuable aid can and should be sought from voluntary workers. It has been found that young helpers, for instance from a church organization, such as Youth Fellowship, make a stimulating contribution in this field.

The continuing observation of the patient discharged from the geriatric unit and the use of the day hospital, day centre and all-day club, have been of great value in preventing social isolation. It is worthwhile to invite a close relative to the hospital ward to see exactly what the patient can do and to appreciate what cannot be done. Stroke clubs and relative consultation clinics are of value.

The importance of a predischarge home visit by the physiotherapist and the occupational therapist was emphasized by Akhtar & Garraway (1982). If the hemiplegic patient and caring relatives are present at that time, a demonstration of the capabilities of the hemiplegic greatly improves the morale of the relative. It may be necessary also for the consultant to guarantee readmission if the condition of the patient deteriorates or the caring relative can no longer cope.

Complications resulting from a stroke

Oedema of the affected limb

Almost one of every six patients with hemiplegia shows oedema of the affected limbs, especially the upper limb. This oedema fluid has been shown to have a high protein content. Alteration in posture may relieve the swelling of an arm. Massage and passive exercises are also of value. In persistent oedema of a lower limb the patient when sitting up should place the leg on a stool. Diuretics may also help to alleviate the condition of persistent swelling of one leg and a crêpe bandage applied from the foot up may also be of use. Controlled intermittent compression therapy with an air-filled inflatable splint may be helpful in reducing oedema. This technique is usually supervised by the physiotherapist for sessions lasting for 20–40 minutes once or twice daily. Contraindications to this form of treatment include evidence of cardiac failure or venous thrombotic disease of the limbs. Every effort must be made to get rid of the swelling as a heavy limb is a great handicap to the patient and hinders his progress in rehabilitation.

Hypothermia

When ischaemic infarction is the cause of a stroke, the illness tends to occur in the early morning. The patient may fall, become unconscious and is immobile perhaps in a cold environment. Watch should thus be kept for hypothermia and appropriate therapy given (p. 274).

Bedsores

On occasion a bedsore develops very rapidly in a stroke patient in spite of every nursing precaution. This is often a sign indicating a bad prognosis and associated with a failing circulation. In the early stages of the treatment of a patient with a stroke a constant watch must be kept to prevent the development of bedsores and the patients must be turned frequently from side-to-side with regular nursing attention to the back and the use of the alternating pressure mattress. Seriously ill or immobile elderly patients are especially liable to develop pressure sores and the nurses may require to change the patient's position 2-hourly day and night. The patient should avoid the semi-reclined position and adopt the upright sitting position whenever possible to avoid shearing pressure on the sacral area. Heels should be protected equally carefully. Bed cradles are useful in reducing the pressure of the bedclothes on the feet, and nurses should be warned not to drag heavy patients up the bed as this may pull skin from the sacrum and heels. The patient should be out of bed as soon as possible. Care should be taken that the patient has adequate nutrition and that anaemia, if present, is corrected and constant soiling of the skin area that is exposed to pressure should be prevented.

The phenothiazine group of drugs may render a patient immobile and should be used with caution in patients at risk.

Treatment of established pressure sores

As mentioned above, general measures are indicated to correct any anaemia present and to overcome protein depletion by giving a high protein diet to bring the patient into a positive nitrogen balance; concern for cleanliness, nutrition and hydration are the main pillars of therapy. Antibiotics, where necessary, should be administered.

The patient should be nursed in such a position as to avoid as far as possible further pressure on the area of the bedsore. This may involve turning a patient very frequently. The patient is nursed on an alternating pressure mattress, but this does not mean that the general nursing procedures can be relaxed. For light patients some prefer to use a water bed.

The local measures adopted vary widely and so many, often bizzare, applications have acquired a reputation in the management of sores that the principles are worth describing. Regular daily debridement, packing, cleansing and expressing of pus when pocketing occurs are the most important parts of local management. Three preparations have been found of use:

1   Thovaline, a cod liver oil ointment which is of value in prevention, being applied when two skin surfaces are in contact, e.g. under the breasts, and in the treatment of superficial bedsores as an emollient.
2   Ilonium, an ointment containing a mixture of volatile oils which helps in the separation of necrotic tissue.
3   Acriflavine 1 : 1000 solution is of value as a local application where the sore is clean.

Plastic surgery when available speeds the healing of granulating bedsores.

Parotitis

Parotid or submandibular salivary gland inflammation occurs occasionally in severely ill patients who have had a stroke, and in such people particular attention should be paid to oral hygiene. Patients on phenothiazine derivatives may develop a dry mouth and fluids should be pushed and particular attention paid to oral cleanliness in such patients. The development of parotid or submandibular swelling is again often associated with a poor prognosis. The condition once established is very painful and the patient may need to receive an analgesic such as dihydrocodeine tartrate 30 mg orally every 4 hours and, in addition, full doses of an appropriate antibiotic.

Bullae

On occasion, bullae that resemble a burn appear on a hemiplegic hand or arm. There is usually no inflammation around the edge of the bullae and they are very similar to those seen in phenobarbitone poisoning. These bullae are usually treated by aspirating the fluid carefully, leaving the skin intact, and applying an antiseptic. They have considerable medicolegal implications as the relatives may assume that the patient has been burned, and this is not so. They should be treated as a burn and dressed with strict aseptic precautions.

Contractures of hand

In healthy subjects the flexor muscles are stronger than the extensors and in hemiplegic patients the tone in the flexor group is always greater than in extensor groups while recovery tends to occur first in the flexor and later in extensor muscles. It is very important to try and prevent flexion deformity because if fine movements of fingers are going to recover it is usually late rather than early. Thus, if irreparable contracture of the fingers occurs before recovery of power the functional capacity will be grossly impaired.

Prevention

1 *Physiotherapy.* Passive movements of fingers and wrists are commenced even when the patient is unconscious from the onset of the illness. Active treatment comprises the training of the patient to put his wrist and fingers through a full range of passive movements with the good hand, following this with graduated exercises when recovery begins. Hand splints may be employed and many different forms of splinting are available. Most people believe now that the use of splints of any kind is rarely necessary and that the fundamental need is for the hand to be put through a full range of movement daily.

2 *Occupational therapy.* The best type of work is that which extends the fingers and wrists and which exercises the prime movers for extension.

Basket work is recommended and simple games such as 'find the penny in a bowl of sand' are beneficial.

Nursing care and medical attention. If flexion deformity of the fingers has occurred, it is essential to perform routine cleaning of the palm of the hand and the condition can be helped by combining passive finger extension and applying night hand splints. Particular attention must be paid to the finger-nails by the nursing staff to prevent them from cutting into the hand. In very severe spastic contractures, consideration, on a very rare occasion, may have to be given to amputation of the fingers. Where the hand has contracted, instructions may be given to the nursing staff to insert pads of increasing bulk composed of Sorbo rubber wrapped in Elastoplast.

Management of the 'useless' hand. When the patient has had a disturbance of body image and of sensation, he may not be aware of the position of the arm and hand in space. In such cases rehabilitation is delayed unless the arm and hands are placed in a sling so that the patient is not thrown off balance. Oedema of the hand may be controlled by elevation and elastic arm 'stockings'. For the ambulant patient a canvas web sling is available. Tubigrip also controls mild oedema and where vasomotor control is deficient affords warmth for the limb. The ambulant male hemiplegic finds that the useless hand inserted under the jacket above the lower button or in the jacket pocket brings the appearance of normality.

Footdrop in the hemiplegic patient

While footdrop can occur in peripheral neuropathies it is most commonly seen in older people following a stroke. The hemiplegic patient may develop inversion of the foot and plantar flexion which can be accentuated by the weight of bedclothes. This undesirable complication may be worsened by apraxia, hemianaesthesia or disturbance of body image. It is essential that every precaution be taken to avoid footdrop and inversion as these make rehabilitation more difficult.

Prevention. The unconscious patient should be examined and, if a cerebrovascular incident has occurred, at this stage a pillow wrapped in a drawsheet can be arranged to prevent footdrop. The ends of the drawsheet are tucked under the mattress at the sides of the bed. Sandbags can be used to fulfil the same purpose and at home a padded wooden box placed against the foot of the bed is a good substitute. If the patient is going to be bedfast for some time, plaster casts with back slabs or polythene foot and back splints may be employed though the risk of pressure necrosis must be appreciated. A bed cradle should be used to relieve the weight of the bedclothes.

Treatment. At first the physiotherapist concentrates on passive movements but as the condition of the patient improves active exercises for the foot and ankle should be started.

The advice of an orthotist may be required in patients with footdrop with or without inversion of the foot. Plastic back splints allow sufficient support, are flexible enough to permit some movement to encourage muscle recovery and are not seen if appropriate clothing is worn. For the sake of improving morale it is vital to ensure that the individual with a footdrop does not look disabled.

Occasionally, for irremediable footdrop the surgeon should be consulted as the operation of lengthening the tendo calcaneus may be of value.

Venous thrombosis

Deep venous thrombosis is common after stroke usually occurring on the hemiplegic side and the incidence increases with age. Pulmonary embolism may be found following the deep venous thrombosis. Prolonged pressure on the calf may cause vein wall damage and initiate thrombosis.

Emotional disturbance

This is a common complication in hemiplegia, and it is worth giving relatives advice that this should be ignored as far as possible. The patient readily changes from laughter to crying without any reason or on occasion starts crying for no apparent cause. If this emotional lability is ignored it usually goes away and reassurance and encouragement to the patient and the relatives are of great value in treating this condition.

Care of the eyes

Particular attention must be paid to care of the eyes in patients who have had a hemiplegia. On occasion, the eye is vulnerable, and it is recommended that an eye pad be worn if there is any evidence of damage to the fifth or seventh cranial nerves. A neuropathic keratitis denotes corneal degeneration following a lesion of the fifth cranial nerve producing corneal analgesia; this may be followed by secondary infection.

The precautionary measures include, as mentioned above, wearing an eye pad and also the instillation of medicinal liquid paraffin. If any inflammation develops atropine drops and an antibiotic ointment, e.g. chloramphenicol ointment, may be used, a culture being taken from the eye before treatment is commenced so that the appropriate antibiotic may be applied later if necessary. Caution must be used not to instil atropine if there is any possibility of glaucoma. In a flagrant keratitis tarsorrhaphy is indicated. In such cases the opinion of the ophthalmolgist must be sought.

Mental barriers

It is characteristic of these mental barriers to recovery that the clinical picture presented by the patient varies from day-to-day, and that it is the relative, nurse or physiotherapist who directs attention to the patient's difficulties and not the patient himself. Some of these barriers to recovery are a defect in comprehension where a patient may respond correctly to a simple request but fail completely with a more elaborate instruction; neglect of hemiplegic limbs despite good recovery of motor power and sensation; denial of disease where the patient states that his limb is normal when it is obviously paralysed or when he rejects ownership of a limb. Other difficulties encountered include disturbance of body image, space-blindness where the patient cannot appreciate the layout of a ward although he can see clearly, apraxia where there is loss of ability to initiate purposive movements in limbs not paralysed, perseveration, memory loss, synkinesia, loss of confidence, true depression, sustained inattention, emotional lability and catastrophic reaction complete the list.

Persistent pain in arm or leg following hemiplegia

For many years it has been accepted that the thalamic syndrome is the cause of persistent pain in hemiplegic limbs. Exact diagnosis is frequently rendered difficult by the inability of the patient to give an accurate account of the pain. Certainly pain and stiffness of the shoulder joint, the frozen shoulder, is a common complication of hemiplegia. Pain, however, also occurs in the lower limb. When it is recalled that the right-sided hemiplegic may be aphasic and that a left hemiplegia is frequently associated with disturbance of body image, the lack of an accurate history is understandable. This means that the patient either cannot say what is wrong or is unable to localize the pain.

When the diagnosis of painful fixed shoulder is made and before therapy is commenced, it is essential to x-ray the shoulder and the cervical spine. Accuracy in diagnosis is necessary before treatment and care must be taken to exclude fracture or dislocation of the shoulder. With the frozen painful shoulder the supreme need for prevention is seen. This condition should no longer occur, and can usually be prevented by the prompt initiation of full-range passive movements by the physiotherapist and by active exercises performed by the patient under supervision. If, however, the condition has developed short-wave diathermy may be used and pulley exercises may help; the affected arm being pulled up by the good hand and arm. Infiltration of the stiff shoulder joint with 5 ml of 2% procaine solution may render movement possible.

A fixed shoulder joint means that dressing and undressing a patient becomes extremely difficult and when the joint is also painful it becomes a great liability to the old person.

If the pain following the stroke is in the lower limb then careful examination should be made including x-ray to make certain that no fracture has occurred.

There are many causes of pain in hemiplegic limbs; sometimes it is due to coincidental cervical spondylosis, occasionally to osteoarthritis or to sensory epilepsy but it is clear that an effort must be made to secure an accurate diagnosis, and apart from analgesic drugs which may be essential no therapy should be given until an accurate diagnosis or list of diagnoses has been made.

Prevention of stroke

A number of risk factors for cerebrovascular disease have been recognized (Table 13.7).

Primary and secondary prevention of stroke are important aspects of the management of cerebrovascular disease in the elderly. The doctor should advise the patient to adopt relevant changes in lifestyle and this

Table 13.7 Risk factors for stroke.

Age
Hypertension
Atrial fibrillation
Cardiac disease
Transient ischaemic attacks
Carotid bruits
Peripheral vascular disease
Diabetes mellitus
Alcohol
Smoking
Lipid abnormalities
Polycythaemia
Cranial arteritis

should include advice on smoking, alcohol intake, diet and exercise. The association between stroke and cigarette smoking, hypercholesterolaemia or haematocrit are less strong in the elderly than in young patients.

In hypertensive stroke survivors, after 6 weeks, gradual reduction of the blood pressure should be considered. The physician should aim to lower the blood pressure to values of 140–160/85–95 while avoiding unwanted effects (*see* Chapter 7).

Atrial fibrillation and other dysrhythmias or conduction defects should be controlled with appropriate drugs or a permanent pacemaker (*see* Chapter 6). Long-term anticoagulation with oral warfarin should be considered in selected elderly patients who have rheumatic atrial fibrillation or a prosthetic cardiac valve thought to be the source of embolic stroke. A CT scan to exclude cerebral haemorrhage as the cause of stroke must precede the use of anticoagulant therapy.

Cardiac failure, diabetes mellitus, polycythaemia and cranial arteritis should be appropriately managed.

Transient ischaemic attacks (TIA) are temporary focal episodes of neurological dysfunction of vascular origin lasting usually up to 15 minutes which leave no residual disability after 24 hours. In the type due to ischaemia of the carotid supply, a hemiparesis or hemianaesthesia develops with dysphasia or dysphagia and in those with vertebrobasilar ischaemia, ataxia, blurring of vision or diplopia may occur with neurological signs involving both sides of the body. The commonest cause of TIA is thought to be platelet emboli from the heart, aorta or major extracranial vessels including the carotid bifurcation. Other causes of such attacks must be excluded, e.g. those due to cardiac disease, anaemia, severe hypertension, cervical spondylosis or postural hypotension. Patients with TIA have a yearly stroke risk of approximately 5%. Antiplatelet treatment with aspirin reduces the risk of stroke by approximately 30% in patients with TIA or a previous stroke (Antiplatelet Trialists' Collaboration 1988). Although most studies have used 900–1300 mg aspirin daily, there is concern about using such high doses in the elderly. Low dose aspirin may be equally effective in preventing stroke and TIA but reduce significantly the risk of gastrotoxic effects. Aspirin 300 mg daily in a single dose in the enteric-coated form should be prescribed for elderly patients with a history of cerebrovascular disease. However, aspirin should be avoided in patients who have a history of dyspepsia, peptic ulceration or a bleeding tendency. There appears to be no advantage in prescribing other platelet antiaggregant agents in addition to aspirin for the secondary prevention of stroke or TIA. Bruits over the carotid vessels may be due to stenosis of the internal or external carotid or subclavian arteries. Other causes include bruits transmitted from the arch of the aorta or heart or increased blood flow due to high cardiac output states, e.g. fever, anaemia or thyrotoxicosis. In asymptomatic carotid disease the risk of stroke or TIA is 2–3% per year and the relatively high mortality rate associated with carotid bruits is due mainly to a high incidence of heart disease. The carotid vessels can be investigated using non-invasive ultrasound techniques which will demonstrate any significant disease or stenosis. There is currently no indication for arteriography or surgery if an elderly patient has a carotid bruit with or without symptoms. Operations such as carotid endarterectomy and extracranial–intracranial arterial bypass have been used to treat patients with symptomatic carotid stenosis. However the role of surgery in stroke and TIA remains unclear in view of the considerable postoperative morbidity and mortality (Grotta 1987).

REFERENCES

Adams G.F. (1974) *Cerebrovascular Disability and the Ageing Brain*. Edinburgh, Churchill Livingstone.

Akhtar A.J. & Garraway W.M. (1982) Management of the elderly patient with stroke. In *Neurological Disorders in the Elderly* (Ed. Caird F.I.) Bristol, John Wright.

Antiplatelet Trialists' Collaboration (1988) Secondary prevention of vascular disease by prolonged antiplatelet treatment. *British Medical Journal* **296**, 320.

Dennis M.S. & Warlow C.P. (1987) Stroke. Incidence, risk factors and outcome. *British Journal of Hospital Medicine* **37**, 194.

Frithz G. & Werner I. (1987) The effect of glycerol infusion in acute cerebral infarction. *Acta Medica Scandinavica* **198**, 287.

Gelmers H.J., Gorter K., De Weerdt C.J. & Wiezer H.J.A. (1988) A controlled trial of nimodipine in acute ischaemic stroke. *New England Journal of Medicine* **318**, 203.

Grotta J.C. (1987) Current medical and surgical therapy for cerebrovascular disease. *New England Journal of Medicine* **317**, 1505.

House A. (1987) Depression after stroke. *British Medical Journal* **294**, 76.

Hurwitz L.J. (1969) Management of major strokes. *British Medical Journal* **3**, 699.

Leading Article (1987) Steroids in haemorrhagic stroke. *Lancet* **1**, 547.

Wolf P.A., Kannel W.B. & McGee P.C. (1986). Epidemiology of strokes in North America. In *Stroke: Pathophysiology, Diagnosis & Management*, Vol. 1. (Eds. Barnett H.J.M. *et al.*) New York, Churchill Livingstone.

14
Other Common Neurological Disorders

PARKINSONISM

Parkinson disease

This condition is among the common neurological disorders and it affects older people in particular. It makes a major impact on the lives of sufferers and those of their relatives. Parkinsonism is the term used to describe the clinical syndrome that consists of rigidity, involuntary tremor and poverty of movement (akinesia). It is usually associated with a disorder of balance, posture and autonomic function.

Causes

Parkinsonism has a variety of causes but only the drug induced form and that of unknown cause (idiopathic parkinsonism) are numerically important. The form of the disease that followed epidemic encephalitis is now rare as the sufferers from the last major epidemic in the 1920s and early 1930s progressively die. The prevalence of parkinsonism increases with age. It is rare under the age of 40 and almost half of the sufferers of the disease are over 70 years of age. The prevalence of the drug induced form is not known and difficult to measure but it is increasingly common in elderly people (Williamson 1984) (*see* Table 14.2). Although the majority of patients with drug induced parkinsonism improve on withdrawal of the drug, signs of the disorder may persist for as long as 2 years after the causal drug has been stopped.

There are many rare causes of parkinsonism, eg. after carbon monoxide or manganese poisoning, viral infections, e.g. coxsackie or herpes zoster, brain tumours, syphilis or trauma.

Clinical features

The main features of parkinsonism are rigidity, tremor and akinesia. Rigidity is of the lead pipe variety, in contrast to the clasp knife rigidity of pyramidal tract lesions and this means that resistance to passive movement is felt throughout the whole range of movement. The cog-wheel type

220

of rigidity is seen when rigidity is interrupted by tremor. The muscles of the face, neck and trunk are more severely affected than those of the limbs. The rigidity and akinesia together cause:

1 Slowness of movement, including inability to turn in bed.
2 Monotonous speech.
3 Mask-like face.
4 Disorders of movement including gait.

The patient presents with a stooping posture, a gait that is slow and shuffling and when asked to walk the patient takes small steps, sometimes leaning forward as if trying to catch up with his centre of gravity. Festination is the term applied to the involuntary quickening of the pace which accompanies this effort to avoid falling. A slight push applied to the front of the chest causes some patients to walk backwards: retropulsion.

In walking the feet look as if the patient is standing on soft tar and cannot lift his feet from the ground. This difficulty with voluntary movement is due to akinesia. This can be used as a diagnostic test for borderline cases in the elderly. The patient is asked to walk slowly and then turn around and as he turns his gait changes to a burst of short, shuffling steps and he becomes unsteady looking as if he was going to fall, and assistance should be available in case he does; as the patient walks there is usually no swinging of the arms. A fall can be serious as the patient with parkinsonism cannot move quickly enough to break his fall; the postural reflexes are defective. The patient with this disease can, however, climb over obstacles and sometimes finds walking on an uneven surface easier. The face is expressionless and does not react briskly to emotion while profuse salivation may be noted. The patient may be very kyphotic or kyphoscoliotic. A tremor of pill-rolling variety may be seen with a slow frequency about 3–5/sec and this tremor ceases when a purposeful movement is performed. The legs may be noted to be cold due to vasomotor disturbance. Postural hypotension is common in the elderly patient with parkinsonism as are defective bladder control and constipation. Autonomic symptoms such as seborrhoea, heat intolerance and wide-eye facies can mimic hyperthyroidism. Depression may occur often associated with loss of appetite, nausea, vomiting, general apathy and a weepy state, accompanied sometimes by delusions.

Crises

In postencephalitic parkinsonism an oculogyric crisis occurs more frequently in women and the onset is often preceded by emotional upset. The eyes during the attack are rotated upwards or upwards and laterally and are usually kept open. When fully developed, voluntary movement of the eye downwards is impossible and the pupils are dilated. Another form of crisis associated with profuse sweating can occur and a respiratory crisis with disorders of the rhythm and rate of respiration may be found.

Marked deformities of arms, legs and spine may be noted and a wide variety of these is seen. The main differences between postencephalitic parkinsonism and the other forms are:

1 Oculogyric crises occur only in postencephalitic parkinsonism.

2 Rigidity is more marked in this illness.

3 Tremor is not as prominent in the postencephalitic form.

4 Tics are more usually seen in postencephalitic parkinsonism, for example recurring movements of mastication.

5 Profuse salivation is more marked in the postencephalitic form.

6 Postencephalitic parkinsonism usually commences before the age of 30.

Diagnosis

This may be very difficult in early cases and instructing the patient to walk and then to turn smartly may be of value. The head dropping test of Wartenberg consists of getting the patient to lie completely flat in the supine position with no pillow. Complete relaxation is encouraged and the examiner then suddenly raises the patient's head and allows it to fall back. A soft fall with a slow downward movement is diagnostic of parkinsonism. In the normal healthy person the head falls quickly. The glabellar tap test is not specific for parkinsonism since it is present in one-third of neurologically normal old people.

Patients with parkinsonism can suddenly become much worse and develop a parkinsonian crisis. This can occur on transfer from their own home to hospital or after stopping antiparkinson drugs abruptly and also with acute infection. The patient becomes more rigid and does not speak. The skin feels warm, there is usually a history of decreasing mobility and intake of food and fluid and there may be a rise in temperature especially at the beginning of the illness, but no leucocytosis unless infection is the precipitating factor. If levodopa either singly or in combination with other drugs has been stopped by the patient it is often wise to observe the individual for a few days while making certain of adequate fluid replacement. The same drug can then be started again in a smaller dose. This rapid deterioration in such cases can be associated with the removal of a patient as mentioned above from familiar surroundings. People with this illness become very accustomed to their own home, their relatives and their friends and this change of surroundings can be accompanied by the rapid formation of bedsores due to the immobility described associated with depression. When arranging admission to a geriatric unit either for treatment or to give the family a rest it is wise to warn the relatives of patients with parkinsonism that there is a risk of this occurrence as well as the usual dangers of infection of any patient admitted to hospital. Much acrimony can be avoided if the family is told of the risk before admission. It is essential for the doctor in hospital to obtain an accurate account of the exact drug regimen being given at home. Doctors and nursing staff should be warned of the need for extreme care in the treatment of such patients in the first few days after admission.

Prognosis

The natural history of untreated Parkinson disease is generally slowly progressive over a decade or more with increasing disability. Death is usually due to respiratory complications and in particular infection. In a small number of patients the disease is rapidly progressive over 1 or 2 years and occasionally sufferers may have little apparent progression of the condition over many years. With modern drug treatment about one-third of patients will remain free from major disability after 10 years (Pentland *et al.* 1982). The most serious complication of the disease, whether treated or untreated, is the development of intellectual impairment. Dementia does not respond to antiparkinson drug treatment and will occur in 30% of patients after 7–10 years.

Treatment

Drug therapy. None of the drugs used in the treatment of parkinisonism are thought to slow or prevent the progression of the underlying pathology of the disorder (Table 14.1). If these drugs are withdrawn the patient will relapse back to a parkinsonian state as bad or worse than before treatment started.

Table 14.1 Drug treatment of parkinsonism.

Mild	Symptoms without disability	Anticholinergics (Artane etc.) Amantadine (Symmetrel)
Moderate	Disabled but independent	Levodopa/Decarboxylase inhibitor combination (Sinemet or Madopar)
Severe	Dependent	Sinemet or Madopar Bromocriptine (Parlodel) Selegiline (Eldepryl)

In the last 30 years a range of synthetic agents have been prescribed as 'anticholinergic preparations' in Parkinson disease. These drugs will usually slightly improve the patient by producing a minor reduction in tremor and rigidity. No single anticholinergic drug is more useful than another, and all of them have side effects which can be very troublesome in elderly patients. The introduction of levodopa revolutionized the treatment of patients of all ages with parkinsonism. The much greater effectiveness of levodopa has been amply demonstrated and there has been a slight resultant increase in the life expectancy of parkinsonian patients. Combination therapy with levodopa and a peripheral dopadecarboxylase inhibitor such as carbidopa or benserazide has greater efficacy and fewer side effects than levodopa alone. Before prescribing any antiparkinson drugs the physician should review the patient's existing drug regimen and withdraw any drug which might be causing or aggravating the parkinsonian state (Table 14.2).

Table 14.2 Drugs which may cause parkinsonism.

Phenothiazines	Chlorpromazine
	Promazine
	Thioridazine
	Prochlorperazine
Butyrophenones	Haloperidol
	Droperidol
Reserpine	
Methyldopa	

Anticholinergic preparations. These agents, e.g. benzhexol (Artane) or orphenadrine (Disipal) may be of value in the early stages of the disease but in the later stages of the condition they should be prescribed with great caution as they may cause or aggravate memory loss and dementia (Gibberd 1987). These drugs are therefore not usually advisable in the treatment of elderly patients with parkinsonism.

Amantadine (Symmetrel) has a modest antiparkinson effect and should be prescribed in the elderly patient with mild parkinsonism. This drug should be started in oral doses of 100 mg daily and this may be increased to 100 mg twice daily if necessary. Side effects may include insomnia, anxiety, dry mouth and ankle oedema. Tolerance may occur but many patients with minor degrees of parkinsonism may be successfully treated with this drug for years. On rare occasions, combined therapy with low doses of amantadine and levodopa compounds may be of value in elderly patients.

Levodopa preparations. All elderly patients who have significant disability due to parkinsonism should be treated with a levodopa combined preparation given cautiously and with a careful watch for any possible unwanted effects (Table 14.3).

Table 14.3 Unwanted effects of levodopa preparations.

Peripheral	Nausea and vomiting
	Hypotension
Central	Dyskinesia
	On/off attacks
	Drowsiness
	Confusion
	Hypomania
	Depression

Sinemet Plus (levodopa 100 mg and carbidopa 25 mg) should be prescribed in oral doses twice daily and this can be titrated to four to six tablets daily in divided doses with 5-day intervals between dose changes. Madopar 62.5 (levodopa 50 mg and benserazide 12.5 mg) and Madopar 125 (double strength) should be prescribed as one lower dose capsule twice daily and gradually increased to give total levodopa daily doses of 400–600 mg. The patient's mental state is the most significant determinant of the response to levodopa. If intellectual impairment is absent or slight the prognosis for treatment is usually good but if there is significant dementia present drug treatment rarely produces much benefit and it often aggravates the psychiatric disorder. Mild extrapyramidal signs may occur in elderly patients with non-vascular or vascular forms of dementia and these rarely benefit from antiparkinson drug treatment.

Nausea and vomiting are the important gastrointestinal adverse effects, and with the regimens described commonly occur in the first week of treatment. If the dose of levodopa is reduced, or the drug given after meals, they rapidly disappear, and after a short delay further cautious increases can be made.

Postural hypotension is the most important cardiovascular adverse effect. A considerable proportion of elderly patients with parkinsonism have postural hypotension before treatment is begun, and this should always be carefully looked for. Postural hypotension is manifest by dizziness on standing, and commonly develops within the first few weeks, reaches a maximum after 8–10 weeks of treatment, and then tends to disappear. As with nausea and vomiting, it commonly responds to a small reduction in dosage, combined with a slower subsequent increase.

The central nervous system manifestations of overdosage are extremely important, because they are the common adverse effects limiting maintenance dosage. The psychiatric manifestations include drowsiness, which may complicate the treatment of patients with significant intellectual impairment, restlessness, and abnormal movements, either dyskinetic movements of the face and tongue, or choreoathetoid movements of the limbs. Abnormal movements of the face are commonly the earliest seen, and should not by themselves lead to a reduction in dosage, unless they distress the patient. Choreoathetoid movements should always lead to a reduction in dose, and they usually then disappear. Confusion, delirium visual hallucinations and psychosis are dose-related adverse effects of levodopa.

Some elderly patients become incontinent of urine for the first time soon after levodopa is started, or pre-existing incontinence may worsen. This should be regarded as an indication for reducing the dose since the incontinence invariably improves if the drug is continued.

The increased mobility given to elderly patients by levodopa may result in two serious complications, fractured femur, consequent on a fall resulting from increase in mobility but not in safety in walking, and the development of angina or occasionally cardiac failure in those with severe co-existent heart disease. The former is difficult to guard against, except by careful attention to safety in walking, and the latter should only be expected in those whose heart disease is clearly apparent on simple clinical examination, assisted by electrocardiography and radiology.

The 'on–off' effect is not common in elderly patients on low-dose levodopa therapy alone. Progressive physical failure may also be noted with disorders of gait and balance while mental function may become worse without symptoms of levodopa toxicity and despite continuing benefit of levodopa on other parkinsonian symptoms. Chronic levodopa therapy in the elderly is associated with the increasing occurrence of vivid nightmares, visual hallucinations and paranoid delusions as well as acute confusional states. Such phenomena can occur when the patient is off all therapy and are probably part of the Parkinsonian syndrome in the elderly (Broe 1982).

Bromocriptine (Parlodel). If patients are poorly controlled with maximal doses of a levodopa preparation, bromocriptine may be added in small doses and this may produce overall better control of parkinsonian features. Low oral doses of 1 mg at night should be introduced and titrated gradually to maximal daily amounts of 10–15 mg in three divided doses. This drug may produce a higher incidence of confusion and paranoid states than levodopa in the elderly.

Selegiline (Eldepryl). This drug may be useful in addition to levodopa compounds to control end-of-dose akinesia. Oral daily doses of 5 mg or

10 mg may be effective. Side effects are similar to those of levodopa or bromocriptine.

The most important *other measure* is the recognition and proper treatment of depression. This is a common accompaniment of parkinsonism, and the elderly are not exempt. Patients with parkinsonism lose some of their ability to communicate their feelings and emotions, in particular because of their facial immobility. Any clues to the presence of depression should be energetically looked for, so that this important complication can receive proper treatment. Once recognized, depression should be treated with an antidepressant drug, either mianserin in an initial dose of 30 mg at night, or imipramine or amitriptyline 25 mg twice or three times daily. It is a frequent experience to see a patient whose progress with levodopa and physiotherapy has ceased, show further functional improvement, once depression has been treated and relieved. All who attend to patients with parkinsonism should realize that their intellectual capacity may not be altered, that their difficulties with speech do not imply difficulty with cerebration, and that they cannot help their slowness and poverty of movement. Very few patients with parkinsonism are lazy.

Surgery. Before the introduction of levodopa, the technique of stereotactic thalamotomy was widely used in the treatment of Parkinson disease. This approach is now only occassionally indicated in early Parkinson disease if the patient has severe tremor which does not respond to drug therapy. Recent attempts have been made to transplant adrenal tissue into the brain of patients with Parkinson disease in the hope that the transplant might generate small amounts of dopamine. Further evaluation of this approach is necessary before it can be included in the recommended range of treatments for Parkinson disease (Leading Article 1987).

Despite optimal drug therapy, the disabled parkinsonian patient will also benefit from assessment by members of the rehabilitation team including the occupational therapist, physiotherapist and speech therapist.

Occupational therapy. The occupational therapist has an important role in advising the parkinsonian patient and his carers about activities of daily living and lifestyle changes which may be necessary to cope with many aspects of the disease. Patients will benefit from assessment at home and from the provision of aids to assist in feeding, bathing and toileting (Beattie & Caird 1980).

Physiotherapy. The parkinsonian patient may suffer from difficulty in turning in bed, rising from a chair, particularly if it is low, starting to walk and in turning corners. The physiotherapist can offer advice to the patient and his carers about ways of maintaining adequate trunk posture, preventing loss of mobility and improving gait. Initiating movement may be improved by placing the patient in a sitting position and encouraging, attempts to turn his trunk from side to side, then twisting and looking as far round to the other side as possible. This manoeuvre is repeated three or four times to each side and this action may release the degree of immobility. The tendency to fall backwards during standing or walking can often be helped by a small (2–2.5 cm) elevation of the heels. Difficulty in moving in bed can be helped by the use of a rope ladder attached to the foot of the bed, which enables the patient to pull himself into the sitting position and so swing his legs over the bed.

Speech Therapy. Communication or swallowing difficulties may be present in up to 50% of parkinsonian patients. Speech difficulties may include reduced intensity of the voice, reduced variability in pitch, stress and rhythm and abnormal rates of speaking. Intelligibility of speech is affected and this may give the impression that the patient is demented, depressed, apathetic or cold and unfeeling. The term prosody describes the correct placement of pitch and stress on words and syllables. Hence this element of communication is largely responsible for the emotional content of speech. Parkinsonian patients are often unable to appreciate prosodic aspects of their own and other people's speech or the emotional content of facial expressions. These communication disorders may respond to speech therapy techniques including prosodic exercises (Scott *et al.* 1985).

Huntington chorea

Patients with this illness are sometimes found in geriatric units, although it is not a common disease. It is a heredofamilial condition starting at the age of 40 or later, and characterized by involuntary movements and progressive intellectual impairment. The disease advances slowly over 10 or more years, to a final fatal termination. The choreiform movements may be reduced by tetrabenazine (Nitoman) 25 mg three to six times daily. This drug should be started in small doses and increased over a period of 2–3 weeks to its maximum. Drowsiness is the usual adverse effect limiting their effectiveness. Some patients respond better to combinations of small doses of both drugs than to large doses of either given alone.

Brain tumours in the elderly

Turner & Caird (1982) noted that raised intracranial pressure in older people did not always produce headache or vomiting and more common symptoms were apathy, lethargy, confusion and incontinence; even papilloedema was unusual. Treatment in most cases of benign turmour is partial or total removal while malignant intracranial tumours are commonly treated with high doses of steroids.

Facial pain

Successful treatment of pain in the face demands correct diagnosis and local and referred pain may be due to inflammation of the antral, ethmoidal or sphenoidal sinuses, dental disease, cranial arteritis, glaucoma or inflammatory lesions of the orbit and malignant disease of the nasopharnyx. Pain referred from the temporo-mandibular joint is one of the most common causes of facial pain in the elderly. Depression is an important cause of facial pain and it is necessary to consider this in patients presenting with neuralgia. Trigeminal neuralgia or tic douloureux is another important cause of paroxysmal facial pain in the elderly.

Trigeminal neuralgia

This is a disease commonly found in the 65 to 75-year-old age range. The patients, more commonly women, present with unilateral intermittent excruciating facial pain, usually limited to the course of the second and third division of the trigeminal nerve. The pain is usually initiated in response to stimulation, such as speaking, chewing, drinking fluids, or a loud noise, but seldom comes on during the night. Physical examination is not helpful; some have described a unilateral furring of the tongue. When these patients come to the doctor analgesics such as aspirin and paracetamol have usually been tried and found to be unsatisfactory. Carbamazepine (Tegretol) is recommended in an initial dose of 100 mg/day increasing rapidly to 100 mg three times daily if there are no adverse effects and this is usually effective. The maximum dose advised is 200 mg three times per day. The adverse effects reported have been dizziness, drowsiness, dryness of the mouth, nausea and vomiting, and skin rashes. Leucopenia and other blood diseases have been noted rarely.

Carbamazepine should not be prescribed with monoamine oxidase inhibitor drugs or when such substances have been used recently.

If treatment with carbamazepine is not successful, phenytoin (Epanutin) in a dose of 100 mg three times per day is worthy of trial. If this is unsatisfactory supplementary doses of carbamazepine can be added, i.e. 100 mg three times per day. Turner & Caird (1982) have recommended, as an alternative drug, clonazepam 2 mg twice per day. If the patients do not respond to drug therapy, surgical intervention is indicated and modern methods enable the pain to be relieved without causing total anaesthesia of the face or facial paralysis. Glossopharyngeal neuralgia is less common in the elderly and may also respond to carbamazepine. If this fails surgical treatment may be necessary.

Postherpetic neuralgia

Postherpetic neuralgia is another painful illness of the elderly, and it is estimated that one patient in every ten infected by herpes zoster who has clinical shingles suffers from postherpetic neuralgia. The pain may precede the rash and reach its height when the rash is in its vesicular stage. Once the condition has developed it may last for 6–18 months and in this time pain should be relieved by analgesics. Treatment by transcutaneous stimulation can relieve pain in such patients especially if combined with drugs such as amitriptyline and perphenazine.

Head injuries

Head injuries occur equally in elderly women and men. Most are due to falls and they are less often the result of an assault or road traffic accident. Alcohol is the cause of injury in half of the men. Most of the elderly with a head injury have a medical condition which may be obscured by the head injury but the medical condition can also obscure the head injury. A hemiparesis may be wrongly attributed to a stroke and a traumatic intracranial haematoma may be missed as a result. As in younger patients, great benefit may be gained by vigorously correcting extracranial disorders and detecting and treating an intracranial haematoma (Galbraith 1987).

REFERENCES

Beattie A. & Caird F.I. (1980) The occupational therapist and the patient with Parkinson's disease. *British Medical Journal* **280,** 1354.

Broe G.A. (1982) Parkinsonism and related disorders. In *Neurological Disorders in the Elderly* (Ed. Caird F.I.) Bristol, John Wright.

Galbraith S. (1987) Head injuries in the elderly. *British Medical Journal* **294,** 325.

Gibberd F.G. (1987) Management of Parkinson's disease. *British Medical Journal* **294,** 1393.

Leading Article (1987) Brain transplant for Parkinson's disease. *Lancet* **1,** 1012.

Pentland B., Matthews D. & Maudsley C. (1982) Parkinson's disease: long term results of levodopa therapy. *Scottish Medical Journal* **27,** 284.

Scott S., Caird F.I. & Williams B.O. (1985) *Communication in Parkinson's Disease.* London, Croom Helm.

Turner J.W. & Caird F.I. (1982) Other neurosurgical problems. In *Neurological Disorders in the Elderly* (Ed. Caird F.I.) Bristol, John Wright.

Williamson J. (1984) Drug induced Parkinson's disease. *British Medical Journal* **288,** 1457.

15
Mental Disorders

The physician caring for the elderly sees many patients who are obviously unable to answer questions clearly and who have no idea where they are and who may not recognize their own nearest relatives. This mental illness sometimes presents very acutely especially following a sudden change of environment and alarms and worries all who are interested in the patient. In general, people are frightened and apprehensive of dealing with the mentally disordered and relatives not less than patients require advice and sometimes therapy.

The importance of diagnosis must be reinforced as treatment cannot be successful unless a clear understanding of the patient's illness and of his difficulties is reached. The psychiatrist can be of the greatest help and his advice should be sought early when any difficulty in diagnosis occurs. Doctors and relatives alike are sometimes slow to consider psychiatric help and it is a wise physician who realizes that failure to seek expert advice may well delay and sometimes impede his patient's chances of recovery. The outlook for many confused old people is excellent and the most remarkable and unexpected improvement may occur. It must never be forgotten that organic physical disease and mental disorder are commonly found in the same patient. If hospital admission is necessary many studies of elderly confused people have shown the importance of referring these patients to the appropriate and correct units. Those afflicted primarily with mental disorders have a much higher recovery rate if admitted to a mental hospital, while those with mainly physical illness make more rapid progress and have a better prognosis if sent to a geriatric unit. The importance of making determined efforts at diagnosis in the patient showing the sudden onset of mental confusion must be emphasized. The old man who during the night becomes mentally confused may well have a pneumonia, a distended bladder or a cerebral infarction. The established hemiplegic who refuses to co-operate with the physiotherapist and makes no effort to improve may be deeply depressed. There is no problem so fascinating as the disentanglement of this mixed skein of physical and mental disorder. Some of the expressions that are used in the description of mental illness may be defined as follows:

Confusion: disordered awareness of the environment which may be revealed by disorientation for time, place or persons.

Dementia: not merely a symptom but a syndrome consisting of progressive deterioration of intellect which may in certain situations lead to confusion.

Delusions: erroneous beliefs occuring in patients who are capable of normal intellectual functioning: they are not due to genuine mistakes and the patient is not open to reasoned argument on the topics concerned.

Benign senescent memory loss: this condition is not an illness, is not obviously progressive and there is no mental confusion or disorientation. It can be accepted as part of the ageing process.

The classification of mental disorders assumes that each case is clear-cut, easily defined and unassociated with other illness. Unfortunately, this is not so and yet in recent years each new advance has made it possible to add another diagnosis to the causes of mental disorders and has helped to make effective therapy possible. The classification that is of value to the physician interested in the elderly is as follows:

1   acute brain failure
2   chronic brain failure
3   affective disorders
4   paranoid syndromes
5   personality changes

Acute brain failure

The use of the words 'brain failure' is intended to stimulate a search for the cause of the brain's inability to carry out its function in the normal way. Acute brain failure manifests itself in the sudden onset of mental confusion and this may be the presenting symptom of the development of many physical illnesses in the elderly. The features are clouding of consciousness and a fluctuating level of awareness. Defects to short-term memory may be accompanied by impairment of recall from long-term memory and by visual hallucinations and misinterpretations (RCP Report 1981). This group comprises almost 8% of mental disorders seen among the over-60s in mental hospitals.

The causes of acute brain failure are many and can be related to the greater vulnerability of the ageing brain. When this is due to physical illness the onset is sudden. Conditions causing acute brain failure are structural damage to the brain such as cerebral infarction, haemorrhage, tumour or subdural haematoma. Disorders of blood supply to the brain as in congestive cardiac failure or severe anaemia; metabolic brain disease as in uraemia, diabetes or infective illness, e.g. respiratory infection are other causes. This state may also be induced by epilepsy, endocrine disorders, e.g. myxoedema or hyperthyroidism and drug toxicity from preparations like digoxin, barbiturates, phenothiazines, antidepressants or antiparkin-sonian drugs. Urinary retention or faecal impaction may also cause acute brain failure. Some of the conditions producing these confusional states are irreversible. Hearing or visual defects can predispose to acute brain failure. A confusional state that advances slowly and is accompanied by a change in personality may indicate a brain neoplasm.

These confusional states are conditions where the impairment of understanding can often be eliminated by suitable treatment, so that the patient returns to his normal level of mental functioning. They occur, of course, in the young as well as the old, but more frequently in old people made vulnerable by some degree of chronic brain failure (demen-tia) – thus making a mild or moderate dementia appear to be severe and beyond hope of treatment. Failure to recognize relatives and visual hallucinations may greatly upset the carer. The response to treatment is usually good but the patient may still have his mild dementia after the confused state has cleared. In confusional states there is usually clouding of consciousness in a disturbed patient. It is useful at interview to think in terms of a telephone conversation with the patient and trying to decide whether he has got a good line to an unintelligent caller: dementia; or a bad line to an intelligent caller: a confusional state. Post (1965) believes that the temporary confusion so commonly seen following removal from home, change of environment, may indicate the presence of a slowly progressive mild deteriorative process. It is obvious from the impressive list of some of the causes that the physician's skill in diagnosis is stretched to the full. One of the most difficult disorders to detect is that due to vita-min B_{12} deficiency, and this may present as an acute confusional state.

Treatment

The treatment of the many causes of the acute confusional state depends on the diagnosis. While the reason for the confusion is being sought dehydration commonly present should be treated; adequate nutrition should be ensured, and attention paid to the care of the bladder and bowels. The environment should be made as simple as possible; informa-tion is poorly absorbed and must be presented in large, unequivocal and frequent doses. If a diagnosis has been made the elderly patient kept in their own homes, i.e. familiar surroundings, will recover more quickly. Appropriate drug therapy with adequate sedation to reduce anxiety, agitation and to abolish hallucinations will be of value. Sleep should be ensured as at night symptoms may become worse because sensory input is reduced and the individual may not be able to distinguish reality and dreams. These patients if admitted to hospital should be told at regular intervals where they are. Their bed should not be changed in position, if possible, to give them an opportunity to relate themselves to their surroundings and they should always be called by their own names, not 'grandpa' or 'pop'. Ward routine should be regular and constant encouragement given.

The nursing of confused old people is difficult but within reason they should be allowed as much freedom as is compatible with their physical condition and thwarted as little as possible.

For calming the patient and overcoming the objection of the others in the ward immediate sedation may be required: chlorpromazine intramuscularly may be necessary and the dose should be adjusted to suit the patient. A thin, frail woman often responds to an intramuscular injection of 12.5 mg of chlorpromazine repeated in 30 minutes if without effect. The reason for this suggestion is that some women are sensitive to chlorpromazine and are rendered unconscious rapidly following the administration of the drug. A well-nourished man may need 50–100 mg intramuscularly of the same drug. Haloperidol (Serenace) given by mouth or injection is useful in calming a patient without inducing sleep. Chlormethiazole (Heminevrin) is useful as a hypnotic especially if there is any history of previous alcoholism.

It is worth noting that no confusional state should be allowed to persist without a blood sugar examination. This may help in the most unexpected cases. Watch should also be maintained for disturbance of electrolyte balance. The so-called silent pneumonias and myocardial infarct do occur, and if a specific cause for a confused state cannot be found after investigation it is justifiable on occasion to administer a course of an antibiotic. While specific therapy is being administered small doses of a tranquillizing agent such as thioridazine 10–25 mg three or four times a day may be necessary to control restlessness.

Finally, the role of emotion as an aetiological factor must be borne in mind. Although emotion may be produced by the illness, fear or anger can actually cause confusion, and they should always be looked for where no organic disease is found or where adequate treatment of a physical abnormality is not effective.

Chronic brain failure

This term is synonymous with dementia which was defined in the RCP Report (1981) as the global impairment of higher cortical function including memory, the capacity to solve the problems of day-to-day living, the performance of learned perceptuomotor skills, the correct use of social skills and control of emotional reactions, in the absence of gross clouding of consciousness. The condition is often irreversible and progressive. In elderly people chronic brain failure may be subdivided into two groups:

1 vascular
2 non-vascular

Vascular

This is usually found in patients who have evidence of vascular disease elsewhere in the body, e.g. myocardial ischaemia or peripheral vascular disease. It is said to be more common in males. It may follow a number of previous minor cerebrovascular accidents or there may be a clear-cut history of a stroke or the sudden onset of mental abnormality, i.e. acute confusion due to an acute ischaemic lesion of the brain (acute brain failure becoming chronic). Emotional instability is frequently found and on examination abnormal neurological signs. Intellectual function declines in a series of steps and the illness starts earlier than senile dementia. The out-look is poor if the patient is confined to bed with a stroke, has a myocardial infarct or is presenting with peripheral gangrene.

Prevention

It is hoped that as hypertension is a major risk factor control of hyper-tension in middle age will reduce the incidence of this disease. Smokers are possibly at greater risk and the gradual disappearance of this habit may also have an effect. In addition diets less rich in animal fat may help to cut down the numbers with this illness.

Non-vascular

It is now usual to describe this condition as senile dementia of the Alzheimer type and the genetics of this illness were described by Harris (1982). It is more common in women and usually steadily but slowly progressive. A sudden environmental change, fracture or intercurrent infection may produce an acute delirious episode resulting in rapid intellectual deterioration. The forgetfulness of old age is difficult to differentiate from early chronic brain failure; depression is one of the most common symptoms, and it may be almost impossible to distinguish between depression presenting as dementia (pseudodementia) and true dementia. The patient with depression is aware of the loss of memory and does not attempt to conceal any disability. The patient with dementia has a progressive disorder with deterioration in personality and increasing behavioural change. This condition should never be diagnosed without a complete medical investigation. Multiple and scattered neurological lesions, a high blood pressure, or renal disease would tend to indicate vascular dementia. Before treatment is commenced the diagnosis must be examined critically. Is there a possibility of a remediable illness such as hypothyroidism, vitamin B_{12} deficiency, cerebral tumour, normal pressure hydrocephalus or chronic subdural haematoma? Some use the term subcortical dementia to describe the cognitive impairment associated with progressive supranuclear palsy. This disease is characterized by changes in personality with a slowness in answering questions, often correctly, and by memory loss. Cortical dementia of which Alzheimer disease is an example shows apraxia, aphasia and agnosia, features lacking in subcortical dementia. Alcoholism should also be kept in mind as should Huntington chorea with the typical writhing movements, the flapping tremors of hepatic encephalopathy and rarely Creutzfeld–Jakob disease with myoclonus and rigidity and also the parkinsonian dementia syndrome.

The diagnosis at an early stage is difficult in ladies with social graces who by their kindly and gracious manner can conceal cerebral deterioration with a flow of meaningless pleasantries. Direct questions demanding factual answers will expose their memory loss.

Data from cross-national studies indicate that 5–7% of the population over the age of 65 have dementia; the prevalence rate rises from about 2% at the age of 65–70 to about 20% in those aged over 80 (RCP Report 1981). A general practitioner with 2500 patients has around 19 with dementia (Anderson *et al.* 1982).

Treatment

When a patient has a dementia it is in many instances impossible for her to be nursed at home, and in any event the investigation necessary for a complete diagnosis usually necessitates a preliminary period in hospital. One of the great problems is to discover these patients at an early stage in the illness. All doctors interested in this disease find that the patients are brought when the illness is well established and severe. However, if the illness can be detected at an early stage alteration to the patient's home with the aim of simplifying the acts of daily living may enable a caring relative to cope for a longer time. In other words altering the environment to suit the individual may be of help.

The most careful assessment of the physical state is essential and nursing attention to bowel and bladder given regularly may avoid incontinence or restore control. In hospital it is of some importance that the patient's lounge area is in close proximity to the toilets. When the intellectual failure of patients has reached such a degree of severity that they cannot motivate themselves to go to the toilet nurses must then take them there at stated times. Bedside testing of mental status, e.g. Kahn MSQ helps to determine the presence and degree of cognitive impairment (Kahn *et al.* 1960). In recent years memory clinics have been established to assist in the diagnosis and management of elderly people with impaired memory, to advise patients and their relatives on how to cope with memory problems of everyday life and to arrange appropriate social services support (Van Der Cammen *et al.* 1987). With regard to medical treatment while investigations are being carried out, the patient must be given adequate sleep. This is not a minor matter for sleep patterns in the demented can be significantly distorted. Oswald (1975) observes that such sleep disturbance parallels the deterioration of the brain. With dementia there tends to be a longer time taken to fall asleep, more frequent awakening and less total sleep. A bed is no place for a dementing patient who as the disease progresses tends to desire to move about. Similarly, such a patient should not, without very good reason, be confined to a chair. It is the nurse's function to watch and protect these ill people. Minor accidents due chiefly to falls occur, but this is a small price to pay for the patient's greater freedom. If it is practicable she is allowed to be up during the day and to walk about as much as possible watched and protected by the nurses. As young parents endeavour to tire out a boisterous infant so the well-trained nurse allows her patient as much liberty as is possible. Constant reassurance as evening comes with no tea or coffee but only milky fluids and the use of a chloral hydrate derivative such as syrup of triclofos or temazepam 10–20 mg may secure a night's sleep. Thioridazine (Melleril) in small doses of 25 mg four times a day may be of value in making the patient more biddable. Severe restlessness and agitation may require full doses of chlorpromazine 150–400 mg/day. Women patients may do better with promazine which may be given as an oral suspension 5 ml three times daily or if required as an injection of 50 mg intramuscularly.

In vascular dementia treatment may require to be directed to cardiac, respiratory or renal disease and this may be neglected because of the cerebral symptoms. One of the many problems in caring for the demented patient is the tendency that these people develop to keep on the move. These individuals because of loss of short-term memory may have a definite objective, get up and then forget the plan they had in mind and continue to wander aimlessly. They may be searching for someone deceased many years ago, be lost in surroundings to which they should be accustomed and be looking for the toilet. Nocturnal wandering, often most marked, is commonly due to complete disorientation and associated with insomnia. There is thus a need for improving security in the home or ward. For those who wander out of doors personal information on a label stitched to outer clothing can facilitate a return home. It was said by an experienced ward sister working in a female psychogeriatric ward that a wandering demented female patient never opened a door if it was labelled 'Gentlemen'. Perhaps this works in reverse. Nocturnal restlessness may require chlorpromazine 25–100 mg orally or 12.5–50 mg intramuscularly (depending on age, sex and body build). In patients with a history of inadequate diet or who are thin many physicians recommend intravenous injections of vitamins particularly all the B group. When symptoms of depression are present in vascular dementia it may be found that under-nutrition becomes a danger to life. The risk associated with electro-convulsive therapy should be considered, and if on balance it is re-commended this treatment frequently cures the depression although the dementia is unchanged. Mianserin may be of value as an alternative to electroconvulsive therapy in people too ill for this treatment. The opinion of the psychiatrist should be sought early rather than late, and frequently these people are treated best initially by the joint supervision of the psychiatrist, and physician in geriatric medicine. If the dementia is mild and the affect is happy, some would advise a special home for the mentally frail as the ideal environment provided the relatives are unable to cope. If the behavioural disorder is of such severity as to disrupt significantly ward routine admission to a mental hospital is necessary. Hodkinson (1975) is of the opinion that the choice between admission to a pyschiatric or geriatric ward is determined by the balance of behaviour disturbance on the one hand and immobility or associated physical illness on the other.

It is often the practice to have the name of every patient in large block capitals at the foot of each bed, to have a large clock in the ward telling the correct time and a perpetual calendar giving the day of the week, date and month. The patient who is clear mentally is not always certain in hospital wards of the essential facts. In the case of demented people the nurse with mental training who has rapport with her patient and insight into his condition is of the greatest value. The need to inspire such individuals with the will to dress and feed themselves and to go to the lavatory is recognized by such nurses. The conversation and interests of younger people help these old patients greatly and even although the conversation may be one-sided eventually contact is made. If such demented individuals are being treated at home in an earlier stage of illness the daughter or responsible relative should give a simple domestic task to the patient even if it means buying an inexpensive set of dishes because of breakages. Occasionally a relative has the gift of maintaining at home quite unbelievably difficult parents by this insight and ability to keep them occupied. So in hospital, group exercises and persistent encouragement to dress and be independent are well worthwhile. The more these individuals can be kept active, on the move and talking to each other the better. They are often, even in hospital, in their own minds carrying out tasks for relatives long since departed in the most happy and euphoric state, and in many cases it is the relatives who require psychotherapy. Post (1965) recommends for the elderly dement the value of organized ward programmes with occupational, recreational and work therapy and feels that these activities can be easily initiated and supervised by nurses. Physiotherapy and speech therapy can also be of help to those suffering from locomotor disability and dysphasia. After an acute delirious episode has settled attempts to get the patient home again are often worthwhile. It is likely that these patients deteriorate more rapidly in hospital. It would be wise in our present state of knowledge to be ever-watchful for further elucidation of these dementias in old people. Some would be more correctly diagnosed as dementias of unknown origin and therapeutic advances will no doubt come. It is tempting in any patient whose dietetic history is doubtful or whose symptomatology is of recent origin to give a course of high potency intravenous polyvitamin therapy. In any doubtful case a serum B_{12} level having been taken a course of vitamin B_{12} might be given. There is, however, no place for polypharmacy and these preparations should only be used on the basis of a therapeutic test. Combinations of tranquillizing drugs should be avoided. Hyams (1980) has reviewed the so-called cerebral activators; examples of these drugs are dihydroergotoxine mesylate (Hydergine), cyclandelate (Cyclospasmol) and naftidrofuryl (Praxilene). Conflicting evidence regarding their efficacy has been presented and, if used, a time limit of up to 12 weeks should be laid down, and if there is no evidence of improvement the medication should be discontinued. Judge & Caird (1978) stated that these drugs are too expensive to be used as placebos and in summary no drug is yet of scientifically proven value.

It must be kept in mind that demented patients do not make explicit or comprehensive complaints and thus physical illness may be difficult to detect. A sudden change in a demented patient's physical state should necessitate a review of physical health. Silent infections, cardiac failure, gastrointestinal bleeding or hypothyroidism may complicate the clinical picture. Conditions such as hyponatraemia, hypokalaemia or subclinical osteomalacia may occur. Clinical physical review will often greatly improve the patient's quality of life.

The realization of the need to help the carers of demented people has resulted in increasing availability of psychogeriatric day hospitals and of intermittent hospital admission. In the UK the Alzheimer's Disease Society has been constantly pressing for improved services and drawing attention rightly to the needs of dementia patients and their carers.

Alcohol abuse in the elderly

The patient will present with symptoms such as repeated falls, self-neglect or mental confusion. Apart from the Wernicke–Korsakoff syndrome a chronic confusional state resembling dementia and associated with cerebral atrophy has been described. There may be signs of malnutrition as shown by iron, folate or B_{12} deficiency anaemia. Clinical signs of chronic liver disease or gastrointestinal upsets, e.g. diarrhoea of recurring nature may be noted.

Management demands help from family and domiciliary health and social services and treatment for the specific alcohol related problems.

Affective disorders

Patients with mood disorders constitute about one-third to one-half of admissions to mental hospitals in the over-65 category. Disorders that involve moods of depression or elation are called affective disorders as they involve changes in affect or emotion. The dementias previously discussed are disorders of intellect. Sometimes in the elderly the two conditions co-exist.

Depression in an elderly person may occur alone or in combination with an organic disorder, e.g. a stroke, and the successful treatment of the individual depends on its detection. A degree of apathy and withdrawal, the presence of hypochondriasis, fearful anxiety or complete lack of initiative may indicate this illness. Alarcon (1964) found hypochondriacal symptoms in 65.7% of men and 62% of women when he studied 152 depressed patients over the age of 60. The most common symptom was concern over constipation. It is worth noting that 24.8% of the patients with hypochondriacal symptoms attempted suicide while of those free of such symptoms only 7.3% attempted suicide. Somatic symptoms are frequently present, constipation, as mentioned above, insomnia, headache, anorexia and fear of cancer; other presenting symptoms are dysphagia, dyspnoea, tinnitus, pain in varying sites and sleeplessness. Delusions may be present and this may make the diagnosis difficult. It may well be that at some time in the history-taking the patient says something that gives a clue to deep unhappiness, e.g. 'I wish I were away from it all'. Post (1965) states: 'anxiety and depression themselves as well as the symptoms derived from them are very unpleasant and cause considerable suffering'. He feels that in elderly people affective symptoms tend to respond to modern therapeutic measures and these should not be withheld on account of unresolved diagnostic difficulties. Many elderly people with depression are agitated and paranoid symptoms may be seen. Affective disorders are often an unrecognized factor in chronic physical illness; depression may be noted in myxoedema or thyrotoxicosis or following a viral illness, e.g. influenza. Drugs such as tranquillisers, methyldopa, corticosteroids and some β-blockers may induce depression. Patients with organic disease, e.g. a stroke, may appear depressed when in fact they have an anxiety state and may be helped by a small dose of thioridazine 10 mg two or three times per day.

It is likely that only between 5 and 10% of elderly people referred for the treatment of affective disorder are excited. Mania in this condition is usually noted in a miserable looking patient who may be garrulous and anecdotal but some depression is usually present at the same time. Expert psychiatric advice should be sought early in such cases. Treatment with phenothiazine drugs controls the severity of the maniacal symptoms.

Treatment of the depressive states

Unless the symptoms of illness are mild this is best undertaken by a psychiatrist. It is recommended that treatment is commenced by 2 or 3 days' rest in bed during which a complete investigation should be made to exclude the presence of physical illness of which the patient might be quite unaware. Admission to hospital may improve the patient's outlook perhaps removing him from an environment associated with acute painful memories. If the patient is poorly nourished a course of vitamin therapy may be of use. Mianserin (Bolvidon, Norval) in a starting dose of 30 mg at night with a gradually increasing dose, if necessary of up to 60 mg, helps many people. This drug relieves sleeplessness and after a few days improves mood. Elderly patients show very rarely any adverse effects, but occasionally if this preparation is used in cases after a severe stroke increased excitability occurs without any relief of the associated depression. If mianserin is not successful then imipramine hydrocholoride (Tofranil) 10–25 mg three times per day may be tried, and it is now possible to control therapy by blood levels. The therapeutic effect usually takes 10–21 days, and once the patient feels better the drug like mianserin should be continued for about 3 months and then gradually withdrawn. If symptoms recur then the previously successful preparation should be restarted. Adverse effects with imipramine (and much less commonly and milder with mianserin) are dryness of mouth, postural hypotension, tremulousness and sweating, and the dose may have to be lowered, and in elderly people mild delirious states with visual upsets have been encountered. Liver damage may occur and in the case of mianserin a full blood count is now recommended every month during the first 3 months of therapy and regularly thereafter.

Imipramine is typical of the group of tricyclic antidepressants and other members, such as amitriptyline, may sometimes be preferred because of their sedative or tranquillizing effect (Roth 1964). Many psychiatrists prescribe the major dose of amitripyline (Tryptizol) at night and thus the introduction of Lentizol, a long-acting preparation of the same substance, was a logical step. Lentizol 25 mg at night is equivalent in dose to amitriptyline 25 mg three times per day. This preparation taken at night has been of value to the elderly and 25 mg at bed-time is a suitable dose. The adverse effects are similar to those caused by imipramine. Tricyclic antidepressants, e.g. imipramine or amitriptyline or tetracyclic compounds like mianserin have a reputation of cardiotoxicity. They can be used with caution in patients with mild heart disease but should be avoided in those with heart failure, heart block or who have recently had a myocardial infarction. Antidepressants are commonly given at home, but Mayer-Gross *et al.* (1960) felt that, once an affective psychosis has been diagnosed in old age, patients are preferably treated in hospital. The reasons are the risk of suicide and exhaustion, the need for thorough investigation and the possibility that electroconvulsive therapy requires to be used. If drug treatment fails then electroconvulsive therapy is often very effective, but if this is being considered the advice of a psychiatrist is essential.

Day hospitals have an important part to play in the continued follow-up and care of such patients.

Depression does occur following stroke and diagnosis is difficult. For those who can co-operate the 10 question Short Zung Interviewer-assisted Depression rating scale may be of help. Social factors almost certainly play a prominent part in the development of the depression. For such patients an active rehabilitation programme with reassurance and explanation to the patient and family will improve the situation. Antidepressants if required must be used with caution and initially with a low dosage. Stroke is not a contraindication to electroconvulsive therapy and this can be reserved for unresponsive patients or those considered to be a high risk for suicide. ECT is not advised within 3 months of a stroke (House 1987).

Paranoid syndromes

Paranoid syndromes in the elderly present diagnostic problems and account for approximately one-tenth of admissions to mental hospitals among the over 60s. They may be associated with a senile character-change, with acute confusional states, with depressive illness or dementia or part of a chronic illness sometimes called paraphrenia.

Cases have been described with predominantly paranoid symptoms that show themselves in the 70s and late paraphrenia is a fairly common condition occurring after the age of 55.

Some are chronic schizophrenics who for many years have managed to live outside hospital or who are readmitted in relapse, but in the majority the illness develops in old age. These people are commonly women, often unmarried, with one-third of their number affected by disorders of vision or, more commonly, hearing. Partial deafness is said to be more potent in producing symptoms. Many of them have had paranoid traits throughout their life and now develop delusions connected either with their neighbours, e.g. threats or thefts, or with sex, e.g. being observed while undressing or being molested. Short-lived paranoid reactions are not uncommon in states of exhaustion in people kept awake by pain or dyspnoea. After severe infection paranoid symptoms are probably as common as depressive ones, e.g. in influenza and in hepatitis, and there are many causes of these paranoid reactions among them steroids and vitamin deficiencies, pellagra and pernicious anaemia. As would be expected, the therapy in these cases is basically the treatment of the organic disease. If this condition is temporary it must be remembered that the paranoid symptoms may not end as soon as the physical illness has been cured.

Treatment

The psychological handling of such patients is extremely important. Great care must be taken to avoid saying or doing anything that increases the patient's paranoid mood. The most difficult problem for the doctor or nurse is to avoid being roused by the aggression directed to them personally and to keep in mind that a soft answer turns away wrath. This direction is easy to lay down but very hard to put into practice. If there are problems with vision or hearing, attention should be directed to the provision of suitable glasses or hearing aid.

A phenothiazine such as thioridazine in a dose of 25 mg three times per day and 50 mg at night is usually effective. Much higher doses may be required. In hospital it is often advantageous to change the medication to a long-acting, intramuscular injection tranquillizer, fluphenazine decanoate (Modecate), if oral drugs are ineffective or if the patient is unwilling to continue oral medication. This drug must be used with care as parkinsonian adverse effects may be severe and long-lasting, but it may produce excellent results. The initial dose should be 6.25 mg (0.25 ml) and no more should be given for at least 14 days so that the individual response may be gauged. Thereafter, dosage should be tailored to the individual case and, usually given once per month. The dose required is commonly in the

12.5–25 mg range; parkinsonian adverse effects may respond to drug therapy. Restlessness and disturbed behaviour due to other mental conditions may also be treated in this way when other methods have failed. The treatment may be continued after discharge from hospital if adequate supervision is available. The auditory hallucinosis of the deaf is usually controlled by relatively small doses of tranquillizing drugs; if there are prominent depressive features electroconvulsive therapy is worth trying.

Personality changes

In old age there is found frequently an exaggeration of the slight personality defects that may have been present in earlier life. The tendency for many elderly people to become introspective may be an increase in shyness and timidity. Self-interest and turning inward results in relationships with others becoming even more limited and can lead to dangerous isolation and the risk of becoming completely cut off from the rest of society. This pattern of behaviour has been described as the Diogenes syndrome and is commoner in widows living alone. Perverted sexual conduct with the obvious association of such factors as loneliness, decline of potency and inactivity may be found in old men. A condition called institutional neurosis characterized by apathy, lack of initiative, loss of interest, apparent inability to make plans for the future, lack of individuality and, on occasion, a characteristic posture and gait may be found (Barton 1959). It is important therefore to avoid admission of elderly people into institutions wherever possible. The importance of finding out the numbers of lonely old people especially those actually living alone in a community and in the 75 and over range is of the highest priority. Once the name and address has been ascertained arrangements for regular supervision are necessary to avoid mental and physical ill health. Day hospitals, day centres, all-day clubs for the elderly, lunch clubs and hobbies and craft centres all have a vital function in this preventive plan. Admission to hospital when essential should be arranged with care. If the elderly person has relatives and contact can be made with the patient it should be explained in detail and frequently that this admission is essential to make the correct diagnosis and to improve the physical or mental condition of the patient. If there is understanding and comprehension of this by the old person, usually consent is given to the transfer to hospital and the ever-present fear that this is a permanent move is overcome. The constant plea by all interested in older people is for earlier diagnosis, for quicker transfer to hospital if this is essential and for a plan to be put into operation which the older person can understand. This, of course, cannot be done in every case: a sudden attack of confusion or a crisis produced by a fall at home; these necessitate immediate action.

If institutional neurosis has developed then contacts with family, if any, should be re-established. If there are no relatives, visitors should be encouraged from voluntary organizations. Many long-term hospitals have clubs for older people operating inside the hospital and the patient should be encouraged to attend and also to take an active part in occupational therapy. Every endeavour should be made to try and make the patient lead an independent life again with hypnotics and tranquillizers cut down as much as possible.

Obsessional neurosis is most intractable when it occurs in the elderly, and it is worth trying to find time to let the patient talk at length about the symptoms. The individual may well be aware that when he asks the doctor to inspect a normal stool he is acting in an unreasoning way but he may be unable to stop this. An elderly man complained that he was being tormented by worms which he was passing in his bowel movement constantly. On being asked what they looked like he stated, 'I do not know, I have never seen them'. Thioridazine 10 mg increasing to 25 mg three times per day may help but of more importance is the ability to devote time for reassurance.

General management of mentally ill old people in hospital

While diagnosis and treatment of the mental state is proceeding a plan of physical rehabilitation should be commenced. The patient, if bedridden, should, where possible, be mobilized and providing the physical condition permits, gradual and increasingly active exercises encouraged. The advice of the physician trained in geriatric medicine should be available in the mental hospitals and a team should be organized just as in the geriatric unit with nurses, physiotherapists, occupational therapists and, where necessary, chiropodist and speech therapist all playing a part.

Incontinence improves if the patient can be mobilized and the whole apparatus necessary for successful physical rehabilitation should be available in the mental hospital.

Plans for discharge home if this is 'on' should be commenced early and the social worker brought into the picture.

If discharge is arranged, follow-up and continued supervision should be planned in liaison with the patient and general practitioner. Full use should be made of the social worker, the health visitor and the district nurse according to local arrangements and all possible help should be obtained financially for the patient. Voluntary organizations should be asked to help with regular home visiting and, if practicable, attendance at an all-day club or lunch club arranged.

It must never be forgotten that suicide is now largely a problem of later life, and social isolation, retirement, lack of employment and loss of status in society are important factors in the elderly suicide. Depression is more closely associated with suicide in old age than in youth. Physical illness and bereavement are common precursors to suicide in later life. When an old person expresses suicidal thoughts or makes a suicidal act, psychiatric advice should be sought and in many cases in-patient treatment in a psychiatric unit or mental hospital is needed.

Legal aspects

These vary according to the legislation in the country concerned but in England and Wales the procedure is as follows.

In the majority of cases admissions can be arranged without any legal process, i.e. on an informal basis. A small proportion of patients whose mental disorders are such as to constitute a danger to themselves or others may require compulsory admission.

The categories are listed as described in the Mental Health Act 1983:

Admission to hospital for assessment or assessment and treatment. This lasts for 28 days and the patient must be suffering from mental disorder that warrants detention in a hospital. The patient is detained in the interests of his own health or safety or to protect others.

Application must be made by the nearest relative or approved social worker and the patient must have been seen within the last 14 days.

Medical recommendation is by two doctors (one approved as having 'special experience in the diagnosis or treatment of mental disorder'). They must examine the patient within 5 days of each other.

Compulsory admission of a patient to hospital for treatment. This lasts 6 months and the patient must be suffering from mental disorder appropriate for him to receive treatment in hospital; such treatment must be likely to alleviate or prevent deterioration of the condition; it must be necessary for the health or safety of the patient or for the protection of others that he should receive such treatment and it cannot be provided unless the patient is detained.

Application must be made as for the category above but if the nearest relative objects the approved social worker cannot go ahead with the application. If the objection is considered unreasonable, a county court may order that the functions of the nearest relative should be vested in another person.

The medical recommendation is as for the previous category but the type of mental disorder must be stated.

Emergency admission for assessment occurs when because of the risk to the patient or others there is not enough time to obtain a second medical opinion. This lasts for 72 hours and grounds for admission are as in the first category described with the addition that it is of urgent necessity that the patient be admitted and detained in hospital. Application may be made by the nearest relative or approved social worker either of whom should have seen the patient in the last 24 hours. Only one medical recommendation is required and if possible this should be by someone with knowledge of the patient.

A patient already receiving treatment in hospital as an in-patient may be detained for 72 hours provided it appears that an application for the patient's compulsory admission to hospital should be made for the health or safety of the patient or others that he should be detained until such an application can be made; the recommendation can be made by the doctor in charge of the case or his nominated deputy.

A patient already receiving treatment for mental disorder in hospital can be detained, until a doctor is found, for 6 hours although the holding power ceases on the arrival of the doctor. It must appear to the nurse that the patient is suffering from mental disorder to such a degree that it is necessary for his health or safety or for the protection of others that he be immediately restrained from leaving hospital and that it is not practical to secure the immediate attendance of a doctor. A registered nurse must record the decision in writing and deliver it to the hospital managers (Briscoe & Harris 1987).

The Mental Health (Scotland) Act, 1960 differs slightly. Compulsory admission requires an application by the nearest relative or a Mental Health Officer, two doctors, usually the family doctor and a psychiatrist, and the approval of a Sheriff. In cases of urgent necessity a single medical recommendation, and when practicable, consent of a relative or Mental Health Officer allows for 7 days of compulsory care.

Response to treatment is usually so rapid that compulsory care for periods for as long as 28 days is rarely necessary and every effort should be made to treat patients informally.

In most cases assessment of the patient by a psychiatrist prior to admission obviates the need for compulsion.

REFERENCES

Alarcon R. de (1964) Hypochondriasis and depression in the aged. *Gerontologia clinica* **6**, 266.
Anderson W.F., Caird F.I., Kennedy R.D. & Schwartz Doris (1982) *Gerontology and Geriatric Nursing.* London, Hodder & Stoughton.
Barton R. (1959) *Institutional Neurosis.* Bristol, John Wright.
Briscoe M. & Harris B. (1987) Compulsory detention in hospital under the Mental Health Act 1983. *British Medical Journal* **294**, 1141.

Harris R. (1982) Genetics of Alzheimer's disease. Leader. *British Medical Journal* **284,** 1065.

Hodkinson H.M. (1975) Psychological medicine: the elderly mind. *British Medical Journal* **2,** 23.

House A. (1987) Depression after stroke. *British Medical Journal* **294,** 76.

Hyams D.E. (1980) Cerebral activating drugs. In *The Treatment of Medical Problems in the Elderly* (Ed. Denham M.J.) Lancaster, MTP.

Judge T.G. & Caird F.I. (1978) *Drug Treatment of the Elderly Patient.* Tunbridge Wells, Pitman Medical.

Kahn R.L., Goldfarb A.I., Pollack M. & Pick A. (1960) Brief objective measures for the determination of mental status in the aged. *American Journal of Psychiatry* **117,** 326.

Mayer-Gross W., Slater E. & Roth M. (1960) *Clinical Psychiatry.* London, Cassell.

Oswald I. (1975) Sleep response and mental illness. Editorial. *Psychological Medicine* **5,** 1.

Post F. (1965) *The Clinical Psychiatry of Later Life.* Oxford, Pergamon Press.

Roth M.J. (1964) Prophylaxis and early diagnosis and treatment of mental illness in late life. In *Current Achievements in Geriatrics* (Ed. Anderson W.F. & Isaacs B.) London, Cassell.

RCP Report (1981) Organic mental impairment in the elderly. *Journal of the Royal College of Physicians of London* (London) **15,** 141.

Van Der Cammen T.J.M., Simpson J.M., Fraser R.M., Preker A.S. & Exton-Smith A.N. (1987) The memory clinic. *British Journal of Psychiatry* **150,** 359.

16
Musculoskeletal Disorders

Rheumatoid disease

This illness is a constitutional disease in which there are inflammatory changes throughout connective tissues of the body. The most common manifestation is a polyarthritis of smaller joints, e.g. the hands and feet. Once the disease has become established the distribution tends to be symmetrical. The arthritis is produced by a chronic proliferative inflammation of synovial membrane which can cause irreversible damage to the joint capsule and articular cartilage. Rheumatoid arthritis affects 15% of women and 5% of men over the age of 65 years, but the female preponderance reduces in the very old. Most elderly patients have inactive or burnt out disease as a legacy from earlier years, but occasionally the arthritis occurs as a very acute late onset problem with marked systemic upset associated with severe functional disability. The prognosis is, however, generally benign with a good return of function and resultant deformities tend to be less severe. Extra-articular manifestations are less common in the elderly.

Fatigue with weight loss, fever, pain, swelling and stiffness of joints are common findings. In a few patients splenic enlargement is discovered on clinical examination and iritis and episcleritis are sometimes found as complications while in longstanding cases amyloidosis may occur. Patches of scleritis may occur and usually signify severe disease and bad prognosis, while kerato-conjunctivitis sicca (Sjögren syndrome) with destruction of salivary and lacrimal glands may be noted.

Treatment

The physician must judge for himself the methods of therapy appropriate to the stage of the illness at which his patient first presents. His main tasks are to relieve pain, to prevent or correct deformity, to improve joint function and to find out and treat any factors, e.g. anaemia, hindering recovery.

Rest in bed is always a risk in elderly people, but if acute illness is present with fever a preliminary period of complete immobilization may be essential. Prolonged bed rest for more than 7–10 days should if possible be avoided because of the risk of bedsores and deep vein thrombosis.

During this time investigation and complete assessment of the patient can be carried out, bearing in mind the mental health and social environment of the individual. For each case a plan must be evolved, and the personal attention of the physician who shows himself keenly interested in the elderly person acts as a great stimulus to the apathetic or depressed patient. During this phase adequate pain relief is required. Analgesics, e.g. paracetamol, alone may be satisfactory in mild cases but most patients will require analgesic anti-inflammatory agents viz. non-steroidal anti-inflammatory drugs (NSAIDs). A wide range of NSAIDs are available and the individual patient's response may vary considerably with different agents at different times. Most of these drugs have similar side effects including gastrointestinal discomfort, nausea and bleeding, hypersensitivity reactions, headache, vertigo and hearing disturbances. Fluid retention may occur and this can precipitate heart failure in the elderly with underlying heart disease. NSAIDs should be used with caution in patients with gastric ulceration, allergic disorders and renal or hepatic impairment. Most patients tolerate some NSAIDs better than others and several compounds may be tried before the most appropriate one is discovered. Aspirin may be given in a dose of 1 g four times a day. Many elderly people tolerate soluble calcium aspirin better than plain aspirin. Keratin coated preparations such as Nu-Seals Aspirin may diminish the likelihood of gastrointestinal bleeding. Ibuprofen (Brufen) should be given in divided doses to a maximum of 2.4 g daily. Naproxen (Naprosyn) can be given in a dosage of 250 or 500 mg twice daily. Piroxicam (Feldene) has the advantage that it only has to be given once daily in a dose of 20 or 40 mg. Sulindac (Clinoril) is given in a dose of 100 or 200 mg twice daily after meals.

During this initial stage attention should be paid to the comfort of the patient in bed. A firm mattress, a cage to remove the weight of the blankets from the legs and the feet, a foot-board across the lower end of the bed to support the feet and as correct a posture as the patient's condition permits are all nursing essentials. Improvement usually occurs and, as soon as the temperature has declined and the patient is better, steps should be taken to commence mobilization. Elderly patients are prone to develop contractures so light splints may be required to correct deformity and once the pain relieving drugs have taken effect the wrist should be put in slight dorsiflexion, the foot midway between dorsi- and plantar-flexion, and the knee in extension. These splints should be reviewed daily and local heat may be of value in easing joint pain. At this stage if progress is retarded by persistent pain and swelling in one joint, e.g. the knee, intra-articular hydrocortisone may be of value, e.g. 25 mg into a knee on three occasions at intervals of 1 month. Weight bearing would not usually be encouraged

if the patient had been bedridden during these injections as disorganiz-
ation of a joint has been reported either due to prolonged injections or
excessive exertion.

Once a subacute stage has been reached attempts may be made by
radiant heat, short-wave diathermy, wax baths, ice therapy and hydro-
therapy to improve or maintain joint function. The place of corticosteroids
in rheumatoid disease remains controversial. In patterns with uncomplicated arthritis steroids should be avoided apart from intra-articular
injections (*see above*). These drugs may however be useful in elderly
patients with severe arthritis (Scott & Coppock 1987). Unless there are
contraindications to the use of steroids such as a history of or current
cardiac failure, peptic ulcer, diabetes mellitus, tuberculosis, osteoporosis,
mental illness, an intercurrent infection or marked hypertension, it is
worth trying these drugs especially where stiffness or gross limitation of
movement are present. Prednisolone in a 10–15 mg once daily dose
should normally be given in addition to an NSAID. The dose should be
reduced to below 7.5 mg daily as soon as the desired effect is achieved. In
patients who show a marked response to prednisolone the daily dose may
be reduced by 1 mg each week until the minimum dose required to
maintain control of symptoms is reached. Second line drugs (Table 16.1)
are slow acting and not recommended for acute attacks of rheumatoid
disease. They are indicated in patients with severe disease which fails to
respond to NSAIDs or progressive disease with radiological rheumatoid
changes. These agents should normally be commenced in addition to
NSAIDs in subacute or chronic joint disease and their use should be
supervised by a specialist rheumatologist.

Hydroxchloroquine (Plaquenil) in a dose 400 mg daily may be used
but care must be taken to avoid the development of corneal opacity,
retinopathy or macular degeneration.

Gold therapy may be useful in the treatment of rheumatoid arthritis
in selected elderly patients but this form of treatment is not generally
recommended as the elderly have a greater liability to toxic reactions.
Penicillamine has been shown to be effective in the management of
elderly patients with rheumatoid disease, although the toxicity is significantly greater than in younger patients. Skin rashes and marked abnormalities in the ability to taste are more likely to occur in the elderly (Kean

Table 16.1 Second line drugs for rheumatoid disease.

Anti-malarials (e.g. chloroquine, hydroxychloroquine)
Gold (e.g. sodium aurothiomalate)
Penicillamine
Sulphasalazine
Dapsone

---

et al. 1982).

An initial dose of 125 mg daily before food is given for 1 month and increased by this amount every 4–12 weeks until remission occurs or until a maximum daily dose of 750 mg is reached.

Third line or cytotoxic drugs, e.g. methotrexate, azathioprine or cyclophosphamide may be indicated when second line drugs fail to control the activity of the disease and in particular when extra-articular manifestations, e.g. vasculitis or pleurisy are present.

The attack on rheumatoid arthritis is a team effort with doctors, nurses, physiotherapists and occupational therapists all playing their part. The surgeon should not be omitted from this co-operation effort.

The place of surgery in rheumatoid arthritis

Surgical intervention is often considered at too late a stage in the rehabilitation of the elderly arthritic patient. The surgeon aims to relieve joint pain and to correct deformity to promote improvement in function. Age is not a contraindication to operative management, but the patient must be very well assessed by the physician and surgeon and other non-articular problems must be corrected in the preoperative period. Anaemia and cardiovascular disorders should be treated and the renal function and fluid balance should be assessed. The mental state of the patient should be carefully noted and active physiotherapy should be prescribed to increase muscle power and joint stability. Adrenal function should be screened in patients who have been on long-term maintenance steroid therapy.

Synovectomy is the most frequent surgical procedure performed in rheumatoid arthritis and at an early stage of the disease good results can be obtained in the knees, shoulder, elbow and ankle. Tenosynovectomy of the wrist may prove valuable and may prevent further joint and tendon damage. If, however, articular damage is advanced or synovectomy has failed then arthroplasty is the operation of choice. Arthrodesis of the knee produces very little benefit and total joint replacement is indicated. Osteotomy occasionally benefits those patients with a genu varum deformity and patellar excision may be helpful if the patellofemoral compartment is involved.

The use of prosthetic replacement has the advantage in the elderly of a short period of immobilization. Replacement of the hip and knee are the usual arthroplasties while silastic finger joint implants are more commonly used in younger age groups. It is essential to ensure that the haemoglobin level is satisfactory as this falls after prosthetic replacement. Infection is the other complication and many surgeons give routinely antibiotic cover.

During this specialized therapy for rheumatoid arthritis attention must be paid to the general condition of the patient. For those underweight, a well-balanced diet with an adequate supply of protein, vitamins and minerals, and for those obese a similar diet but designed to promote weight reduction, should be given.

Physiotherapy

Physical methods of treatment are valuable adjuncts in the treatment of rheumatoid arthritis. Before any treatment is ordered, a specific aim must be defined and the treatment must be adapted to individual requirements and in a changing disease this must be kept constantly under review. Physiotherapy falls into three categories: the maintenance of joint movement and prevention or correction of deformity; the strengthening of muscle groups by remedial exercises; walking re-education with instruction in the use of aids such as walking sticks.

Occupational therapy

Occupational therapy is of the greatest value in the rehabilitation of the patient when the active phase of the disease has passed and, in conjunction with physiotherapy, improves movements and muscle tone. It also provides a great psychological stimulus in demonstrating to the patient that he can do something useful. The occupational therapist also shows the patient how to use the appropriate aids to daily living and makes the endeavour to render the patient independent. A spring seat is available which is of great help in patients who have difficulty in rising from a chair and yet when up are ambulant. Local authorities help in this way; some provide occupational therapy at home and all modify houses to suit the requirements of the disabled person.

Anaemia in rheumatoid disease

Anaemia is extremely common in patients with rheumatoid disease. It is usually in the form of the anaemia of chronic inflammation where the haemoglobin level is about 11 g%. This anaemia is normochromic or mildly hypochromic. Iron deficiency anaemia may also be present and this may be due to a variety of causes including poor diet and chronic gastrointestinal blood loss as a side effect of treatment. Bleeding may occur into actively inflamed joints. Serum iron and iron binding capacity levels may be diffcult to interpret and bone marrow samples may help to clarify the haematological diagnosis. The serum ferritin levels are raised in inflammatory states and usually reduced in iron deficiency states. Pernicious anaemia may co-exist with rheumatoid disease. Hypersplenism and anaemia may occur in Felty syndrome. Here the patient has splenomegaly in addition to rheumatoid arthritis. Splenectomy is indicated if recurrent life-threatening infections are occurring.

Rheumatoid neuropathy

In most patients occlusion of the vasa nervorum by vasculitis is thought to be the cause of neuropathy. Two main forms of neuropathy occur. A mild, mainly sensory form occurs mostly in females and the prognosis is relatively benign. A more severe sensorimotor neuropathy occurs mainly in men and in association with destructive nodular rheumatoid disease. Motor signs predominate with mild sensory symptoms. No specific therapy influences the course of rheumatoid neuropathy but loss of muscle power must be treated by appropriate support and physiotherapy as deformities may become permanent unless contractures are prevented by splinting.

Entrapment neuropathies may occur and these include median nerve compression (carpal tunnel syndrome), posterior tibial nerve compression (tarsal tunnel syndrome) and ulnar nerve compression at the elbow. These disorders can usually be treated satisfactorily by surgical decompression.

Osteoarthritis

Osteoarthritis or osteoarthrosis is radiologically but not necessarily clinically present in the majority of the population over 60 years of age.

It is regarded by some as due to a constitutional defect in the patient's articular cartilage which is thereby rendered excessively sensitive to slight degrees of trauma. This arthritis, especially if knees are involved, is aggravated if not induced by obesity and weight reduction could be regarded as a preventive measure. Previous injury to a joint or malalignment of a fractured long bone and continued trauma associated with occupational strain are predisposing causes. Change of occupation might be of value in prevention in certain cases. As people grow older an attempt should be made to put their joints through as full a range of movement as possible every day. Restricted movement of a joint would seem one possible factor in aetiology. Osteoarthritis is found in many hips in which there was congenital dislocation apparently successfully treated many years previously. The joints most frequently affected are those of the spine, hips, knees, elbows and, in women, terminal joints of fingers.

Pain is the first symptom, intermittent and aching, and appearing especially after the joint has been used. If the hip joint is affected the pain is sometimes felt in the knee. Movement of the affected joint becomes limited by muscular spasm and by loss of joint cartilage and formation of osteophytes. Muscular wasting is noted, crepitus is felt or heard and stiffness and deformity occur. In women the generalized form affecting many joints is common with the terminal interphalangeal joints of the fingers usually affected. The Heberden nodes (cartilaginous or bony outgrowths) may appear on the fingers giving rise to considerable deformity of joints but little disability. In men the disease is usually confined to the hips or the knees. One of the fascinating unsolved features of this illness is the lack of correlation between the symptoms complained of by the patient and the degree of degenerative changes seen in the x-ray film.

Treatment

For the elderly patient with osteoarthritis, therapy is directed most frequently to the hip and knees and is dependent on the stage of illness at which the patient is first seen. The only exception to this statement is that obesity must always be treated. Weight reduction is an essential factor in preventing further damage and in helping recovery. If there is severe persistent pain in the joint, and this is sometimes found in both knee joints, then a preliminary period of rest in bed is required. There is often a degree of inflammation in many cases of osteoarthrosis and therefore drugs with an anti-inflammatory action are usually preferable to simple analgesics. One or other form of aspirin is still the most commonly recommended first choice if the patients can tolerate salicylates and doses of up to 3 g or more daily may be required to control symptoms. Other forms of salicylates including soluble and enteric-coated tablets may be more acceptable. In patients who cannot tolerate salicylates or in whom pain relief is inadequate, one or other of the NSAID may be beneficial. Whenever the pain is under control active non-weight bearing exercises should be started.

Physiotherapy has an important part to play and massage and heat may help to reduce the pain. It is, however, the active exercises that the patient can undertake which are most important. If a very elderly frail person has already some flexion deformity of the knee it may be necessary to build up the heels rather than spend time correcting the deformity. With built-up heels much better contact is made with the ground and exercises with a Zimmer walk-aid or with two-, three- or four-legged sticks may encourage a patient previously confined to a chair to walk; wasted muscles may require building up.

The analgesic effect of heat may be attained by use of diathermy or short-wave therapy in deep-seated joints such as the hip or spine.

treatment of this condition. Manipulation under a general anaesthetic may be of value in selected cases where there is considerable pain and limitation of movement but only moderate bony changes. Three surgical procedures are of value in osteoarthritis: arthrodesis, osteotomy and arthroplasty. Arthrodesis is indicated in unilateral disease with severe pain in, for example, the knee joint with evidence of gross radiological destruction. A satisfactory operation can be expected to relieve pain completely. Osteotomy is useful for patients who have pain, e.g. in an osteoarthritic knee that has significant lateral angulation. The aim is to obtain a straight leg which can flex. Arthroplasty can relieve pain and improve mobility. This is a most useful and helpful operation in hip-joint disease. The patient should be mentally normal, co-operative and anxious for operation. The quality of life can be improved immensely by a successful operation. The primary indication for surgery is severe pain which cannot be relieved by conservative measures. The choice of operation must of course be left to the orthopaedic surgeon.

In the very elderly the main treatment of osteoarthritis involving hip and knee certainly initially is active, graduated and supervised physiotherapy; correction of deformity may not be the most important aim but active movement culminating in independent walking is of prime importance. Even in advanced age the opinion of the orthopaedic surgeon should be sought if pain is constantly severe and unyielding to medical treatment.

Gout

Hyperuricaemia tends to occur in the elderly as a secondary phenomenon and is associated with the use of thiazide diuretics, small doses of salicylates or renal or haematological abnormalities. Clinical problems with gout in these patients, however, are relatively uncommon.

Clinical gout occurs much more frequently in men, but gout beginning in old age is characterized by an increased female incidence. The condition usually presents as an attack of acute arthritis with a tender inflamed joint, commonly the metatarsophalangeal joint of the big toe. There is usually an associated constitutional disturbance with mild pyrexia and leucocytosis. The illness comes on in middle age and is episodic until in old age a chronic arthritis exists with several joints involved which undergo occasional exacerbations. Trauma, exposure to cold and surgical operation may be the trigger mechanism that precipitates an attack. Tophi on the helix of the ears or on elbows are sometimes found, and x-ray shows translucent areas in the bones of the hands and the feet. The serum uric acid level is above 7 mg/100 ml (0.42 mmol/l) but acute attacks of gout may be associated with a normal serum level. The diagnosis of urate gout should be confirmed by finding intraleucocytic crystals in the synovial fluid aspirated from an inflamed joint, particularly if the knee is involved.

Treatment

Severe dietary restriction is unnecessary in gout but the patient should be advised to avoid purine-rich foods like sweetbreads, kidney, liver, meat extracts and heavy wines while obese patients should also take a reducing diet. The acute attack is relieved by colchicine in a dose of 0.5 mg 2-hourly by mouth until relief has been obtained, or a maximum of 8 mg has been given or diarrhoea or vomiting occurs. In the treatment of subsequent attacks the total amount of colchicine advised should be 2 mg less than the quantity that in the previous instance produced diarrhoea. After the acute pain is relieved colchicine should be continued in a dose of 0.5 mg after each meal three times per day for a few days. Pain during the acute bout should be relieved by an NSAID, e.g. indomethacin (indocid), orally in divided doses of up to 150 mg daily. A useful alternative is azapropazone (rheumox) orally in divided doses of 900 mg daily after food. During this phase rest in bed may be necessary and the weight of the bedclothes should be kept from the feet by a bed cradle while ample fluids should be given.

After an acute attack of gout has been relieved the question of long-term management must be considered. Indications for lowering the serum uric acid include chronic tophaceous gout, frequent acute attacks, gout with evidence of renal damage or gout accompanied by a consistently raised serum urate concentration, that is 8 mg/100 ml (0.48 mmol/l) (Scott 1980).

Serum urate reduction is achieved by use of the drug allopurinol. This drug is usually given in a maintenance dose of 200–400 mg daily, but smaller doses may be indicated if there is renal impairment. Concurrent administration of colchicine or an NSAID should be given for the first few months of allopurinol therapy. Allopurinol is a safe drug with infrequent adverse effects but occasionally rashes may occur and in these patients an alternative regimen might include one of the uricosuric agents, e.g. probenecid or sulphinpyrazone.

Where joints have been deformed, physiotherapy as for rheumatoid arthritis should be recommended.

Pseudo-gout

Symptoms in this condition are due to the deposition of crystals of calcium pyrophosphate and the diagnosis can be confirmed by polarizing microscopy which reveals intraleucocytic positively birefringent crystals of calcium pyrophosphate in fluid from the affected joint, e.g. the knee. X-ray will show articular calcification in the fibrocartilage (chondrocalcinosis). Treatment is similar to that of gout while if the acute episode occurs in the knee aspiration often aborts the attack.

Cervical spondylosis

This is a degenerative disorder of the cervical spine leading to narrowing and protrusion of the intervertebral discs with its greatest incidence in the 60–70 age range. The disc changes cause pressure upon the spinal nerves in the foramina and on the spinal cord. This disease is more common in men than in women and the symptoms are due to involvement either of the affected nerve roots or of the spinal cord itself. The first group of symptoms consists of hyperaesthesia, root pain or muscle wasting with acroparaesthesia (an unpleasant tingling in arm or fingers), and these symptoms usually occur at night. The pain may be made worse by moving the neck or pulling on the arm; coarse fasciculation may be seen in the affected muscles and the tendon reflexes of the involved muscles are diminished or lost. The second group of symptoms, i.e. those due to pressure on the spinal cord, may be initiated by numbness and weakness of the hand or increasing weakness of one or both legs. Muscular weakness of lower motor neurone type may found in the upper limbs and spasticity of upper motor neurone type in the legs, with sensory loss in the upper limbs, but not the lower limbs. The bladder is rarely involved. Rarely cervical spondylosis can produce syncope and vertigo, these symptoms being brought on by movement of the head causing compression of the vertebral arteries. The diagnosis in elderly people is not simple as so many of the over 60s have gross changes in the cervical spine with no symptoms of disease. A straight lateral x-ray of the cervical spine is not sufficient to confirm the diagnosis, and certainly before any operative procedure myelography would be necessary to demonstrate the actual points of pressure.

Treatment

For the elderly patient appropriate analgesics such as aspirin should be given and in more severe pain an NSAID may be required for a period of 2–3 weeks. If tension in the cervical muscles is a problem, small doses of diazepam may be useful. A collar holding the chin up is of help. To start with the collar should be worn night and day but as symptoms improve it should gradually be left off, at first at night and then during the day as well. Once the severe pain is gone the patient should be encouraged to undertake active exercises for the neck and shoulders combined with heat treatment. In early cases the fluid intake should be increased as on occasion symptoms disappear on this regimen alone. An extra 3 pints (1.75 litres) of fluid per day as water should be taken. Where there is the possibility of compression of the vertebral arteries or spinal cord the opinion of the neurosurgeon should be sought.

Lumbar and thoracic spine

Degeneration changes are also found in the thoracic and lumbar spine. The osteophytes rising from the edges of the vertebral bodies are due to primary degeneration of the intervertebral discs with consequent narrowing of the space between the vertebral bodies. Injury, heavy lifting and obesity are all causative factors and backache of intermittent character, becoming worse as the patient grows older, is the usual symptom.

Treatment

The fitting of a spinal support may be of value but in an acute attack pain may be so severe that the patient requires an initial phase of rest in bed with heat applied locally and salicylates or other NSAID given to relieve the pain. When pain is acute, limitation of movement is noticed and this is associated with some degree of spasm of the spinal muscles.

Neuropathic joint disease

This is a chronic progressive degeneration of one or more joints occurring most frequently as a complication of tabes dorsalis but also found in syringomyelia, in diabetic neuropathy and following repeated intra-articular injections of hydrocortisone into large joints. The patient usually complains of progressive swelling of a single large joint with increasing instability of this joint. There is little pain as a rule but marked hypermobility of the affected joint, which usually reveals the presence of fluid, while x-ray of the joint shows destructive and hypertrophic changes. In tabes dorsalis the joints affected are more often the knee, hip and ankle and the lumbar and lower dorsal spine. In diabetic neuropathy changes occur most frequently in the tarsal and metatarsal joints, less commonly in the ankles and rarely in the knees. The shoulders and elbows are the usual sites of joint degeneration in syringomyelia.

Treatment

This is usually unsatisfactory but splints and braces may make walking possible after a course of careful and graduated physiotherapy. When the ankle or foot is affected amputation is sometimes recommended as the only practical solution.

Connective tissue disorders

These disorders as a cause of arthritis in the elderly should not be forgotten, especially when the arthritis is accompanied by symptoms that are referred to many different systems of the body, e.g. respiratory system as pleurisy, cardiovascular system as pericarditis or kidneys as renal disease. Rheumatoid arthritis has been discussed elsewhere (p. 249) and the less common disorders include systemic sclerosis, systemic lupus erythematosus and polyartertis nodosa.

Systemic sclerosis

This condition has its highest incidence over the age of 65 years. The majority of patients are women and present with Raynaud phenomenon, skin ulceration or necrosis of the fingers associated with telangiectasia and half of the affected individuals have oesophageal strictures. Most patients have a benign form of the disease and the prognosis is generally favourable, but the condition may be rapidly fatal (Williams & Gumpel 1981); treatment is largely symptomatic. Steroid therapy may be helpful in the more severe forms of this condition, but expert rheumatological advice is required.

Systemic lupus erythematosus (SLE)

This condition predominantly affects females and it may develop at any time between early childhood and old age, although it is more frequent during the second and third decades. Clincial manifestation may include arthritis, neuropsychiatric disorders, skin rashes and renal disease. Most affected patients have detectable anti-DNA antibodies in their serum. Management includes NSAID and most patients require corticosteriod drugs at some stage during the illness.

Polyarteritis nodosa (PAN)

The clinical manifestations of this disorder are due to partial or complete arterial occlusion, haemorrhage and tissue necrosis. The peak incidence is in the fifth and sixth decades and males are predominantly affected. Arthralgia and myalgia are associated with multi-system involvement. Renal involvement may progress to renal failure and this is the most common cause of death in this condition. Steroid therapy should be considered but expert rheumatological supervision is required.

Paget disease of bone

This illness is seldom found in people under 50 years of age and affects both sexes. It is occasionally restricted to one bone but more commonly lesions are found in pelvis, skull, humerus, spine, femur or tibia. This condition is frequently discovered as a result of an x-ray for some other reason and can thus be symptomless. However, pain in bones may be severe and the affected areas can be tender on pressure and warm to the touch. Deafness and headaches may occur when the skull is involved but rarely is vision affected. Compression of the spinal cord may take place giving a paraplegia and fractures may be noted spontaneously or after minor trauma but usually heal normally. Osteogenic sarcoma is an uncommon late complication of this disease. When widespread bone lesions are found cardiac enlargement and failure may appear. The serum calcium and phosphorus concentrations are normal except during periods of rest in bed when they may be considerably raised. Serum alkaline phosphatase is usually increased and may rise to very high levels and this estimation is a useful index of activity.

Treatment

Pain is the most common symptom of Paget disease of bone and this can often be controlled by analgesics or NSAID.

Calcitonin therapy is indicated in patients who have pain that does not respond to analgesics (Hosking 1981), neurological complications particularly paraplegia, osteolytic lesions particularly in the long bones, immobilization hypercalcaemia and in the preparation of elderly patients for orthopaedic surgery. The pain of Paget disease of bone, however, must be differentiated from the pain of Paget arthritis in the joints or degenerative arthritis before calcitonin therapy is commenced.

Calcitonin may improve paraplegia and although it does not improve deafness it may prevent its progression. Calcitonin may reduce the cardiac output in patients who have a high output cardiac failure in response to widespread disease of bone, but this complication is fortunately rare.

Calcitonin may be administered in the porcine form or in a synthetic salmon preparation. This agent is given by subcutaneous or intramuscular injection and the dose varies between 100 international units daily and 50–100 international units three times a week. Osteoclastic bone resorption and bone turnover are reduced and this is associated with symptomatic relief of bone pain. Adverse effects of therapy may include nausea, flushing, tingling in the extremities and a metallic taste in the mouth. When pain is the indication for calcitonin it should be given for an initial period of 6–8weeks, and if there is no improvement the calcitonin should be stopped. If there is relief of pain associated with a satisfactory biochemical response then the agent can be continued for up to 1 year and then stopped. Further courses of calcitonin may be required if symptoms recur.

Diphosphonates may be used as an alternative to calcitonin and they are effective in oral form. Disodium etidronate is usually given in a daily dose of 5–10 mg/kg of body weight for 6 months or up to 20 mg/kg of body weight for 3 months. Higher doses can cause diarrhoea.

Osteoporosis

This condition is common in old people, especially in women, and the term implies a reduction in bone mass without change in chemical composition. Postmenopausal osteoporosis in females is multifactorial in aetiology and important factors include oestrogen deficiency, normal ageing, reduced exercise and subnutrition. It is associated with kyphosis and a liability to fracture with minimal trauma. This bony rarefaction can be caused by corticosteroid therapy and aggravated by bed rest. Pain occurs in the back and may radiate round the chest or trunk or into the legs; when pain occurs search should be made for fracture. The diagnosis is difficult to make at an early stage in the illness as the bony rarefaction comes on gradually. Three diagnostic features are described on radiography: a ghost-like appearance of bones; the upper and lower borders of the vertebral bodies are biconcave in shape; and the width of the cortex is reduced in the long bones. This illness can be suspected clinically when there is obvious kyphosis and the distance between the head and the symphysis pubis is found to have diminished with appearance of a fold of abdominal skin. Compression fractures of vertebral bodies are common and are often multiple.

Osteoporosis of this variety is not associated with any characteristic changes in blood chemistry.

Treatment

The aims of therapy are to prevent the loss of bone mass and to restore bone mass when fractures have occurred. Many treatments have been advocated, but the short- and long-term benefits have not yet been established (Smith 1987). At present there are available a number of agents which may slow bone loss by reducing bone resorption, for example anabolic steroids, fluoride, calcitonin and diphosphonates, but there are few therapeutic regimens which appear to restore bone loss and there are no recommendations for their use in elderly patients.

Oral calcium supplements have a known short-term benefit in reducing bone loss and the diet of the average elderly female is deficient in calcium. Vitamin D supplementation is a useful addition to the regimen if osteomalacia co-exists. Oestrogen therapy prevents bone loss in postmenopausal women and this will reduce the incidence of osteoporotic fractures. The benefits of this hormone therapy are greatest just after the menopause and there is no proven indication for commencing this form of treatment for the first time in elderly females (Arnaud *et al.* 1987). There are as yet no recommendations for the routine use of fluoride, anabolic steroids or calcitonin in elderly patients with osteoporosis. Exercise protects against bone loss and walking and swimming are safe forms of muscular activitiy in the elderly.

A firm corset or light spinal brace may help to prevent backache and the patient should be encouraged to be as active as possible.

Neurological complications of spinal osteoporosis are so unusual that it is not justifiable to limit the patient's mobility and, for this reason alone, such people should not be confined to bed. Bed rest encourages further decalcification. When evidence of a recent fracture, e.g. a tender vertebra with positive x-ray findings present, 10–14 days' bed rest with adequate analgesia is indicated.

A warning should be given to relatives or nursing staff when the diagnosis of osteoporosis has been made that great care must be exercised in handling the patient. If the old person is returning to live alone then every precaution should be taken to render the house as free from the possibility of a domestic accident as possible. Advice on accident prevention and help in this should be implemented by a home visit paid by the social worker, occupational therapist or health visitor.

In an endeavour to encourage earlier diagnosis, part of any screening test of older patients should include a lateral radiograph of spine and this should certainly be taken in any person who complains of back pain; this symptom should not be attributed to rheumatism or fibrositis without investigation.

Osteomalacia

This disease is characterized by a failure of calcium salts to be deposited in newly formed osteoid. Intestinal malabsorption, renal tubular defects and nutritional vitamin D deficiency are recognized causes. The incidence of osteomalacia is particularly high in old women especially those living alone, who do not go out of doors and may have an insufficient diet and in patients who have had a gastrectomy or who take anticonvulsant therapy on a long-term basis.

It is now realized that in the elderly lack of exposure to sunlight is the key factor in the aetiology of osteomalacia. In the elderly this illness may co-exist with osteoporosis and must be considered when there is a raised serum alkaline phosphatase but this is not always present.

Diagnosis

The elderly at risk patient may have a history of vague muscular aches and weakness. The main radiological abnormality is bone rarefaction and only occasionally are the diagnostic features of a pseudofracture (Looser zone) noted, in femur, pelvis or scapula. Biochemical tests on venous blood can sometimes confirm the diagnosis and should show a normal or low serum calcium and a low serum phosphorous or a low serum calcium and a normal serum phosphorus, increased alkaline phosphatase and normal serum creatinine, protein, electrolytes and blood urea. Urine tests should reveal a low calcium : creatinine ratio, a high phosphate clearance, a low percentage tubular reabsorption of phosphate and a high phosphate excretion index. Unfortunately, in patients with osteomalacia in the upper age range (over 70 years) the urinary indices not infrequently are of little diagnostic help in cases with equivocal blood chemistry. Faecal fat test excludes steatorrhoea as a cause of osteomalacia. Serum vitamin D is invariably low in osteomalacia.

Treatment

The correct therapy depends on the cause of the osteomalacia but if it is nutritional and found in the elderly who do not have much opportunity for getting sunlight, then a small daily dose of up to 10 000 units of calciferol is of great help. Steps should be taken to correct the factors that have caused the illness. If the bone disease has been due to other causes, e.g. previous partial gastrectomy or some form of malabsorption, then much larger doses may be required.

Many now advise a larger dose of vitamin D (50 000 units per day) initially, especially in patients with bone pain and the dose is reduced to a maintenance dose of 5000–10 000 units daily when clinical or biochemical evidence of relief of osteomalacia is obtained. If this regimen is adopted, the serum calcium should be determined at least once per month to avoid the possibility of hypervitaminosis D. It is probably wise to prescribe a high calcium intake as for osteoporosis. Once treatment is commenced bone pain and tenderness are relieved within a few days if the diagnosis is correct.

Metastatic lesions

Secondary tumour can be overlooked in elderly people unless the possibility is considered, and the spread of tumour can occur many years after a primary has been treated surgically. When there is a history of operation for malignant disease great care should be taken before a patient admitted to hospital bedridden is mobilized. The reason for the deterioration in the patient's general condition that precipitated hospitial admission may have been the secondary spread of neoplasm. A careful clinical examination for metastatic lesions should be undertaken and the long bones of the legs should be x-rayed before the patient is permitted to stand. Hard bony tumours may be found clinically from a primary lesion of breast, prostate, lung or thyroid and myelomatosis may be responsible for widely scattered bone lesions. The vertebral bodies are the most common site of metastatic growth. Other bones frequently affected are the proximal femur, pelvis, ribs, sternum, scapula, humerus and skull. Pathological fractures are frequently seen.

Malignant arthropathy

A generalized arthritis resembling rheumatoid arthritis may be found in patients with carcinoma of stomach, colon, ovary and lung. Hypertrophic pulmonary osteoarthropathy may be noted in cases with carcinoma of lung. This, when it involves wrists and fingers, may also simulate rheumatoid arthritis.

Polymyalgia rheumatica

This illness is characterized by widespread muscular pain and symptoms of a mild constitutional upset affecting middle-aged and elderly people. It is more common in women and presents often abruptly with pain and stiffness in the neck and shoulder muscles spreading to the lumbar, gluteal and thigh groups. Disability is caused by stiffness and pain, but tenderness is slight and muscle weakness is not present. The patient also has headache, mild pyrexia, sweating, anorexia, malaise and depression. Disorders of taste and generalized itching may also be noted. Symptoms of temporal arteritis may appear at any time during this disease and tenderness over the large vessels such as the carotid and brachial arteries may be noted. The erythrocyte sedimentation rate is elevated and normochromic anaemia with an increase in serum globulin is usual. The illness is, in most cases, of a few months' duration but the course of the disease can fluctuate with recurrence and exacerbations. An initial short period of rest in bed is advised with aspirin for relief of pain. Corticosteroid treatment usually gives dramatic symptomatic relief. Prednisolone should be prescribed in a daily dose of 10–15 mg until the symptoms and the ESR are controlled. Maintenance prednisolone therapy, often with doses as low as 3 mg, may be required however for several years before the patient is free from the disease.

Giant cell arteritis (temporal arteritis)

This condition may co-exist with polymyalgia rheumatica. The elderly patient often has a short history of headache with a reddened tender superficial temporal or occipital artery. Other presentations can include transient ischaemic attacks and visual involvment due to ischaemic optic neuropathy which may present as irreversible unilateral blindness. The diagnosis rests on the history associated with a high ESR and the classical histological appearances on serial sections of an urgent biospy of a clinically affected superficial scalp vessel. If the diagnosis is suspected prednisolone should be started immediately in daily doses of 60 mg. This dosage should be reduced when the ESR and symptoms are controlled. A maintenance dose of 5–10 mg daily is usually reached within 4–8 weeks of therapy. Maintenance therapy is continued with regular monitoring of the patient's clinical state and ESR. Steroids can be gradually withdrawn if the patient has had no symptoms and a normal ESR for 2–3 years. Relapses are common and some patients require lifelong treatment.

Fibrositis

This term is now not so widely used and the name *non-articular rheumatism* is more popular. Both are equally uninformative as to the aetiology of the condition. Pain and stiffness occurring in the occipital region, along the upper borders of the trapezius muscle, below the scapulae, over the sacroiliac joints, on the inner aspects of the knees and in the legs are the usual symptoms. Marked tenderness may be found in these areas and small nodules may be felt, especially over the sacroiliac joints. Extreme pain is elicited on pressing the musculotendinous junctions at the back of the ankle or at the base of the skull. On occasion a trigger area can be found, pressure on which causes the typical pain. Precipitating factors are cold, fatigue, trauma, incorrect posture and obesity. In certain endocrine disorders, e.g. hypothyroidism and hypopituitarism, painful tender areas in muscle and subcutaneous tissues are common. This illness is thought by many to occur in sensitive people emotionally unstable and very conscious of bodily function. Careful examination to exclude other causes of pain is essential, but once a diagnosis of fibrositis has been made the condition should be treated with energy and enthusiasm. This approach encourages and helps the patient to whom the pain is serious and who is in much need of reassurance.

Treatment

Aspirin is of value for the relief of pain and local heat in the most suitable form encourages muscular relaxation. The nodules may be dispersed by physiotherapy and can be injected with 0.5 ml of 1% procaine. Many patients are helped by wearing a flannel body belt and by trying to avoid sudden chills and fatigue. It is also necessary to put an obese patient on a reduction diet and to make sure that weight is lost. The posture if faulty should be corrected, and if the symptoms are acute and severe, treatment may have to be initiated with a short period of rest in bed. There should be no hesitation in investigating thoroughly by x-ray any patients who fail to respond to the above measures as disease of the spine must be excluded.

Painful shoulder

Reference has been made in the section on rehabilitation to the necessity to avoid this condition following a hemiplegia. The shoulder may be very painful when attempts are made to move it for the first time following a stroke. However, with the aid of analgesics, persistent efforts should be directed to prevent the formation of adhesions. Passive movements throughout the full range of the joint should be attempted by the physiotherapist and the patient should be encouraged to move the shoulder joint actively with her good hand by gripping the forearm or hand on the affected side. Occasionally, manipulation of the shoulder under general anaesthesia may be necessary but in this case x-ray of shoulder should always be taken first to exclude the commonly missed fracture, or inferior dislocation. Injections of hydrocortisone round the capsule may be of value. Early passive movement in hemiplegic patients prevents this condition.

Rupture of the supraspinatus tendon

Complete rupture of this tendon occurs in middle-aged and elderly people as a result of a sudden fall or severe muscle strain. Some hours after this, acute pain develops in the shoulder and over the deltoid muscle. Little or no limitation of passive movement is found but active abduction of the shoulder is limited in spite of a palpable vigorous contraction of the deltoid. External rotation is often also weak due to an associated tear of the infraspinatus tendon. Incomplete rupture of supraspinatus tendon can also occur and here the arm cannot be held abducted to shoulder level against resistance. This type of injury should be treated by the orthopaedic surgeon, and both diagnosis and treatment are difficult.

Inflammation and degeneration of the tendons of the supraspinatus, subscapularis, infraspinatus, teres minor (rotator cuff) can be involved in the aetiology of a painful shoulder as can subacromial bursitis or osteo-arthritis of the acromioclavicular joint. X-rays often show accumulation of calcium just above and lateral to the acromion which is also seen in patients without a sore shoulder. The differential diagnosis may be difficult and the advice of the orthopaedic surgeon should be sought.

Supraspinatus tendonitis

Apart from the possibility that repeated trauma may have some bearing on the aetiology of this condition, no causative factor is known. The condition usually comes on suddenly and acute pain, felt at the upper end of the humerus, is the presenting symptom. This pain may radiate up to the neck and even down to the fingers. It is provoked and increased by movement, particularly abduction or external rotation of the shoulder. The arm is usually held fixed in abduction to the side of the body with the forearm flexed. Tenderness is noted at the lateral area of the head of the humerus below the acromion and often at and above the insertion of the deltoid. In the acute case, fever, leucocytosis and elevated ESR may be found. Calcareous deposit in the supraspinatus tendon may be seen on x-ray of the shoulder as a large dense opacity lying above the outer aspect of the head of the humerus and extending under the acromion process. It may be an associated subacromial bursitis which is responsible for the symptoms. It is certain that the clincial symptoms and radiological findings do not bear a constant relation to one another.

Treatment

The shoulder should be immobilized and aspirin or an NSAID should be prescribed. Codeine may be added to this therapy if the pain is still unrelieved and the symptoms may be of such severity as to demand the adminstration of opiates. Hydrocortisone acetate may be given intra-articularly in a suspension in doses of 1–2 ml (25–50 mg of hydrocortisone) at standard concentration marketed for intra-articular injection every 3–10 days if needed. This may be followed by local application of heat to allow graduated exercises to be started. The opinion of the surgeon is required if no improvement follows this therapy, and it is wise to consult with a surgical colleague on any painful condition of the shoulder with no apparent aetiology.

Pain in the shoulder or upper humerus may, of course, be due to fracture; the history obtainable may be so inaccurate that no consideration has been given to this possibility. An elderly person walking about with a dislocated shoulder, which is painful but has been accepted as a cause of stiffness without the doctor being consulted, is discovered on rare occasions.

The shoulder–hand syndrome is sometimes found following cardiac infarction and in association with epilepsy. Pain and stiffness develop in the shoulder and the hand may become hot, swollen and painful. This condition may recover spontaneously or with the help of the physiotherapist. A short course of cortisone in a total daily dosage of 50–100 mg given in divided doses orally may cure the more resistant cases. If this therapy fails, procaine block of the stellate ganglion has been recommended.

Disease of the gall-bladder, of the lungs and of the cervical spine can also cause a painful shoulder; this condition is often a test of the doctor's diagnostic skill.

Painful heel

It is not uncommon to find an elderly person unable to walk because of pain on the sole of the foot under the heel. There is usually marked tenderness under the anteromedial aspect of the heel corresponding to the medial process of the calcaneal tuberosity. The aetiology of this condition is not clear and no history of trauma is obtainable in most cases. The complaint is of severe pain on putting weight on the foot and the illness lasts about 6 weeks. Analgesics such as paracetamol may be of use but an NSAID may be more effective. This condition usually passes off without treatment so that cutting down weight-bearing itself helps. However, if the pain is very severe, an injection of hydrocortisone acetate BP 25–50 mg

(1–2 ml), after the use of a local anaesthetic, into the point of greatest tenderness has been found useful. Usually only one or two treatments are required.

Care of feet

Many elderly people cannot reach their feet, and even if they could they do not have the vision or the steadiness of hand necessary to cut their toe-nails and the assumption can readily be made that foot care is not adequate. It is essential to ensure that older people do not slip quietly into bed and become bedridden because of painful lesions of their feet. As people grow older the feet tend to become smaller due to loss of subcutaneous fat and atrophy of the fibro-fatty pads. The skin often becomes dry and lesions are apt to occur over the pressure points of the feet. Nails are thickened and hard and with lack of cleanliness accumulation of dirt and debris aggravates the condition.

Ulcers between the toes are not uncommonly due to defective peripheral circulation and even corns and bunions can cause great distress. Such minor troubles are often complicated because the patient has rheumatoid arthritis or osteoarthritis.

In view of the vast amount of foot attention needed in the elderly it may be necessary to train district nurses in the elements of foot care, e.g. cutting normal toe-nails and teaching foot hygiene. The chiropodist's skill would then be reserved for corns, bunions and toe deformities. In these foot lesions the chiropodist can help his patient in the most dramatic way using techniques designed to direct pressure away from the painful traumatized area.

In patients showing the more serious conditions associated with circulatory deficiency it may be necessary to advise a short period of rest in bed until the small raw area has healed. In any old person whose symptoms suggest the onset of poor arterial supply the feet should be examined very carefully as broken areas of skin especially between the toes may not be painful and may be overlooked.

Once the initial lesion has healed the feet should be washed at least once per day and then lightly rubbed with cotton wool soaked in surgical spirits, dried thoroughly and then powdered with a baby powder. Constant unremitting attention to the hygiene of the feet is a wise procedure when the blood supply is poor. Even when a small ulcerated area has appeared it can usually be healed with a short spell of bed rest as mentioned above and, with adequate hygiene, no more trouble may occur. A nightcap of whisky may be helpful in some cases if the feet are very cold at night and bed socks are of use. Any stockings worn, however, should be loose fitting and should not cause any tightness round the leg; it is wise to avoid the use of hot water bottles.

Chilblains can be treated by applying 5% compound benzoin tincture in hydrous wool fat ointment and by making certain that the feet are not allowed near a fire or radiator.

Public propaganda as a measure of health education should be directed especially towards the elderly, advising them to take care of their feet. The consequences of foot disease are often dire indeed for the old.

The need for skilled attention to the feet of the older person has been proved beyond doubt and much benefit follows the advice and treatment of the state registered chiropodist.

REFERENCES

Arnaud C.D. *et al.* (1987) Consensus development conference: prophylaxis and treatment of osteoporosis. *British Medical Journal* **295**, 914.

Hosking D.J. (1981) Paget's disease of bone. *British Medical Journal* **283**, 686.

Kean W.F., Anastassiades T.P., Dwosh I.L., Ford P.M., Kelly W.G. & Dok C.M. (1982) Efficacy and toxicity of D-Penicillamine for rheumatoid disease in the elderly. *Journal of the American Geriatric Society* **30**, 94.

Scott D.G.I. & Coppock J.S. (1987) The treatment of rheumatoid arthritis: a symposium. *Prescriber's Journal* **27**, 13.

Scott J.T. (1980) Long term management of gout and hyperuricaemia. *British Medical Journal* **281**, 1164.

Smith R. (1987) Osteoporosis: cause and management. *British Medical Journal* **294**, 329.

Williams P.L. & Gumpel J.M. (1981) Scleroderma in the elderly. *British Medical Journal* **282**, 948.

17

Accidental Hypothermia

Hypothermia is generally defined as a core body temperature of below 35°C. The term accidental is used to distinguish this type from therapeutic and primary hypothermias which occur when normal individuals are exposed to extremely low temperatures such as prolonged immersion in sea water.

Cold winters in Britain are associated with an increased morbidity and mortality from cardiovascular and respiratory disorders in the elderly. The total number of cases and deaths due to environmentally induced hypothermia is probably quite small (Collins 1987). Mortality figures may be distorted by a failure to recognize hypothermia. Sublingual temperature readings often give a false low indication of the body core temperature in cold surroundings.

Hypothermia is uncommon, usually secondary and not always an important complication of a serious underlying condition. In one London hospital in the winter of 1985 only 0.04% (three cases) of patients presenting at an accident and emergency department had a core temperature of less than 35°C (Coleshaw *et al.* 1986).

The causes of accidental hypothermia are most conveniently considered under the headings:

1 exogenous
2 endogenous

Exogenous

Exposure to cold is of course, a prime factor in the production of hypothermia. Many elderly people have homes which are badly constructed, poorly insulated and inadequately heated. A high proportion have no heating in their bedrooms and the majority still live in homes without central heating (Collins 1986). The recommended room temperature for the elderly according to a department of health and social security publication is 21.1°C. A common story is of the old person who falls while attempting to get out of bed at night, and remains on the floor. It should be remembered that hypothermia can occur under much less extreme conditions, not being unknown even in hospital.

Endogenous

The main causes are due to:

1   Thermoregulatory mechanisms which are frequently impaired in the elderly. Older people often appear not to be aware of lowering temperatures (Collins *et al.* 1981) and have impaired shivering responses.

2   Drugs active on the nervous system can further impair physiological mechanisms. Phenothiazines not only cause vasodilatation and abolish shivering but may also reduce awareness of falling external temperatures. Alcohol, sedatives, hypnotics and antidepressants have all been reported as causing hypothermia.

Other factors include:

3   Neurological disorders: cerebrovascular accidents, lesions in the proximity of the hypothalamus.

4   Mental impairment.

5   Acute infections and circulatory collapse.

6   Conditions associated with immobility, e.g. paraplegia, parkinsonism, severe arthritis.

7   Endocrine disorders, e.g. hypopituitarism, hypothyroidism, diabetes mellitus.

Clinical features

General appearance. The patient is often pale with a puffy face and a husky voice and may be thought to be myxoedematous. Occasionally, however, the skin is abnormally pink and the appearances are suggestive of fever. The most significant feature is the extreme coldness of parts of the body which are normally covered, e.g. abdomen.

Central nervous system. Below 32°C there is progressive clouding of consciousness leading to coma. At this temperature shivering is absent and is replaced by generalized muscular rigidity. Reflexes are sluggish and may disappear below 26.7°C.

Cardiovascular system. Pulse rate and blood pressure fall progressively. At low temperatures ventricular ectopic beats are common and ventricular fibrillation is one cause of sudden death. The J waves seen in the left ventricular leads in about 30% of cases are pathognomonic of hypothermia.

Respiratory system. Slow and shallow respirations. Brochopneumonia is common but clinical signs are few.

Alimentary system. Bowel sounds may be absent or diminished and abdominal distension may occur. Occasionally there is abdominal pain due to pancreatitis.

Investigations

Blood biochemical investigations may reveal hyperglycaemia or hypoglycaemia. Acidosis is usually present. The serum amylase and muscle enzymes are commonly raised. The diagnosis of a hypothyroid state should be made by radio-immunoassay of the serum levels of T_3 and T_4.

Thrombocytopenia may be due to hypothermia or it may reflect evidence of disseminated intravascular coagulation.

Diagnosis

If all cases of hypothermia are to be recognized it is necessary to record rectal temperatures with a low reading thermometer as a routine. Core body temperature can also be determined from the temperature of freshly voided urine. A urine temperature of 34.8°C is equivalent to a rectal temperature of 35°C. The most reliable method of measuring the core temperature is by a rectal thermoelectric probe inserted to at least 80 mm depth.

Management

Most elderly patients who present with hypothermia have a severe underlying illness and the clinical course during rewarming varies between patients (Emslie-Smith 1981). Rapid rewarming in an old person is liable to cause circulatory collapse and an after-drop of core body temperature. The patient is best nursed in a comfortably warm room (25–30°C) with no active rewarming procedure. In these conditions deep body temperature should rise at a rate of about 0.5–1°C per hour, if the patient is insulated against heat loss by one or two blankets. Metallized plastic space-blankets may increase the rate of rewarming. The process should be slowed if the blood pressure drops.

The following additional measures may be required:
1   Administration of oxygen if hypoxaemia is present.
2   Correction of dehydration, acidosis and hypoglycaemia by appropriate intravenous fluids.
3   Parenteral prophylactic administration of broad-spectrum antibiotics.
4   Management of complications, e.g. ventricular fibrillation or pulmonary oedema.

There is no good evidence that benefit accrues from the routine use of steroids, vasoactive drugs or thyroid hormones.

Prognosis

In established hypothermia the prognosis must always be guarded. The mortality rate among elderly hypothermic patients is disappointingly high and most of the patients die of the underlying medical disorder rather than from hypothermia itself. Where the initial temperature is below 30°C the expected mortality may be as high as 70%.

Prevention

Hypothermia is a serious condition and efforts must be made to prevent its occurrence. The elderly living alone are especially at risk and regular visiting of such people is a social duty of the community. No nation-wide serious effort has yet been made either to ascertain where all the elderly people who are isolated are living or to arrange visits by voluntary or statutory workers. This is by no means an impossible task and is already an accomplished fact in many communities. It has, of course, far wider implications than the prevention of hypothermia but the warning signs of this condition can be explained to voluntary visitors. Elderly people should be given advice on the correct type of clothing: light in weight, closely woven and not restricting. It is also essential that the bedroom should not be too cold at night and if money is not available for such necessities application should be made to the Department of Health and Social Security. Adequate nutrition and good warm housing are also factors which help to prevent this condition. Fox *et al.* (1973) emphasized that priority should be given to identifying old people who through lack of money cannot protect themselves from the cold in their own homes. They suggested also the use of low-wattage electric under-blankets designed to prevent hypothermia, and that there should be a programme of education both for old people and those responsible for their welfare.

REFERENCES

Coleshaw S.R.K., Easton J.C., Keatinge W.R., Floyer M.A. & Garrard J. (1986) Hypothermia in emergency admissions in cold weather. *Clinical Science* **70**, 93.

Collins K.J. (1986) Low indoor temperatures and morbidity in the elderly. *Age and Ageing* **15**, 212.

Collins K.J. (1987) Effects of cold on old people. *British Journal of Hospital Medicine* **38**, 506.

Collins K.J., Exton-Smith A.N. & Doré C. (1981) Urban hypothermia: preferred temperature and thermal perception in old age. *British Medical Journal* **282**, 175.

Emslie-Smith D. (1981) Hypothermia in the elderly. *British Journal of Hospital Medicine* **26**, 442.

Fox R.H., Woodward P.M., Exton-Smith A.N., Green M.F., Downison D.V. & Wicks M.A. (1973) Body temperature in the elderly. A national study of physiological, social and environmental conditions. *British Medical Journal* **1**, 200.

18
Nutrition

People eat less as they grow older and a study of nutrient intakes and energy expenditure in men of different ages found that the total calorie requirements diminished with age and that there is a disproportionate drop in fat intake with age (McGandy *et al.* 1966). This may explain a decrease of 15 mg/100 ml in serum cholesterol between the age of 50 and 70 years. This decrease in total caloric intake was accounted for by decrements in basal metabolism and in energy expended in physical activity.

In the report *Recommended Daily Amounts of Food Energy and Nutrients for Groups of People in the United Kingdom* (DHSS 1979) intakes recommended assuming a sedentary life were as follows (DHSS 1969 figures in brackets):

For men aged 65–74: 2400 (2350) kcal, and for those aged 75 and over: 2150 (2100) kcal.

For women the corresponding intakes were 1900 (2050) kcal and 1680 (1900) kcal.

In Glasgow mean intakes were less in women than men, and these fell slightly with age. The differences were abolished by expressing the intakes on the basis of lean body mass. Mean intakes of energy were 2300 kcal for men and 1750 for women. These were people over 65 all living at home (MacLeod *et al.* 1974a).

The most important cause for the lower intake in the older group is due to a rising incidence during the 70s of disease and physical disability that reduce appetite and energy expenditure in some of the subjects in the older group (Stanton & Exton-Smith 1970).

Low intakes of nutrients are shown to be associated with impairment of health by studying the nutrition of housebound old people (Exton-Smith *et al.* 1972). The intakes of the housebound were compared with those of age-related active people and for women the difference amounted to 15% less for carbohydrate to 40% less for vitamin C. For the housebound group as a whole there was no decline in intake with age. Indeed some of the youngest people had the lowest intake. This is because for the housebound, in contrast with the active people, disability was just as severe and as frequent in the younger as in the older people. Thus disease and disability had a greater effect on nutrient intake than age alone. Nutrient intakes therefore are maintained into extreme old age provided the person remains active.

Many factors begin to operate more frequently with increasing age and these may lead to nutritional deficiencies. Some factors leading to nutritional deficiency in old age may be decline of bodily health, difficulty in obtaining and preparing food, the changed economic circumstances resulting from retirement, social isolation and loneliness, depression following bereavement, and ignorance as to what constitutes a balanced diet, especially in the widower who must often cater for himself for the first time.

In a nutritional survey of the elderly (DHSS 1972) a report was published of the dietary habits of 879 men and women aged 65 and over living alone or with their spouses or others but outside institutions in six areas of England and Scotland. A diagnosis of malnutrition was made in 3% of the elderly population; usually on the grounds of excessive thinness. In the majority of cases an underlying medical condition was responsible. In the absence of overt malnutrition, socio-economic factors may be of importance, since it was noted that men aged 75 and over who were living alone fared worse than their fellows in respect of a large number of nutrients, and this was in some measure reflected in the numbers recorded as having biochemical values below certain arbitrary limits, for example 30.8% of those living alone had leucocyte ascorbic acid levels below 7 $\mu g/10^8$ WBC compared with 7.7% of those living with a spouse. For both men and women there was a statistically significant higher incidence of anaemia in those living alone compared with other groups. In the main the dietary pattern was very similar to that of the normal adult population but smaller quantities of the various foods were taken. Some evidence was found of the statistical relationship between raised serum alkaline phosphatase and low bone mass in women over 75.

Symptoms of sufficient severity to induce an old person to consult his doctor are not often due to malnutrition but present indications are that a phase of subclinical malnutrition may affect some people leading to poor health, apathy and loss of interest and when illness supervenes frank deficiency may be provoked. Some such individuals complain of lassitude or apathy and these symptoms call for further investigation. As well as anaemia these symptoms may indicate sideropenia, potassium deficiency or deficiency of vitamin C, B_{12} or folate. Such symptoms are of course not specific and may be present in incipient cerebrovascular disease, intercurrent acute infection or depression.

Subnutrition in the elderly is still a subject of debate and the use of nutrient supplements is controversial. Individuals with, for example, biochemical evidence of osteomalacia should be given calciferol; the injection of vitamin B complex may be of help in confusional states, in acute illness or after a proximal fracture of the femur. In hip fractures protein supplementation has been given by nasogastric tube to counteract the catabolic effects of trauma (MacLennan 1986).

Old people do not always buy wisely so that income may be sufficient but spent on inappropriate food, and it is extremely difficult to change the food habits of elderly people. It is recognized that if any miscalculation in budget occurred the economies are made in food and it is suggested that local authorities could improve the nutrition of the elderly by seeking the advice of dieticians in the instruction of home helps and in the preparation of food for the meals-on-wheels service. The sensation of taste is diminished in the elderly and this may alter the choice of food.

There exists a high risk group of people over 65 who spend, for various reasons, less than they should on food. Some are depressed and apathetic, perhaps recently bereaved, some have a constant fear of poverty, others are mildly confused and a few have esoteric food habits. There are those immobile because of physical disease who depend on others for food and these should be included in this at risk group as should those who require long-term analgesic therapy, especially with aspirin.

The diets, clinical condition and social circumstances of 60 women over the age of 70 years living alone were investigated in two London boroughs (Exton-Smith & Stanton 1965). Some diets were ill-balanced and provided too little vitamin C, vitamin D, calcium, iron or protein and a striking deterioration in health and nutrition was found in the late 70s. From these findings it was concluded that special care was needed to preserve health in the early 70s. The recommendation was made that meals designed for the elderly should contain a high proportion of protein with an adequate supply of calcium, iron, and vitamin D presented in such a way that the whole meal is eaten. The meal should be supplied three or four times a week and vitamin C might require to be provided separately as the food must be kept hot for long periods in a meals-on-wheels service. From the social aspects of the survey the main points to emerge were the importance of home helps for shopping, especially for the housebound or in times of bad weather, the use of small refrigerators and the great need for informed and kindly advice on budgeting and choosing nutritious meals. The most valuable help would be that given by a known and trusted person such as a health visitor or a dietician.

Protein, fat and carbohydrate

There seems to be little protein deficiency among the elderly in Britain.

The Department of Health and Social Security's recommendations (1979) with the 1969 figures in brackets were 60 (59) g daily for men aged 65 to 74, and 54 (53) g daily for those over 75, and for women 47 (51) g and 42 (48) g respectively.

In Glasgow the mean protein intake of male subjects was 78 g/day, and of the women 60 g/day. Protein contributed 14–15% of calories; this reflects the current dietary habits in the United Kingdom where at least 10% of total energy intake comes from protein. These levels appear satisfactory; a figure of 0.8 g/kg of body weight per day is a generally accepted minimum (MacLeod *et al.* 1974).

Further increases in proteins, vitamins and minerals are required during acute illness, e.g. pneumonia, which in the elderly may precipitate acute nutritional deficiency. Similar increases are required following surgical operations and trauma. Old people who know that protein is required tend to think of it as meat or that they cannot chew meat or that meat is too expensive to buy. They may admit that they cannot be bothered cooking meat, especially if they live alone. In survey work at Rutherglen in people over 65, not one patient was found who was unable to chew meat and this finding is in agreement with previous work. If the diet contains one egg this replaces 30 g (1 oz) of meat. One pint of milk provides the protein equivalent of 60 g (2 oz) of meat. Four ounces of cooked dried peas, haricot beans and lentils and 30 g (1oz) of cheese are together approximately equivalent to 30 g (1 oz) of meat.

The protein in the diet of old age pensioners receiving meals-on-wheels was surveyed (Davies *et al.* 1975). The mean protein content was 28 g with a range of 8 to 58 g. Over one-third of the delivered meals provided less than the 25 g protein that is recommended as being the minimum for a domiciliary meal. The mean daily intake of protein for men and women was above the recommended daily intake (DHSS 1969) and showed no appreciable change on the days when meals-on-wheels were delivered.

Fat intake presents no problem since it is difficult to devise a simple diet that does not contain an adequate amount and in one survey it was 107 g/day for men and 86 g/day for women and contributed 42% and 44% of energy intake respectively (MacLeod *et al.* 1974a).

Carbohydrate intake according to the same workers averaged 265 g/day in men and 194 g/day in women, and the main point about this nutrient is its restriction since carbohydrates are cheap, attractive and require little or no preparation. Excessive carbohydrate intake is of great medical importance at the present time in view of the large numbers of people who are overweight with consequent morbidity and mortality.

Dietary fibre

Fibre is that part of plant material taken in diet which is resistant to digestion by the secretions of the gastrointestinal tract. It can absorb and hold water and is thus a valuable bulking agent as it increases stool weight. Gut transit time is shortened if prolonged and if rapid decreased. Fibre has proved of value in the treatment of constipation, irritable bowel syndrome in which constipation predominates, diverticular disease, haemorrhoids and anal fissure.

Dietary fibre may be protective against the development of colonic cancer and by modifying intestinal absorption may improve metabolic control in diabetes mellitus, hyperlipidaemia and possibly liver disease. It, by its metabolic changes, may be of benefit in improving the prognosis in ischaemic heart disease and gallstone disease. Bran may help to reduce weight in obesity because of the sensation of fulness it produces (Taylor 1984). Too much fibre may result in a deficiency of calcium, iron or magnesium.

The simplest way to take additional fibre is to eat a less refined, mixed diet with reasonable quantities of fruit, vegetables and cereals. For the elderly it may be easier to include in the diet two slices of wholemeal bread plus two bran biscuits plus two desertspoonfuls of bran spread throughout the day's meals (Webster 1980).

Vitamins

On occasion frank vitamin deficiency diseases are seen in elderly patients admitted to hospitals; in the case of scurvy this is primary and results directly from inadequate diet; alternatively, as in osteomalacia, the deficiency can be associated with intestinal malabsorption. The question of subclinical vitamin deficiency is controversial and the incidence is difficult to assess. Apart from scurvy, deficiency of a single vitamin rarely occurs and some of the classical signs of vitamin deficiency disease are the result of lack of several different food factors.

With regard to vitamin A, there is no good evidence of deficiency in the elderly. This may be because this vitamin is stable in cooking and occurs in cabbage and lettuce as well as in fruits and vegetables. Fat-soluble vitamin D present in milk, eggs, butter and vitaminized margarine is also synthesized in the skin following exposure to sunlight. In many countries the elderly do not consume enough dairy produce, may be housebound, live in industrial cities and consequently rarely get enough sunshine. Thus osteomalacia may ensue; in addition for various reasons malabsorption of vitamin D is relatively common and this may again produce osteomalacia.

Thus inadequate dietary intake, lack of exposure to sunlight, and minor degrees of intestinal malabsorption are probably the most important causes of vitamin D deficiency in the elderly. Summer sunlight is an important and possibly chief determinant of vitamin D nutrition in Britain (Stamp & Round 1974); the amount of vitamin obtained in this way varies with latitude and environmental conditions and cannot at present be assessed (DHSS Report 1979). Thus housebound old people may be at the greatest disadvantage since they lack exposure to sunlight and often have very low dietary intakes. Forty-eight per cent of housebound women aged 70–79 years had a dietary intake of less than 30 i.u. (0.75 μg cholecalciferol)/day compared with 13% of active women of similar age (Exton-Smith *et al.* 1972). Twenty-five per cent of men and 33% of women 65 and over took less than 50 i.u./day of vitamin D (MacLeod *et al.* 1974b).

The not infrequent occurrence of osteomalacia in the elderly has been demonstrated (Anderson *et al.* 1966; Aaron *et al.* 1974). This condition should always be considered in the differential diagnosis of bone pain, especially backache in the elderly. Six housebound old people who sustained a fracture of the femur had a lower mean daily intake of vitamin D than that for the whole housebound group (Exton-Smith *et al.* 1972). The elderly in long-stay geriatric wards have a low dietary intake of vitamin D (1.2 μg of cholecalciferol) (Corless *et al.* 1975). There is a recommendation from the DHSS of an intake of 10 μg of cholecalciferol daily (1969 figure was 2.5 μg) for adults with inadequate exposure to sunlight. Older patients in geriatric wards should be encouraged to seek sunlight on balconies or verandahs. Adding fish especially herring or kippers and margarine with added vitamin D are ways of improving intake of this vitamin.

Water-soluble vitamin C is found in citrus fruits and Brussels sprouts while a small amount is present in potatoes, but because the elderly eat large amounts of potatoes these vegetables form the principal source of this vitamin in the old people's diet. Unfortunately the quantity of vitamin C is reduced in cooking and the amount of this substance in potatoes falls off with storage. This explains the increased incidence of scurvy during the late winter and early spring months. Low levels of leucocyte ascorbic acid have been reported by many workers, and there is a moderate correlation between vitamin C intake and leucocyte ascorbic acid levels and in Edinburgh leucocyte ascorbic acid levels were significantly higher in July to December compared with the rest of the year. Slightly more than half the subjects had intakes of less than 30 mg daily, and the significantly greater proportion had low intakes in the months of October to March compared with the months April to September (Milne *et al.* 1971). Other dietary surveys have revealed that there is an appreciable number of old people with an intake of less than 10 mg/day which is known to be the amount required to prevent or cure scurvy. The recommended allowance of 30 mg/day takes into account the considerable individual variations and requirements and the increased requirements due to stress.

Some old people avoid vitamin C containing foods and give as reasons, expense, fruit like oranges difficult to peel, fruit juice stings gums and lips and pips difficult with artificial dentures; poor cooking methods result in loss of vitamin C (Davies 1981). The destruction of a considerable amount of vitamin C during the preparation of meals-on-wheels has been revealed and it has been shown that vitamin C intake is often lower on those days when meals-on-wheels are supplied. Suggestions have been made to improve this (Davies 1981). This author has also recommended that older people could improve their vitamin C intake by sucking sweets containing ascorbic acid, e.g. Blackcurrant Flavour Drops (Boots).

Scurvy

This disease is found in elderly men who live alone and less commonly in women with the exception of those who are food faddists. Scurvy is characterized by subcutaneous ecchymosis, anaemia and delay in wound healing. When an elderly person is edentulous, ulceration and haemorrhage of the gums does not occur. The haemorrhages tend to occur in the thighs and round the ankles and perifollicular petechiae are also found. Sheet haemorrhages may present as a woody leg or in the form of pseudogangrene of the feet with bullae and warm extremities. When haemarthrosis is noted it is often the result of minor injury and these patients are usually found attending orthopaedic clinics. Two useful physical signs are the presence of corkscrew hairs and of sublingual petechial haemorrhages which must be distinguished from small sublingual varicosities which are of no significance.

Treatment

The treatment consists in the administration of 1 g of ascorbic acid by mouth daily for 10 days followed by an intake of 30 mg or more ascorbic acid per day. The daily regimen and diet of the patient should be investigated and a suitable diet commenced. Scurvy may well be associated with anaemia and this may require correction with the appropriate haematinic (p. 138). To prevent scurvy the diet should contain 30 mg ascorbic acid per day.

Vitamin B

Thiamine is widely found in all animal and plant tissue; it is extremely soluble and may be thrown away with the cooking water or destroyed by boiling in alkaline solution. Deficiency manifests itself as beriberi and this is occasionally seen and should be considered in the differential diagnosis of high-output cardiac failure, especially in alcoholics. There is marked cardiac enlargement and the onset of failure may be sudden. Rapid improvement occurs with parenteral thiamine.

Wernicke–Korsakoff syndrome

This disease was first described in alcoholics and is due to thiamine deficiency and can occur with dietary deficiency quite independently of alcohol, in any disease seriously interfering with nutrition. Clinical features are ophthalmoplegia, postural hypotension, intellectual impairment and memory disturbances. Thiamine is given initially parenterally 25 mg for 3 days and thereafter 10 mg three times per day orally until the patient is better. Recovery is not usually complete and the erythrocyte transketolase test is a guide to prognosis.

Changes in the mucous membranes of the tongue and lips in elderly patients have been reported due to deficiency of B vitamins (Griffiths *et al.* 1967; Brocklehurst *et al.* 1968). When these studies were repeated it was shown that when single vitamin supplementation was given for 1 year riboflavine produced an improvement in cheilosis and nicotinamide in the appearance of the dorsum of the tongue (Dymock & Brocklehurst 1972). These findings have not been confirmed.

Nicotinic acid found in yeast, bran and meat, is also formed in the body from its pro-vitamin tryptophan. Deficiency of nicotinic acid results in pellagra which is occasionally seen in older people with its classical manifestations of dermatitis, diarrhoea and dementia. The dermatitis is an erythema on exposed parts of the body and over areas of friction and is not unlike severe sunburn. A red, swollen, painful tongue may be found in milder forms of the disease. Like thiamine deficiency the clinical effects of nicotinic acid lack are usually found in chronic alcoholics or in patients with serious illness associated with vomiting, e.g. carcinoma of the gastro-intestinal tract.

Riboflavine is present in liver, milk, eggs and green vegetables and is highly soluble being lost in cooking and destroyed by exposure to sunlight. The classical findings of riboflavine deficiency are angular stomatitis, corneal vascularization, cheilosis, the magenta tongue and the orogenital syndrome. These, however, are non-specific and tend to arise from multiple deficiencies. On occasion, they respond to treatment with riboflavine but multiple vitamin therapy should be given along with a good diet. Riboflavine deficiency creates a problem in diagnosis because blood levels of this nutriment cannot be correlated with the patient's clinical state, and further investigations are required to find out if riboflavine deficiency exists in the elderly as a separate entity.

Low serum levels of vitamin B_{12} are relatively common in the elderly not because of lack of intake in the diet, which rarely occurs, but because of the increasing frequency of atrophic gastritis in old age and the consequent achlorhydria and lack of intrinsic factor. B_{12} deficiency should be considered in the differential diagnosis of peripheral neuropathies, myopathies and obscure neurological disturbances whether or not anaemia is present. Patients who have had a partial gastrectomy are at special risk and clinical and laboratory signs of neurological disease have been found many years after this operation. Vitamin B_{12} deficiency occurs but only those with signs of subacute combined degeneration of the cord respond to treatment with vitamin B_{12}. Psychopathic disturbances are unresponsive to this therapy. The association between mental disturbance and deficiency of vitamin B_{12} and folic acid is at present not clearly defined. Three cases illustrating a variety of psychiatric symptoms that might occur in avitaminosis B_{12} in the absence of subacute combined degeneration of the cord or any abnormality of the peripheral blood and marrow have been described as have two patients with advanced dementia who had megaloblastic anaemia due to folate deficiency (Strachan & Henderson 1965; 1967). Screening for vitamin B_{12} deficiency on 1004 consecutive new patients over 50 years admitted to a mental hospital led to the diagnosis of only two cases of pernicious anaemia; the incidence of this illness being slightly lower than that in a general population of comparable age groups prompted the conclusion that such assays were not justified as a routine until fully automated techniques become available (Murphy *et al.* 1969). The psychiatrist should be alert to the possibility of vitamin B_{12} deficiency in three situations: patients thought to be at risk clinically, e.g. anaemic or postgastrectomy patients; patients with unexplained fatigue; and those with confusional states or dementia of unknown origin.

In most patients with mental symptoms due to vitamin B_{12} deficiency, changes are found in the peripheral blood or the bone marrow. The haemoglobin estimation, a full blood count and a film must be checked and the blood film seen by an expert haematologist. Evidence of macrocytosis or of hypersegmentation of the nuclei of the polymorphs indicate that estimation of serum B_{12} and folate levels should be performed. If any neurological abnormalities are discovered, such as peripheral neuropathy or signs of subacute combined degeneration then regardless of the haematological findings serum B_{12} and folate estimations should be made. No evidence has been found that in elderly subjects with low levels of serum B_{12} without a macrocytic anaemia, or neuropathy, vitamin B_{12} therapy is superior to a placebo in affecting an improvement in psychiatric state or general well-being.

An interesting form of localized vitamin B_{12} deficiency occurs in smokers where the cyanide present in smoke converts hydroxocobalamin to cyanocobalamin, which is much less active and as a result of the local deficiency, tobacco amblyopia arises. It is important to recognize this condition since blindness resulting from it can be reversed by treatment with hydroxocobalamin (p. 300).

Low serum folates are frequently found in old people and their significance is still not clearly understood. The folic acid content of food is variable and existing food tables unreliable. In the *Nutritional Survey of the Elderly* (DHSS 1972) 14.6% of subjects had serum folates of less than 3 ng/ml and 3.7% had red cell folate levels of less than 100 ng/ml: levels of 3 ng/ml in serum and a red cell folate of 150 ng/ml are regarded as lower limits of normal. In this study there was no significant relationship between folate levels and the clinician's assessment of the mental state. Folate deficiency might be a feature of chronic infection, chronic skin disease, malignancy, chronic alcoholism, rheumatoid arthritis, malabsorption or following anticonvulsant drugs. Other complicating factors were drugs such as phenobarbitone, phenylbutazone or nitrofurantoin which might interfere with folate metabolism; methotrexate and trimethoprim have also similar effects. The clinical findings are soreness of the tongue which has a smooth atrophic surface; it is occasionally red. Folate deficiency certainly predisposes patients to overt nutritional megaloblastic anaemia if they develop a severe infection or suffer from conditions like myelofibrosis or haemolytic anaemia which increase folate requirements. True folic acid deficiency should be considered in the diagnosis of dementia, peripheral neuropathy, myelopathy and macrocytic anaemia. Since folic acid deficiency often occurs in conjunction with vitamin B_{12} deficiency it is unwise to treat elderly patients with folic acid alone even after full investigation.

ELECTROLYTES AND WATER

The elderly patient is particularly liable to be upset by a low fluid intake or by vomiting or diarrhoea as the homeostatic mechanisms are not as efficient as in younger persons. The descriptions that are given here of the various depletions are intended to illustrate the dangers associated with such conditions in older people.

Early diagnosis of electrolyte and water depletion depends on suspicion based on knowledge of the provocative conditions, since the diagnostic clinical signs and serum changes occur late and in some individuals too late for effective treatment. Treatment of these biochemical abnormalities requires the closest liaison between the physician and the doctor in the laboratory, and advice from the biochemist is essential if appropriate correction of the deficiences is to be made.

Dehydration

The most common cause of pure water depletion is physical illness associated with reduced intake and impairment of the thirst mechanism – oral water deprivation. This condition may develop in dysphagia, for example, in patients with oesophageal obstruction, or in a comatose patient following a cerebral incident, in the depressed or apathetic, or in the elderly person afraid of incontinence who is purposefully limiting fluid intake. In pure dehydration insufficient water is being swallowed but the daily loss from lungs, skin and urine continues. This imbalance may be accentuated by increased insensible loss in pyrexia or hyperpnoea. Similarly excessive loss of water in the urine may result from water-losing nephritis, diabetes insipidus and hyperparathyroidism. Osmotic diuresis occurs in uncontrolled diabetes mellitus when a large amount of glucose being passed in the urine takes with it water in excess – this results in dehydration; this can proceed to hyperosmolar hyperglycaemic non-ketotic diabetic coma. If the patient is conscious thirst is usual, and the tongue is dry, but the blood pressure is unaltered in the early stages. The clinical findings are sunken eyes, dry mucous membranes, decreased salivary and bronchial secretions, loss of elasticity of skin and weight loss. The urine volume is markedly reduced and the specimen is concentrated, in the absence of disease affecting renal concentration. The blood urea is moderately raised and the serum sodium is normal or raised.

Treatment

Treatment will depend on the underlying condition, e.g. diabetes mellitus. In pure water depletion salt-free fluids are indicated and where possible should be given by mouth until hydration is accomplished. Thereafter a routine oral intake of 1500–2500 ml/day should be established. Water itself is excellent in this condition, and suitable amounts of carbohydrate such as glucose may be added to provide some nourishment. If the patient is unable to swallow or is in danger of aspirating fluid into the lungs, intravenous 5% glucose in water should be used; replacement should take place slowly; enthusiastic intravenous therapy can produce cerebral oedema. Alternative to the intravenous route in the elderly is subcutaneous administration, using hyaluronidase. Absorption following subcutaneous infusion is more gradual and less likely to overload the circulation. The quantity of fluid given should be assessed by the urinary output. It must be emphasized that the use of salt-containing preparations is absolutely contraindicated in the rare occasion when there is pure-water depletion.

Salt and water depletion

Pure-salt loss without significant water loss is rare and the usual deficit is a mixed salt and water depletion which occurs in many physical illnesses. The main causes are;
1   Chronic nephritis and pyelonephritis i.e. salt-losing nephritis.
2   Addison disease.
3   Uncontrolled diabetes mellitus.
4   Loss of fluid containing electrolytes by chronic diarrhoea, intestinal fistulae, vomiting; over-zealous diuretic therapy, excessive sweating, exfoliative dermatitis or burns.

Thirst sensation appears diminished and there is failure of total renal conservation. As more salt than water is lost in such conditions the extracellular fluid becomes hypotonic, and to lessen this the volume of water excreted by the kidneys is increased so that there is an increase in the associated water loss and some of the water from the hypotonic extracellular fluid migrates into the cells. These conditions produce a diminution in volume of extracellular fluid while the actual water content of the cells increases. The clinical findings are dry tongue and a diminution of intraocular pressure. Unlike the water-depletion syndrome, thirst is not a prominent complaint. An initial polyuria may occur but this is followed by oliguria. The pulse rate increases, postural hypotension may develop, then later the blood pressure falls, the skin becomes cold and vomiting may be noted. The blood urea begins to rise and is higher than in pure-water depletion and in severe cases the serum sodium concentration may be reduced to 130 mEq/l or less. In this type of depletion urinary chlorides are reduced while it is usual in pure-water depletion to find no diminution of chloride in the urine.

Treatment

Minor degrees of salt depletion are remedied by the addition of salt to the diet with ample fluids. The salt is given in capsules in a total daily dose of about 6 g for a few days. These capsules should be well distributed throughout the day and swallowed with ample amounts of fluid: a teacupful per capsule. In more severe cases, intravenous administration of isotonic saline is required and 2 litres of such solution or preferably 5% glucose in normal saline may be given in 24 hours. For elderly people who so commonly have a mixed salt and water deficit, the use of normal saline by subcutaneous drip with hyaluronidase can be of the greatest value and 2 litres can be given in 24 hours by this method. On occasion it may be of value to give 500 ml of normal saline and follow with 500 ml of 5% glucose while the biochemical estimations are being performed. There is much to commend the subcutaneous drip in older patients as this can be continued during a restless phase and has not the associated dangers of either an intragastric or an intravenous drip. The best indication of the amount of salt required is the restoration of the blood pressure. The lung bases should be examined frequently to avoid any possibility of overloading the circulation. If such overload is anticipated and intravenous infusion is imperative, it should be remembered that the central venous pressure gives early warning of impending disaster. It must be emphasized again that while these depletions are described as individual entities it is likely that acid base balance will be upset and potassium depletion may also be present. Biochemical investigation, including serum electrolytes, urinary electrolytes and fluid balance studies are required.

Potassium deficiency

Potassium deficiency is relatively common in the elderly. Average daily losses in urine, faeces and sweat are in total approximately 60 mEq/day, whilst many elderly people consume less than this in their diet. A dietary intake of less than 30–35 mEq/day is almost certainly the critical level. Nutritional deficiency of potassium is important and not uncommon; it may remain undiagnosed until a crisis is precipitated by the use of diuretics. The elderly person in good health requires about 60 mEq/day of potassium. One frequent manifestation of hidden potassium deficiency is sensitivity to digoxin, common in older people.

In patients with a marginal potassium intake deficiency can be produced by intercurrent disease. The symptoms of potassium deficiency are apathy, depression, impaired intellectual function and vague weakness with often faecal impaction. Later widespread loss of power of intestinal, cardiac and skeletal muscles occurs and these symptoms and signs are often mistaken for a psychological disorder in a withdrawn elderly patient.

In the early stages of potassium depletion the serum potassium may be normal since in whole-body potassium there is migration from the intracellular compartment. Later the serum potassium drops and the bicarbonate and pH rise. The urine is alkaline and contains little or no potassium, unless a potassium losing renal state is present. The ECG changes correlate poorly with the potassium status but classical changes of prolongation of the Q–T interval, S–T depression, flattening of the T wave and increase in size of the U wave may occur.

In studying dietary potassium intake and muscle strength in older people, Judge & Cowan (1971) found in 50 men and 50 women aged 65 years and over, picked by chance selection, that 60% of the women and 40% of the men had an inadequate daily intake of potassium, i.e. less than 60 mEq/day; all these subjects had normal serum levels of potassium. Serum potassium levels bear little relationship to the potassium status of an individual and when dietary potassium and handgrip pressure were correlated there was found to be a decrease in handgrip pressure from the expected value when the dietary intake decreased. With a decreased dietary potassium there is a decline in muscle strength, although serum potassium levels were normal.

In a nutritional study of elderly people caring for themselves at home, this group ate a diet containing less potassium compared with a group of young adults (Judge & MacLeod 1968).

Dall, Paulose & Ferguson (1971) in a study of two groups of eight geriatric patients who were not acutely ill, found a dietary intake of potassium that was below normal, while studies in convalescent surgical patients over the same period as one group of geriatric patients revealed that a normal intake of potassium was possible from the diet supplied. When given an oral diuretic the geriatric patients became hypokalaemic readily. A supplement of 24 mEq potassium (1800 mg Slow K) daily appeared to be adequate replacement therapy maintaining serum potassium levels during treatment with a diuretic.

Dall & Gardiner (1971) found that if geriatric patients, taking a diet poorer than the average adult intake in potassium, had drunk a full pint of milk (23.5 mmol of potassium) each day as part of their diet all would have reached a low level of normal standard potassium intake. Milky coffee is to be preferred to sweetened tea while orange juice or a banana are also recommended.

Causes of hypokalaemia in the elderly are nutritional deficiency, intake of oral diuretics, including those which contain potassium supplements, persistent use of purgatives or enemata, prolonged fluid loss through vomiting, diarrhoea, intestinal fistulae, diabetes mellitus and insipidus, potassium-losing nephropathy and corticosteroid administration. Hypokalaemia may develop during treatment of megaloblastic or iron deficiency anaemia.

As a prophylactic measure, adequate potassium supplements should be given to patients receiving diuretic therapy. Possible exceptions to this rule are triamterene, spironolactone and amiloride which still require continuing laboratory control of potassium levels because of a possible rise. Thus, where practicable, all elderly people receiving any form of diuretic therapy require laboratory supervision. The patient given diuretics with added potassium supplementation may drift slowly into potassium depletion because of inadequate potassium therapy and such medication should be controlled by a watchful eye on suggestive symptoms and repeated estimations of the serum potassium level. It is important to remember that patients with potassium depletion are unduly sensitive to preparations of digitalis. The renal conservation of potassium is less efficient than that of sodium.

Treatment

This should be directed at correction of the underlying cause, where possible, at increasing the dietary intake and at specifically replacing the missing factors. It is now reasonably certain that replacement of both potassium and chloride is necessary. Normally the main dietary sources of potassium in the elderly are from dairy produce and potatoes, but concentrated sources are citrus fruits, meat, wheat germ, instant coffee and milk chocolate. If the deficiency is moderate and particularly if the serum level is normal, oral therapy is satisfactory. Suitable preparations are effervescent potassium chloride (Kloref Cox Continental and Sando-K Sandoz) or if the patient can swallow solid preparations (Slow-K Ciba). Unfortunately the solid potassium chloride preparations of the enteric-coated preparations have been shown to cause small bowel ulceration. Where serious deficiency has been found, parenteral therapy is essential. Such therapy should never be used if the serum potassium is normal. One 10 ml ampoule potassium chloride BP, containing approximately 20 mEq of potassium and 20 mEq of chloride may be added to 500 ml of ½N saline and administered subcutaneously (such a solution is only marginally hypotonic), or added to 500 ml of N saline or 5% glucose may be given intravenously. Either therapy is contraindicated if anuria or oliguria is present; in any case, frequent estimation of the serum potassium level is essential.

Potassium intoxication

This condition is usually found in association with severe oliguria or anuria such as may be found in circulatory failure from blood loss, acute renal failure, diabetic coma, the terminal stages of glomerulonephritis and severe Addison disease. The patients are weak and often confused with the development of flaccid paralysis, the features being indistinguishable from those due to hypokalaemia. An irregular pulse which becomes slow in rate because of developing heart block is also found. ECG changes include increase in amplitude of T waves, atrioventricular and intraventricular conduction defects and finally ventricular standstill and death.

Treatment

The prevention of this condition in patients with oliguria or anuria must be kept in mind. Potassium excess is virtually impossible in the normal healthy subject. Success in treating potassium intoxication depends on two factors:
1   Any further increase in extracellular potassium must be prevented.
2   Accumulated potassium must be eliminated.
  Potassium by mouth must be immediately restricted and this can be done by avoiding foods containing large amounts of potassium such as fruit, fruit juices and foods rich in protein. Any concomitant water or water and salt depletion must be corrected, and an ionic exchange resin such as Resonium A absorbs potassium and hastens its excretion. A dose of 7.5–15 g Resonium A in suspension in water is administered by mouth up to three times per day, and if vomiting prevents oral medication the substance may be given as a retention enema. This route of administration is not without complication and reference should be made to the manufacturer's instructions. In addition, glucose 50 g by mouth followed by 20 units of soluble insulin subcutaneously lower serum potassium level. Caution is the rule in patients who are digitalized and who may experience acute digitalis intoxication in the course of potassium removal. Some advise calcium gluconate 10 ml of 10% solution by intravenous injection and the same dose repeated in 3 hours. This form of therapy is reputed to reduce the toxic effect of potassium on the heart. The treatment of each patient, however, is linked basically with the disease causing the condition and adequate therapy for this is essential.

Calcium deficiency

The exact role of calcium deficiency in producing disease in the elderly is not clearly defined as there is usually also deficiency of vitamin D or some degree of malabsorption present. Calcium intake however tends to be low in the elderly population and calcium absorption decreases with age. About 1500 mg should be taken daily (Heaney *et al.* 1982). Prolonged intake of anticonvulsant drugs can produce calcium deficiency.

Iron

Iron deficiency in the elderly does occur; this mineral is found in meat, vegetables and eggs and is almost always deficient in carbohydrate diets.

Low serum iron levels associated with raised total iron-binding capacity and thus low iron saturation are common in elderly patients admitted to acute geriatric units and suggest widespread iron deficiency. It is commonly due to gastrointestinal blood loss not to an inadequate iron intake alone. Conditions such as hiatus hernia, diverticulitis, and long-term consumption of aspirin are frequently found. These factors increase the need for iron in the diet.

Magnesium

A minimal daily intake of 8–12 mmol is advised and depletion is more common than presently recognized. The normal serum magnesium is 1.4–2.5 mEq/l and foods containing this substance are bread, cow's milk, cereals, meats, vegetables and fruits.

Magnesium deficiency is established if there are typical clinical findings with confirmation of serum magnesium lower than 1.4 mEq/l (Nandi & Lewis 1985). Clinical presentation includes tremor of limbs and tongue, convulsions, ataxia, nystagmus, dysphagia and vertigo. The Chvostek and Trousseau signs may be positive if calcium deficiency also exists; carpopedal spasm may be noted. Depression and hallucinations may occur while tachycardia and ventricular arrhythmias may be found. There is often associated hypocalcaemia and hypokalaemia and this hypokalaemia may be resistant to treatment with potassium supplements unless magnesium is also given.

The causes of hypomagnesaemia include severe diarrhoea, malabsorption, prolonged gastrointestinal aspiration, chronic pyelonephritis and diuretic therapy. Sick old people often have a low dietary intake of magnesium and thus are at risk if given a diuretic. Self-neglect, alcoholic cirrhosis and malignant disease are other causative factors. The asymptomatic patient with an inadequate intake should be advised to increase the consumption of foods with a high magnesium content e.g. fruits, cereals, milk and vegetables. If the symptoms are minimal four bananas per day may provide sufficient supplementation. In established depletion with marked symptoms parenteral magnesium is advised given slowly and with great care in renal insufficiency. It is worth noting that potassium sparing agents have also a magnesium sparing effect.

The side effects of parenteral magnesium include flushing, sweating and minor T wave changes in the ECG. If parenteral magnesium therapy is used serum magnesium levels and deep tendon reflexes should be monitored.

Hypermagnesaemia is found in chronic renal failure, in the acute stages of renal failure and in adrenal failure. There is also a progressive decrease in glomerular filtration rate with increasing age. Thus this condition may be noted if too much magnesium is taken in, for example, magnesium containing antacids.

The clinical features are drowsiness, feeling of warmth and unsteadiness. The tendon reflexes are diminished and with higher levels of magnesium nausea, vomiting and hypotension occur with serious arrhythmias. Plasma levels of magnesium may be above 6 mEq/l. Asymptomatic hypermagnesaemia needs no treatment and if the patient is drowsy with only decreased tendon reflexes stopping the source of the magnesium will suffice. When the symptoms are severe, e.g. coma and respiratory depression, a slow intravenous injection of 10–20 ml of 10% calcium gluconate is advised; the last remaining therapy is dialysis.

Zinc

The main dietary sources of zinc are meat, seafoods and dairy products. The recommended daily allowance is 15 mg of elemental zinc per day (Smith 1987). There is no functional body store of this substance and serum zinc is a poor indicator of zinc status. Lower levels of zinc in the serum have been found in low-income groups and may be a reflection of nutrition. Leucocyte zinc concentration is lower in long-stay elderly patients than in age matched controls in the community. Deficiency of zinc may be associated with delayed healing of wounds and ulcers. There is some evidence that patients with lowered serum zinc concentrations show accelerated wound healing by zinc supplementation. No improvement has been demonstrated when diets are adequate in zinc.

Clinical symptoms of anorexia and abnormalities of smell and taste have been described. These may respond to zinc. Zinc deficiency leads to a defective cell-mediated response so that infections regarded as commensals are common in zinc deficiency and it has been suggested that the occurrence of candida infections and intertrigo should lead to an investigation of zinc status (Golden 1980).

The unaided efforts of old men and women over 80 are associated with the worst diet, with men faring appreciably worse than women when cooking for themselves. Married people fare better but the best results are achieved when meals are prepared wholly by someone coming into the house, paid or otherwise.

The elderly in the community are in a marginally satisfactory nutritional state; they are liable to suffer from nutritional deficiency because of added physical, psychological or social difficulties. Alcoholism should not be overlooked. In many forms of nutritional deficiency in the elderly the factors responsible can be identified and the problem of improving nutrition is that of early ascertainment and correction of needs in vulnerable groups of the elderly population. Those old people especially at risk are the socially isolated, those with physical disability, impairment of the special senses, the recently bereaved, old men living alone, and those with mental disorders and deep depression, while poverty and ignorance are other important factors. This supports the belief that people 75 years and over should be visited regularly by a health visitor who should have received some training in the dietary problems of old people.

By simple scoring systems based on the number of main meals and the frequency of consumption of certain foods containing protein, meat, bread, eggs, cheese, and milk, a health visitor can obtain a rough guide to the quality of the diet. From the survey of Davies (1981) the following risk factors emerged: fewer than eight main meals eaten in a week, less than one-half pint of milk drunk daily, virtual absence of fruit and vegetables, wastage of food, long periods in the day without food, depression or loneliness, unexpected weight change, shopping difficulties, low income and indication of other factors or disabilities including alcoholism. If malnutrition is suspected the diagnosis can be confirmed by the general practitioner who may refer the patient to the hospital, for example if osteomalacia is suspected, for more specialized investigation.

Encouraging old people to attend a day centre for meals, improving the meals-on-wheels service, and making the standard of such meals better, are other ways to help. Food education through radio and television also helps. Nothing can replace, however, the home visit by the health visitor to individuals 75 years and over. Doctors should be aware of the risks of diuretic therapy and should be informed of the need for supplementation of diet in certain situations, e.g. following serious or long continued illness, surgical operation, accident or bereavement.

REFERENCES

Aaron J.E., Gallacher J.C., Anderson J., Stasiak L., Longton E.B., Nordin B.E.C. & Nicholson M. (1974) Frequency of osteomalacia and osteoporosis in fractures of the proximal femur. *Lancet* **1**, 229.

Anderson I., Campbell A.E.R., Dunn A. & Runciman J.B.M. (1966) Osteomalacia in elderly women. *Scottish Medical Journal* **11**, 429.

Brocklehurst J., Griffiths L.L., Taylor G.F., Marks J., Scott D.L. & Blackley J. (1968) The clinical features of chronic vitamin deficiency — a therapeutic trial with geriatric hospital patients. *Gerontologia clinica* **10**, 309.

Corless D., Beer M., Boucher B.J., Gupta S.P. & Cohen R.D. (1975) Vitamin-D status in long-stay geriatric patients. *Lancet* **1**, 1404.

Dall J.L.C. & Gardiner H.S. (1971) Dietary intake of potassium by geriatric patients. *Gerontologia clinica* **13**, 119.

Dall J.L.C., Paulose S. & Ferguson J.A. (1971) Potassium intakes of elderly patients in hospital. *Gerontologia clinica* **13**, 114.

Davies L. (1981) *Three Score Years . . . and Then?* London, Heinemann Medical.

Davies L., Hastrop K. & Bender A.E. (1975) Protein in the diet of old age pensioners receiving meals on wheels. *Modern Geriatrics* **5**, 12.

Department of Health and Social Security (1969) *Recommended Intakes of Nutrients for the United Kingdom.* Reports on Public Health and Medical Subjects, No. 120. London, HMSO.

Department of Health and Social Security (1972) *Nutrition Survey of the Elderly.* Report on Health and Social Subjects, No. 3. London, HMSO.

Department of Health and Social Security (1979) *Recommended Daily Amounts of Food Energy and Nutrients for Groups of People in the United Kingdom.* Report on Health and Social Subjects, No. 15. London, HMSO.

Dymock S. & Brocklehurst J.C. (1972) *A further investigation into the relationship between clinical findings and supplementation with water-soluble vitamins in long-stay geriatric patients.* Paper given at Meeting of British Geriatrics Society, London.

Exton-Smith A.N. & Stanton B.R. (1965) *Report of an Investigation into the Dietary of Elderly Women Living Alone.* London, King Edward's Hospital Fund.

Exton-Smith A.N., Stanton B.R. & Windsor A.C.M. (1972) *Nutrition of Housebound Old People.* London, King Edward's Hospital Fund.

Golden M.H.N. (1980) Trace elements. In *Metabolic and Nutritional Disorders in the Elderly* (Ed. Exton-Smith A.N. & Caird F.I.) p. 50. Bristol, John Wright.

Griffiths L.L., Brocklehurst J.C., Scott D.L., Marks J. & Blackley J. (1967) Thiamine and ascorbic acid levels in the elderly. *Gerontologia clinica* **9**, 1.

Heaney R.P., Gallagher J.C., Johnston C.C., Neer R., Parfitt A.M. & Wheldon G.D. (1982) Calcium nutrition and bone health in the elderly. *American Journal of Nutrition* **36**, 986.

Judge T.G. & MacLeod C.C. (1968) Dietary potassium in the elderly. *Proceedings, 5th European Meeting on Clinical Gerontology*, Brussels, p. 295.

Judge T.G. & Cowan N.R. (1971) Dietary potassium intake and grip strength in older people. *Gerontologia clinica* **13**, 221.

McGandy R.B., Barrows C.H. Jun., Spanias A., Meredith A., Stone J.L. & Norris A.N. (1966) Nutrient intakes and energy expenditure in men of different ages. *Journal of Gerontology* **21**, 581.

MacLennan W.J. (1986) Subnutrition in the elderly. *British Medical Journal* **293**, 1184.

MacLeod C., Judge T.G. & Caird F.I. (1974a) Nutrition of the elderly at home. I: Intakes of energy, protein, carbohydrate and fat. *Age and Ageing* **3**, 158.

MacLeod C., Judge T.G. & Caird F.I. (1974b) Nutrition of the elderly at home. II: Intakes of vitamins. *Age and Ageing* **3**, 209.

Milne J.A., Lonergan M.E., Williamson J., Moore F.M.L., McMaster R. & Percy N. (1971) Leucocyte ascorbic acid levels and vitamin C intake in older people. *British Medical Journal* **4**, 383.

Murphy F., Srivastava P.C., Varadi S. & Elwis A. (1969) Screening of psychiatric patients for hypovitaminosis B_{12}. *British Medical Journal* **3**, 559.

Nandi S.R. & Lewis Ann M. (1985) The key to restoring magnesium balance. *Geriatric Medicine* Dec, 32.

Smith R.G. (1987) Zinc may be important in the elderly patient's ability to resist infection. *Geriatric Medicine* July, 18.

Stamp T.C.B. & Round J.M. (1974) Seasonal changes in human plasma levels of 25-Hydroxyvitamin D. *Nature* **247**, 563.

Stanton B.R. & Exton-Smith A.N. (1970) *A Longitudinal Study of the Dietary of Elderly Women.* London, King Edward's Hospital Fund.

Strachan R.W. & Henderson J.G. (1965) Psychiatric syndromes due to avitaminosis B_{12} with normal blood and marrow. *Quarterly Journal of Medicine* **34**, 303.

Strachan R.W. & Henderson J.G. (1967) Dementia and folate deficiency. *Quarterly Journal of Medicine* **36**, 189.

Taylor R.H. (1984) Bran yesterday . . . bran tomorrow. *British Medical Journal* **289**, 69.

Webster S.G.P. (1980) Gastrointestinal functions and absorption of nutrients. In *Metabolic and Nutritional Disorders in the Elderly* (Eds. Exton-Smith A.N. & Caird F.I.) p. 97. Bristol, John Wright.

19
Eye Diseases

Changes occur in the eyes associated with ageing and some, such as arcus senilis are symptomless and harmless; others, like cataract, and glaucoma can cause severe visual disturbance.

The following descriptions of eye diseases are given only to bring some conditions to mind. The opinion of the ophthalmologist must be taken and this is better done early than late. An awareness of the possible lesions is essential for the physician interested in the elderly.

Refractive errors

In many men and women over the age of 60 or so refraction remains practically stationary, and the mere passage of years need not imply a change in spectacles. If, however, vision is failing, refraction should be retested and appropriate spectacles prescribed. If vision is still below standard, other causes must be sought. A change in refraction in the direction of myopia may indicate developing nuclear cataract with reading vision actually temporarily improved thereby (second sight).

Cataract

This is the most common disease of the aged eye. The fibres of the lens lose their transparency, and a greyish or brownish opacity appears in the pupil. Treatment is surgical. It is now possible to remove the lens as soon as vision has diminished to the point at which the patient is handicapped in his ability to read or to write, and there is no need to delay until the cataract is 'ripe'. The best results are obtained in patients who can walk, are mentally well, and desire the operation; early ambulation must be encouraged in the elderly and modern methods of suturing make this possible. Some elderly persons may have considerable difficulty in overcoming the optical disadvantages of the spectacles necessary after the operation, however the advent of intraocular lenses (now being inserted in approximately 60% of eyes after cataract extraction in the United Kingdom) overcomes the magnification problem of aphakic spectacles.

Glaucoma

The early symptoms of angle-closure glaucoma are blurred vision in one eye which may clear quickly or may last for several hours classically associated with the symptom of coloured haloes round lights, especially in the evening. Acute glaucoma develops rapidly in one eye or sometimes in both eyes, with loss of vision, aching pain in and around the eye, a steamy cornea, a fixed semi-dilated pupil, and an eyeball firm on palpation. Vomiting may be a feature, which does not mislead the alert clinician.

The open-angle type of glaucoma is usually asymptomatic and vision may be lost before there is realization that anything is much amiss. Any complaint of slight loss of vision in an elderly person indicates the need for a check of intraocular tension. An increasing number of optometrists (opticians) routinely measure intraocular tension and this is to be commended. The prevalence of open-angle glaucoma approaches 8% in people over 80 years of age.

Treatment

This is highly specialized and the patient should be under expert supervision. Acute or subacute glaucoma is an emergency, urgently requiring specialist advice. Initial measures for the typical case include the instillation of 2% pilocarpine drops in the affected eye every 15 minutes for 2 hours and then less frequently, and acetazolamide (Diamox), which reduces the formation of aqueous, in an initial dose of 0.5 g intravenously or intramuscularly followed by a 0.25 g tablet four times daily with potassium supplements. Once the acute attack has subsided, or if it does not promptly subside, the patient should undergo surgery. The fellow eye also requires attention in the form of prophylactic surgery to prevent the risk of an acute closure attack.

Open-angle glaucoma can be treated by drugs such as 1% Neutral adrenaline eye drops (Eppy), pilocarpine 1–4% eye drops, or topical β-blockers. The use of these and the other drugs available is a matter for specialist advice. Surgery is indicated if medical treatment is ineffective or if compliance with the treatment regimen is suspect.

First degree family members of patients with glaucoma are also at risk and should be advised to have a complete ophthalmological examination.

Macular degeneration

In older people macular degeneration causes a loss of central vision so that the part of vision that is clearest and sharpest is affected. The patients cannot read small print or sew, but they may be reassured that they will not go blind and the peripheral fields of vision are not affected. Many other diseases affect the macular area including diabetes mellitus, hypertension, nephritis and vascular conditions; sometimes no cause is found. If detected early laser photocoagulation may be used to limit the disorder, otherwise treatment is unsatisfactory and consists mainly of therapy for any underlying condition and the provision of a low visual acuity aid, if the old person has enough perseverance to use it.

Vascular occlusion

Arterial occlusion may be caused by small emboli from atheromatous plaques in the aorta or carotid arteries or by atherosclerosis of the central retinal artery or its branches. Sudden loss of vision in the affected eye is the dominant symptom. The significance of amaurosis fugax is similar to that of transient ischaemic attacks affecting other cerebral arterial territories.

Treatment

As with any cerebral end artery irreversible damage usually results, but attempts may be made to re-establish retinal flow.

Visual loss may also denote venous occlusion and thrombosis of the central retinal vein is found in elderly people who have hypertension or arteriosclerosis, being commonly associated with disease in the central retinal artery. The effect of treatment is to reduce the risk of the development of thrombotic glaucoma.

Giant cell arteritis

Progressive occlusion of the central retinal artery or its branches may be associated with temporal arteritis. Treatment with prednisolone, 120 mg daily in divided doses, may control the acute symptoms and prevent blindness in the less affected eye. The total daily dose is gradually reduced and the drug is stopped when the disease becomes inactive as judged by the return of the ESR to normal (p. 266). The dangers of developing severe unwanted effects of large doses of systemic steroids are justified if the diagnosis is correct.

Retinal detachment

This condition is by no means limited to older people and presents with a burst of floaters and later by a shadow over part of the visual field. Prompt treatment must be given to forestall involvement of the macula if that has not already occurred. Untreated it can cause complete loss of vision. The important point is that the patient must be able to undergo the general anaesthesia necessary for the surgical correction.

Hemianopia

Homonymous hemianopia, usually from circulatory deficiency affecting the higher visual pathway, is seldom amenable to treatment, but the disability should be recognized and the risk of accident, particularly in road traffic, should be avoided. In addition, if a defect in one field of vision is demonstrated to relatives or other carers, day-to-day management can be much improved, e.g. positioning of cutlery or meals in the patient's intact field of vision.

Bitemporal hemianopia, due to pituitary tumour, is much rarer but may be remediable and can be missed if examination is inadequate.

Tobacco amblyopia

Pipe-smoking elderly men, especially if anaemic, heavy alcohol drinkers or otherwise debilitated, may notice their vision deteriorating, sometimes as a failure to recognize their friends who appear 'pasty-faced'. The bilateral centrocaecal scotoma and a loss of colour discrimination are highly characteristic, and the condition, due possibly to poisoning by cyanide in tobacco smoke, is remediable by abstinence from tobacco or, after identifying and treating any blood disease, by intramuscular injections of hydroxocobalamin (Neo-Cytamen), giving 1000 µg daily for 2 weeks, twice weekly for 4 weeks, and thereafter monthly.

Eyelids and cornea

Many elderly people suffer from laxity of the lower eyelid, which falls away from the eye causing the conjuctival surface to turn outwards (ectropion) and this results in a watery eye due to tear duct malposition. The lower lid may turn inward causing the eyelashes to rub on the cornea and so produce irritation (entropion). Minor plastic operations correct these problems. Similarly, chronic dacryocystitis carries a risk of corneal infection and may be eliminated surgically. Corneal ulceration requires prompt treatment to prevent scarring. A watch should be kept on the eyelids for tumours, such as basal-cell carcinoma.

The eyes must not be neglected as people grow older. Good visual acuity may be maintained to a ripe old age and every effort must be made to avoid the affliction of blindness as an added burden to the aged individual.

20
Skin Diseases

Correct diagnosis is essential as so many dermatological conditions are completely amenable to appropriate therapy, and the advice of the dermatologist should be sought if there is any doubt about the diagnosis.

The human skin as it ages shows changes that are in essence the effect of exposure. The protected skin of the body, for example from the buttock, is histologically young. Verbov (1974) stresses that when the elderly patient presents at the skin clinic he may well have one or more systemic diseases in addition to his skin problem. Skin diseases as they affect the elderly have been reviewed by Marks (1987).

Senile purpura

This occurs from the rupture of unsupported capillaries which are sensitive to minimal trauma. It presents as haemorrhagic patches under the skin and does not require treatment.

Pruritus

The most troublesome complaint of the elderly person is itch, and a generalized pruritus may occur as an idiopathic condition or it may be due to 'winter itch', resulting from excessive defatting of the ageing skin if bathing in cold weather is overdone. Itching is made worse by a hot bath or by sitting too close to a fire. Examination may reveal no physical sign or a dry scaling xeroderma, with patches of eczematous dermatitis and secondary infection. Widespread itching with no skin lesions requires appropriate investigations to exclude systemic disease such as diabetes mellitus, renal or hepatic disease, leukaemia, internal malignancy or gout. It is essential to exclude pediculosis, ringworm or scabies as the cause of the itching.

Treatment

This depends on the diagnosis but if no systemic disease is found baths containing sodium bicarbonate, 120 g (4 oz) to moderately warm bath water help to relieve itching. Promethazine hydrochloride, diphenhydramine hydrochloride and chlorpromazine are useful in controlling pruritus. If antihistamines are used the patients must be warned of possible sedative effects and perhaps impairment of judgement in car driving. It should also be remembered that the actions of alcohol and barbiturates are potentiated by antihistamines. Crotamiton ointment BP (Eurax) or menthol 0.25% in oily calamine lotion BPC frequently relieves the itching. If the itching is in the natal cleft, groin or buttock, it may be due to monilial infection, but care must be taken to exclude diabetes mellitus. The monilial infection can be treated with nystatin ointment (100 000 units/g) or clotrimazole (Canesten) cream.

Eczema

This is an inflammatory condition of the skin (dermatitis) with redness, swelling, vesicles and itching. It may be a contact dermatitis due to sensitization by drugs, household materials or plants. Removal of the allergen, topical steroids and antihistamines given orally cure the condition. Discovering the cause of the allergy may be difficult and patch testing may be needed.

Urinary incontinence and dermatitis

Chronic urinary incontinence may cause an ammoniacal dermatitis of the thighs and genital area. The treatment consists of applications of soothing ointments such as Thovaline or calamine liniment. As candidal infections are so common, combined preparations, e.g. Canesten-HC or Daktacort, are helpful.

Varicose eczema

The skin of the lower half of the inner side of one or both legs in elderly patients with varicose veins is often eczematous and similarly the term gravitational eczema is used to describe that dermatitis associated with longstanding oedema from any cause. These are chronic conditions and from them a general sensitization of the skin may ensue resulting in a widespread eczema. Topical antibiotics should not be used because of the risk of sensitization.

Treatment consists primarily of support by elastocrepe bandages or elastic hose and the feet should be kept elevated as much as possible and Lassar paste with 15% glycerin applied to the inflamed area (Verbov 1974). Oily calamine lotion may be used as an alternative application.

Stasis ulcers

These are also associated with varicose veins and are usually precipitated by mild trauma.

Treatment

The varicose veins should be treated, but if this cannot be done elastic stockings are necessary to overcome the venous hypertension. Complete bed rest may initially be required in severe cases. The treatment of stasis ulcer should aim first at reducing any local oedema and the whole leg should be firmly supported with a bandage such as elastocrepe applied from toes to knee. Tulle gras may be applied locally to the ulcerated area with gauze above. Eusol may be of great value as a local application at the beginning of treatment, and dextranomer (Debrisan) may be of help in removing any slough. When the ulcer is clean the leg can be enclosed from toe to knee with an occlusive zinc paste bandage such as Viscopaste. This should be left in place if possible for 2 weeks between changes. If the patient required bed rest initially, he should be mobilized fairly quickly and encouraged to take light exercise, being warned not to stand too long and when resting to keep his leg elevated on a stool. Graduated compression using stockings such as the Sigvaris type could be helpful in restoring physiological function.

Intertrigo

This condition affects the body folds, where there is skin apposition in areas such as the breasts, axillae, abdominal folds or groins. It is most commonly found in the obese and is often associated with lack of cleanliness. This flexural inflammation is usually due to a combination of friction, sweating and infection. The skin folds should be separated with linen strips and Hydrocortisone clioquinol ointment BPC or calamine lotion and methylated spirits in equal parts are usually effective remedies. When candida intertrigo is present, diabetes must always be excluded and the intertriginous reaction treated with Canesten-HC or Daktacort. After the intertrigo has healed, dusting powder should be applied regularly to the body folds.

Tinea (ringworm)

Tinea pedis involves the skin between the toes and causes a maceration of the skin with itching. Small fissures may form and vesicles may be seen.

This condition is common in the elderly and diagnosis may be confirmed by microscopy and culture. Topical applications of clotrimazole (Canesten) cream are effective. Tolnaftate cream (Tinaderm) and zinc undecenoate (Tineafax) are less frequently used now. While griseofulvin is useful for tinea of body or neck it is unlikely to be of value in eradicating ringworm of the toe-nails in patients over 65.

Sweating and lack of cleanliness can cause maceration of the skin especially between the toes mimicking ringworm and applications of Castellani paint are of use.

Scabies

In the elderly it is frequently extremely difficult to find the burrows and the only diagnostic features apart from itching may be scratch marks and secondary infection. The characteristic sites for burrows are the wrists, between the fingers, the anterior axillary fold, the lower part of the buttock, the female breasts, male external genitalia and the inner sides of the feet. In doubtful cases it is wise to treat for scabies.

The diagnosis of scabies for practical purpose is made on the recognition of burrows, but it can only be considered completely proven if an acarus is identified microscopically.

Treatment

This differs in no way from that in younger age groups and consists in the application of emulsion of 25% benzyl benzoate: this is applied all over the body below the neck after a warm bath. Twenty-four hours later another application of emulsion is repeated but no bath is taken. Forty-eight hours after the first application of the emulsion the patient should have a hot cleansing bath and a complete change of underclothing and bed linen. If hands are washed during the 48-hour treatment it is essential to re-apply the emulsion. All members of the household should be treated and underclothes and bed linen sterilized by laundering and ironing. Gamma benzene hexachloride 1% is another effective remedy and should be applied in a similar fashion over 48 hours. Any residual itchy lesions may be treated with Crotamiton ointment which is also antiscabetic.

Norwegian scabies is commonly seen in homes for the elderly, psychogeriatric units or any institution with large numbers of old people and may be mistaken for eczema or psoriasis. Itch may be absent and the diagnosis not considered until other people or the caring attendants become infested. The same treatment as for ordinary scabies should be sufficient but must be continued for longer.

Pediculosis capitis

Eggs (nits) are laid on the hair and fixed to it by a cement-like substance. This infestation may be asymptomatic and noted during a routine examination or the patient may complain of itching of the scalp, neck and shoulders. This is uncommon in the elderly and is usually associated with severe social problems such as alcoholism or sleeping rough.

Treatment

All infected people in the family must be treated, and if the infestation is severe the hair should be cut short. Malathion 0.5% or carbaryl 0.5% used as lotions are the preparations of choice. These liquids are rubbed thoroughly into the scalp. The hair is left to dry naturally and after 12 hours is washed. The hair is finally cleared of nits using a fine-toothed comb.

It is advisable to repeat such treatments in a week. Another effective remedy is gamma benzene hexachloride application BPC and this should be rubbed into the entire scalp. The hair is not washed for 24 hours. It must be emphasized that this agent does not kill the nits and it is advisable to repeat the treatment 1 week later. Previous application of 2% acetic acid or domestic vinegar may assist in the removal of the nits.

Pediculosis corporis

This is another common cause of itching and usually affects the upper trunk and shoulders with crusted scratch marks and patchy pigmentation. Parasites may be noted on the seams of bloodstained underclothing. Treatment consists of lindane or malathion lotions applied to the affected areas. Twenty-four hours later it is removed by washing. In severe cases this procedure can be repeated two to three times. Underclothes and bedclothing should be disinfected by heat and seams of the underclothing ironed with a hot iron.

Psoriasis

This common condition presents with sharply demarcated reddened areas of skin with scaling, and is characterized by remissions, recurrences and exacerbations. Crude coal tar and dithranol are effective local treatments but psoriasis presents in different forms and the treatment varies according to the chronicity and sites of lesions. The advice of a dermatologist should be sought in the management of this chronic recurring disease.

Herpes zoster (shingles)

This illness presents with an intense burning pain in the dermatomes of the affected nerve roots. This may be followed by cutaneous hyperaesthesia and after 2 or 3 days the skin of the affected area becomes red and quickly thereafter vesicles appear. If the ophthalmic division of the fifth nerve is affected the cornea may be involved with subsequent scarring. Vesicles in the external auditory meatus may be noted if the geniculate ganglion is affected, and this may be followed by a facial palsy of lower motor neurone type with loss of taste on the anterior two-thirds of the tongue. Occasionally paralysis of skeletal muscle in other sites is noted due to involvement of anterior horn cells. Old people with shingles are ill and mental confusion can occur.

Treatment

Mild cases are treated with Betadine paint and calamine lotion and analgesics are given. If more severe, paint the lesions with Herpid (5% idoxuridine) four times daily for 4 days and also relieve pain with analgesics. In very severe cases, for example, with trigeminal nerve involvement Acyclovir 800 mg five times daily for 5 days may cut the total duration of the disease and possibly reduce the incidence of postherpetic neuralgia.

Eye involvement demands that the opinion of the ophthalmologist be sought at once as, apart from other considerations, the solution of idoxuridine recommended is not suitable for application to mucosal surfaces such as the eye. While waiting for the opinion of the ophthalmologist, chloramphenical eye ointment and homatropine drops can be used. The occurrence of postherpetic pain is unfortunately still not uncommon although it is claimed that its incidence has been lessened by the use of idoxuridine. This consists in severe burning pain at the site of the former rash. Pathy (1978) recommended that the affected area should be sprayed lightly with ethylchloride for 30 seconds every 2 hours seven or eight times daily for 2 or 3 weeks. Analgesics may be required and carbamazepine may be of value in intractable cases of postherpetic neuralgia; appropriate nerve section may be required in suitable cases.

Seborrhoeic or senile warts

These are flat brown or black small excrescences, raised slightly above the surface and common on the trunk of older patients. These warts give the appearance of being on rather than in the skin. Generally they are symptomless but occasionally itching does occur.

Treatment

Freezing with carbon dioxide snow, liquid nitrogen or cautery are effective.

Actinic keratoses

These warty growths are seen on the exposed surfaces of the skin, rarely occurring unless there has been considerable exposure to the sun throughout life. They may lead to overt squamous carcinoma after some years. The treatment is to freeze them with carbon dioxode snow for 15–30 seconds provided there is no infiltration of the base. In any doubtful case skin biopsy should be undertaken.

Senile lentigo (lentigo maligna)

This can occur as a well-defined brown spot on the face of the elderly individual. It slowly enlarges over the years and eventually the development of invasive malignant melanoma may occur. Treatment is by wide excision if possible. Cryotherapy is useful in patients unfit for surgery.

Malignant tumours

Basal-cell carcinoma (rodent ulcer)

This is found typically on the light exposed areas of face, i.e. below eyebrow level and above the level of the lobe of the ear, but may also be seen on the scalp, aural meatus and other areas of skin. The most common form is a pearly nodule which becomes encrusted and develops into a shallow ulcer with a rolled edge. It may also present, however, as a pigmented or button-like nodule, globular and like a cyst. It is essential to consider this diagnosis if a persistently crusted spot is found on the face of an elderly person. Treatment is by excision when this is convenient but these ulcers are radiosensitive and respond to radiotherapy and this is best employed where the situation renders excision impossible.

Squamous cell carcinoma

This lesion is most common after the age of 60 years and some of these tumours arise from old standing lupus vulgaris or x-ray burns. They present as warty nodules, which ulcerate forming an irregular ulcer with firm everted edges and commonly found on the lower lip, ears, cheeks or scalp; metastases occur. Treatment is by local excision if the lesion is diagnosed early, but block dissection of the glands draining the area may be necessary. Radiotherapy may also be of value and on the lip this is often the treatment of choice. A combination of surgery and irradiation may be required. Bowen disease is a local intraepidermal carcinoma presenting as a flat, oval, slightly raised plaque with a salmon-red colour and psoriasiform scales. These are more commonly found on the lower leg and the diagnosis is made by biopsy. Treatment is by application of fluorouracil (Efudix), by cautery or by irradiation.

Bullous pemphigoid

This disease is more common in elderly people and presents with large, tense subepidermal blisters usually on limbs and abdomen. They are not itchy. Diagnosis is important as the condition responds rapidly to prednisolone 60–80 mg/day. Whenever the blisters stop appearing the dose is gradually reduced.

Drug rashes

These are common in the elderly partly because of the wide variety of drugs that many old people take. The clinical picture varies and the following forms are seen:

1   An urticarial reaction of rapid onset, life threatening if around the mouth or throat, with transient individual lesions which may recur irregularly over a few days. Common causes are penicillin, local anaesthetics, salicylates and opiate alkaloids.

2   Erythema multiforme starts abruptly with a maculopapular eruption and a fever may be present. In cases of intermediate severity the classical target or iris lesions of this condition are found on the distal limbs, palms of the hands and soles of the feet. In the most severe form (Stevens–Johnson syndrome) there is mucocutaneous ulceration and involvement of mouth, eyes and genitalia. This disease may last up to 28 days and the long-acting sulphonamides and the antirheumatic drugs are often the cause.

3   Exfoliative dermatitis with scaling and redness of skin can be induced by gold, antirheumatic and antibiotic preparations.

4   Measles-like rashes can be due to antibiotics, anti-inflammatory drugs or diuretics.

5   Purpuric rashes can be caused by thiazide diuretics and erythema nodosum by sulphonamides, while photosensitivity reactions may be found in bright conditions and occur in sunny weather following the use of sulphonamides, tetracyclines, nalidixic acid or phenothiazines and sul-

phonamide derivatives such as thiazide diuretics.

β-Blockers not infrequently cause a rash like psoriasis.

Treatment

The drug considered responsible should be discontinued immediately; occasionally hospital admission may be essential for correction of fluid and electrolyte balance and for the urticarial type of reaction antihistamines are of value. Systemic steroids may be required for acute explosive lesions.

REFERENCES

Marks R. (1987) *Skin Disease in Old Age*. London, Dunitz.

Pathy M.S.J. (1978) Postherpetic neuralgia. In *Textbook of Geriatric Medicine and Gerontology* (Ed. Brocklehurst J.C.) Edinburgh, Churchill Livingstone.

Verbov J. (1974) *Skin Diseases in the Elderly*. London, Heinemann Medical.

21

Care of the Dying

At the beginning of this century, infectious disease, tuberculosis, and gastroenteritis were the common causes of death of the elderly, but now heart disease, malignancy and diseases of the nervous system are most frequently recorded. Heart disease in old age is commonly due to coronary artery disease, malignancy is usually cancer of the alimentary tract or bronchus, and among diseases of the central nervous system the most frequently recorded. Heart disease in old age is commonly due to coronary artery disease, malignancy is usually cancer of the alimentary tract or myocardial infarction and the atypical presentation of some diseases.

McKeown (1965) reported autopsy findings in a series of 1500 patients, 70 years or more at the time of death, and found disorders of the cardio-vascular system coming first as a cause of death (21%); second was malignancy (20%); and next the nervous system (12%). The high pre-valence of carcinoma of the stomach and large bowel contributed largely to mortality from malignancy. In addition to primary tumour the elderly have a predisposition to host a second or even third primary neoplasm. In an autopsy study 82% of a cohort of 72-year-olds had a second distinct primary tumour and 17% had a third (Lao *et al.* 1978). This finding of multiple primary neoplasm in the elderly has been substantiated by other studies (Spratt 1977).

Of 500 000 deaths each year in the United Kingdom, half take place at over 75 years of age, over 90 000 take place at over 85, and 500 at over 100.

In Sheffield it was demonstrated that no less than 14% of cancer patients dying at home were being cared for by relatives themselves over 70, while 74% of caring relatives were over 50 (Wilkes 1965). In this survey, the general practitioners classed the medical attention needed by terminal cancer patients dying at home as minimal in 27%, moderate in 59%, and heavy only in 12% of cases. Half the patients dying of cancer at home had no real nursing problems or serious suffering. Twenty per cent of patients had real difficulties for a fortnight or less, and 15% had serious trouble lasting 6 weeks or longer. Alderson (1970), in a survey of terminal care in malignant disease found that patients were admitted to hospital in the terminal stages primarily for nursing care, i.e. because the family could not cope; only 30% went in for medical attention.

310

In clinical practice in the hospital setting, women are ill for longer periods of time than men.

Dying patients have been defined as those in whom a diagnosis of incurable disease has been made, and whose doctors expect them to die within a few weeks or months. For what characterizes 'the dying' as a group is the fact that their attendants expect them to die.

The care of the dying can be considered in regard to the patient, the relatives, the nurses, the hospital consultant, the family doctor and the padre.

The first essential is an accurate diagnosis; if this is incorrect then subsequent therapy will obviously be totally incompetent.

The patient

The doctor who sees previously unknown elderly patients must listen to them carefully. A diagnosis may already have been made in this particular individual and it may indicate that the illness is a fatal one. However, while it may be true that this is so, the diagnosis must not be assumed to be correct, and the doctor must keep an open mind. On other occasions, the patient's symptoms may not fit into a previously experienced pattern of disease, and careful thought must be given to the diagnosis. Patients have an uncanny habit of being right, and unusual symptoms should not be classed as hysterical or imaginary. Accurate information about past illnesses and previous operations or medical treatment must be obtained from each elderly person. In old age atypical presentation of a common illness is much more frequently seen than a rare disease and in many individuals multiple pathology is found, while the onset of very serious illness may be insidious and quiet. Many physicians unwittingly consider malignancy as their first choice just because the patient is elderly, and too quickly close their minds.

After a careful history, full clinical examination, bearing in mind the previously recorded facts, may indicate that the patient is indeed dying. Care has to be taken to ensure that the complaints that the patient has are due to this fatal illness and not caused by other relatively minor pathological conditions which may make the individual's life miserable, for example the presence of mouth ulcers or haemorrhoids. The adverse effects of medication with drugs, for example mental confusion or depression, and symptoms such as nausea and vomiting due to previous therapy, e.g. radiotherapy, must also be kept in mind. It may be necessary to admit the older person to hospital so that the diagnosis which has been suggested may be confirmed, as it is essential to have a correct diagnosis as soon as possible. This does not mean that an elderly, weary and emaciated person, obviously in the last stages of life, should be subjected to investigation in order to satisfy scientific curiosity. On the other hand, the amazing and often unexpected ability of older people to recover indicates that where possible accurate diagnosis must be made. It must never be assumed, because the elderly individual looks seriously ill that a fatal illness is present. The elderly, like children, may suddenly appear desperately ill, partly due to their severe reaction to dehydration, and this may be aggravated by impairment of sensation to thirst. When fluid deprivation is restored and electrolyte balance corrected, a sudden and dramatic improvement in general condition occurs.

Treatment may first, however, be curative and active steps, e.g. operation or drug therapy, may be recommended. Stress must be laid on the psychological aspect of the illness and here constant reassurance is necessary. In the United Kingdom, care is required to be taken in the use of the word cancer; to some patients this diagnosis implies that without doubt they are dying. Knowledge and understanding of the individual person help and guide the physician at this time. At some stage in therapy it may be considered, clinically, that the patient is dying and here the treatment, although palliative, must be just as energetic.

After the correct diagnosis has been made and palliative therapy initiated, the management of dying older persons involves the understanding of a complex interplay of physical, mental and social factors.

Physical factors

Pain

The main problem with many dying patients and the one that causes most worry is pain or fear of pain. Rees (1972) found that 44% of his dying patients had continuous pain in spite of his own concern for the problem.

Pain sensation in general changes with age, and it has been suggested that blunting of sensibility to pain is a beneficent process suggesting that with gradual involution and approach to physiological death the warning normally conveyed by symptoms is no longer needed. 13.6% of elderly patients dying in a geriatric unit had pain of moderate or severe nature (Exton-Smith 1961) and this can be compared with the Marie Curie Foundation's study (1952) where 68% of a group of patients with cancer who were of all ages, had moderate or severe suffering. Saunders (1960), in her series of 474 patients admitted to a terminal care unit, found the prevalence of severe pain was 19% in patients of 70 years and over and 37% under that age. Thirty-two per cent of long stay and 41% of assessment patients in a geriatric unit were considered to have been distressed in the last week of life (Wilson *et al.* 1987).

Pain in the elderly, when it occurs, must be controlled and Saunders (1972a) believes that pain-relieving substances should be given regularly according to an invariable 4-hourly schedule. Whatever drugs are used, if pain breaks through, the dose and not the timing should be changed. Thus, once pain has been relieved, theoretically the patient should never suffer from pain again; this requires training and teaching of nursing staff. Many nurses are reluctant to give strong drugs unless they feel the patient is bad enough to require them and analgesics used to control chronic pain must be prescribed on a regular, not as required, basis. People who are felt to be demanding or patients with communication difficulties such as dysphasia, may have to stress their symptoms to convince the attendants of their suffering. Once the pain is overcome then it may be that smaller doses of the pain-relieving drug can be used regularly because the patient's pain threshold and morale have been raised and the fear of pain has been conquered.

Saunders uses oral heroin for pain relief in most of her terminal patients, including those at home, as she finds that this drug causes less nausea and less drowsiness than morphine, and is more potent orally due to better absorption. The usual dose of heroin required by mouth is 10 mg every 4 hours and in Saunders' series (1972b) of 428 patients, only 19% needed more than 20 mg at any one time; long-acting formulations of morphine are now available (MST Continus) and are useful and are equally potent analgesics on a mg/mg equivalent basis.

To control mild pain in the early stages, aspirin or paracetamol may be used. Paracetamol has to be given with caution if there is liver impairment and aspirin enhances the effect of oral anticoagulants. Codeine is another weak narcotic analgesic and Tempest & Clarke (1982) recommend soluble aspirin and papaveretum (soluble aspirin 500 mg and papaveretum 10 mg as a tablet) as a useful preparation in a dose of two tablets every 4 hours in pain of central or peripheral origin. When strong oral narcotic drugs are required to relieve pain diamorphine or morphine can be given in a simple solution of chloroform water. When a suppository is necessary morphine sulphate 15 to 30 mg is available and may be used every 4 hours. Towards the end of life an injectable preparation may be appropriate and diamorphine is the drug of choice. Papaveretum by mouth or by injection may be of special value in the elderly as it does not commonly cause nausea and because of its high solubility. To obviate the need for repeated injections a new lightweight syringe driver may be used to infuse diamorphine and other drugs to ensure adequate symptom control (Oliver

1985; Wright & Callan 1979). Pain and other symptoms are reviewed by Twycross (1986) and a technique for the continuous administration of epidural opoids by a subcutaneous implantation portal system which provides long-term relief in patients with cancer has been described (Cherry *et al.* 1985).

The non-steroidal anti-inflammatory drugs are of value in the relief of bone and other pain, e.g. diflunisal (Dolobid) 500 mg every 12 hours. This drug may enhance the action of the oral anticoagulants. Indomethacin (Indocid) is also of use, but it is a gastric irritant; several non-steroidal anti-inflammatory drugs are now available in suppository form, e.g. flurbiprofen, piroxicam and are useful in the nauseated, vomiting or dysphagic patient. The control of pain with and without drugs was reviewed by Tempest & Clarke (1982).

Many elderly dying patients become weak and unhappy by being made too sleepy during the day and thus prevented from getting out of bed or eating and this, if possible, must be avoided.

Drugs of the phenothiazine group often help to dissociate the patient from his illness, and large doses are not required. Largactil (chlorpromazine) 25 mg, three times per day orally, may be useful, but large doses should be given with care in elderly people as the phenothiazines can cause mental confusion or by reducing mobility can encourage the development of pressure sores. Amitriptyline combined with perphenazine (Triptafen DA) has a useful effect when given at night in producing mild analgesia, sleep and mood improvement.

Insomnia

The patient requires a good night's sleep, and if pain is the cause of wakefulness, pain relief may be enough to ensure this. If a hypnotic is required, temazepam, chloral hydrate or one of the chloral derivatives are recommended. Triazolam is well tolerated by many elderly patients and has a rapid rate of absorption and a short half-life. Residual sedation is rare at a dose of 0.125 mg. For older people who complain of difficulty in getting off to sleep, Heminevrin (chlormethiazole) is of use.

The cause of insomnia should be analysed as it may be that depression, faecal impaction or a bedsore may be the real reason for the wakefulness. For depression, which potentiates pain or causes insomnia, mianserin or imipramine may be of value. Frequency of micturition may disturb sleep and the cause should be sought and appropriate treatment advised.

More important than drugs is the establishment of a warm relationship with a doctor or nurse. The doctor must sit down and listen to the various facets of his patient's distress, without giving the impression that he is too busy, and he must elicit even trivial sounding complaints; after such a discussion pain can sometimes be relieved without resorting to drugs at all. Pathological fracture of the femur may require traction, or a palliative operation may relieve distress, as may radiotherapy in causing shrinkage of tumour. The administration of hormones and cytotoxic drugs, or the action of the neurosurgeon by cutting nerves may be able to reduce suffering. In deciding about the possible use of radiotherapy or chemo-therapy the advice of a clinical oncologist may be of immense help. The disadvantages of all these measures must be assessed against the possible benefits, and especially in elderly patients there must be clear evidence of adequate gain for the individual before any interference is considered; the use of chemical nerve blocking can give pain relief in even the very old and this method should not be forgotten.

If analgesics are required it is essential to give enough of the pain-relieving drug to relieve pain. The dose of morphine, pethidine, or heroin that completely abolishes the pain is the correct dose, and if large amounts are required frequently in the last week or two of a patient's life to relieve pain, this would seem to break no rule, and is an essential phase of the patient's therapy.

Nausea

Nausea is a most troublesome complaint, and the cause for this should be sought. Faecal impaction should always be excluded and then appropriate investigations should be undertaken to exclude tumours or other causes. Biochemical abnormalities, e.g. hypercalcaemia, radiotherapy, cytotoxic treatment or drugs must be excluded as causes. A good fluid intake is essential and this demands constant attention from the nursing staff. Small drinks of cool fluids, especially water, are valuable and only if this fails should a subcutaneous or intravenous drip be employed. Phenothiazines, e.g. chlorpromazine, may be helpful.

Occasionally nausea may be helped by treatment of associated depression with antidepressant drugs, as this symptom may be associated with anxiety.

Vomiting

Intractable vomiting is another problem and in some cases is due to mechanical obstruction by the growth itself; faecal impaction should never be overlooked. In others the vomiting is associated with the drug being given and occasionally there may be a psychological element. Opiates are reported not to cause vomiting so frequently when the patient in pain is in bed.

Antiemetics are of value and if drug control is the therapeutic approach the cause of the vomiting must be clear. If it is central in origin drugs such as prochlorperazine, cyclizine or haloperidol may be used; if it is peripheral, e.g. there is evidence of gastric stasis or oesophageal reflux, metoclopramide or domperidone will be the drugs of choice. Combinations of antiemetics may be required and the drugs may have to be given by injection or as a suppository if such a preparation of the particular drug is available. The butyrophenones, e.g. haloperidol, can be infused subcutaneously in order to control vomiting or nausea. Sometimes a patient tolerates soda water or iced water and occasionally relief of pain relieves vomiting. If persistent vomiting occurs, when the time for any form of surgical intervention is past, it may be worthwhile passing a nasal tube and instituting intermittent or continuous suction to prevent constant retching. The fluid intake can be supplemented by a subcutaneous drip, and this therapy, given in order to alleviate symptoms of dry mouth and thirst, is not prolonging the patient's life unnecessarily, but is relieving uncomfortable and worrying symptoms. It is often of great help to nursing staff and relatives to explain that the act of dying is not being prolonged but rather that the patient may die in comfort.

Dysphagia

When dysphagia is present, if due to oesophagitis, antacids, cimetidine or mucaine may be of use. If monilia is thought to be the cause then nystatin should be given. The patient who has had a Souttar tube passed requires watching in case this becomes blocked. When loss of appetite is the main symptom, 5 mg of prednisolone two or three times per day can improve appetite and is sometimes of use for the widespread aches and pains which are so frequent among many dying people. Steroids also cause euphoria, which may of itself reduce the perception of pain.

Hiccups

These are often most troublesome, being irritating and exhausting. The quickest way to overcome this is to have the patient breathe in and out of a paper bag for a few minutes. If carbon dioxide is available this can be used also as an inhalant, and if the carbon dioxide fails, chlorpromazine by injection may be effective. Another suggested remedy is metoclopramide (Maxolon) 10 mg by injection and thereafter orally.

Cough

Persistent cough is sometimes a great worry, and if a linctus like Ethnine (pholcodine linctus) in a dose of 5–10 ml is given in very hot water this may help. Diamorphine is the strongest antitussive and may eventually have to be given by injection. It should not be forgotten that if the sputum is purulent, a short course of an appropriate antibiotic is helpful.

Periodic re-examination of the dying individual may be unexpectedly rewarding and may reveal new ways of helping the patient; for example if the patient complains of dyspnoea, a pleural effusion may be discovered and may require draining. In malignant effusions particularly those associated with carcinoma of the breast, the effusion should be drained to dryness and a sclerosing agent such as bleomycin 60 mg dissolved in 100 ml physiological saline may be instilled into the pleural cavity and this will usually reduce the rate of re-accumulation of the fluid.

Tiredness

In longstanding illness there is often an increasing sense of tiredness and the use of exercise with or without physiotherapy should be considered. In the elderly, immobility may lead to stiffness and bedsores and the older patient should not be allowed to become bedridden before it is inevitable. In fact, there is much to be said for keeping the patient mobile as long as possible and this cheers him up and helps to prevent apathy, boredom and despair. Pain may prevent movement and when the pain is overcome the individual may be able to be on his feet again. If there has been an old stroke, physiotherapy for this should not be neglected, and the importance of regular chiropody should not be forgotten. Time can hang heavily in certain phases of illness, and time to think may be a mixed blessing. It is well worth finding out if the patient has any particular ability or hobby, and every encouragement to use all remaining faculties should be given.

The undertaking of minor chores in the ward or at home should be encouraged and praise given for work done. The help of the occupational therapist should be obtained and full use of any facilities that are available in her department. The minister or priest at this stage may have much to offer and should be part of the therapeutic team.

The importance of adequate fluid intake, bowel regulation without discomfort, and correction of electrolyte imbalance, must be stressed in the terminal patient as in any other. In dealing with all these symptoms the doctor's enthusiasm and confidence in his therapy, is without doubt transmitted to the patient. While it is necessary to bear in mind that heroic measures are seldom indicated, it is also essential to have the same interest in the patient during this stage of life as in any other. A balance must be struck; terminal dehydration (Leader 1986) is discussed and the point is made that medical and nursing staff may find their attention diverted from the care of the patient and family to the control of electrolytes and fluid balance. It must be stressed that whether the elderly patient is nursed at home, in an institution, or by intermittent admission and discharge there must be continuity of care. The older person must understand clearly that during each phase of illness the doctor knows what is happening and continues to care.

Mental state

It is important to remember that not only must the physical health of the patient be treated, but attention must also be paid to the mental state. Once an elderly person has a diagnosis that indicates a fatal outcome, the physician tends to pass by this individual on the ward round; in general, people tend to turn away from dying patients. Perhaps the doctor feels his time is wasted with someone he cannot cure; he may fear that he may be asked a question that would involve him emotionally in a way for which he is not prepared, as doctors are not usually taught at medical school or elsewhere how to face dying patients. The patient's own doctor is usually the most suitable person to answer the question 'Am I dying?'. This being accepted then it is essential that communication between hospital specialist and general practitioner be prompt and accurate stating exactly what the patient has been told about the illness.

Relatives

Information about the diagnosis, the progress of the illness, the purpose of the therapy and the prognosis should be given to relatives. Judgement must be used in estimating their ability to understand the information given and very detailed points of therapy are often best left out of the discussion. Any idea that treatment of any kind is not being given may arouse, quite wrongly, suspicions of euthanasia or some desire to speed up death.

Time must be made available by the general practitioner or a senior hospital doctor to allow questions to be asked and the psychological handling of near relatives is often much more difficult than communication with the patient.

Nurses

Nursing of the elderly dying patient is of fundamental importance, and the mental health of the nursing staff must be kept in mind. Explanations to the nurses on each stage of care should be given by the doctor and the objective clearly stated.

In the nursing of such older people, adequate care of the mouth is essential. It is often worthwhile re-shaping ill-fitting dentures to cut down discomfort and salivation, and a constant watch must be kept for thrush. When pain-relieving drugs are being used, constipation may occur and this may go on to faecal impaction, which in turn may produce retention of urine. Due regard must be paid therefore to the regular action of the bowel.

Nothing can replace good nursing in the prevention of bedsores, but ripple mattresses may be of value while the danger of the phenothiazine derivatives in causing immobility of the patient should be kept in mind. Good general nursing and regular turning of the patient help to prevent bedsores, as does adequate protein intake, and appropriate measures should be taken if a pressure area becomes red. When the patient is incontinent, part of the regular nursing should be to use a barrier cream over the affected areas whenever the bed is changed. Much argument exists on the treatment of bedsores, but prevention is far more important than waiting until the skin is broken. In early cases a local anaesthetic cream and an antibiotic powder such as Cicatrin may be of use.

Perhaps the most important way a doctor can help the nurse is by ensuring that while being kept free from the pain the patient is not at the same time made too sleepy to eat or move about the bed bearing in mind that drowsiness due to opioids wears off after 2 or 3 days; immobility is a great danger to elderly people. When there is extreme pain on turning the patient with a bedsore in bed, Wilkes (1973) states that this can be controlled by an Entonox machine for inhalation before the turning. This machine delivers 50% nitrous oxide and 50% oxygen and enables the patient to be turned over without pain. Similarly pain invoked by any potentially painful procedure can be prevented by administration of dextromoramide (palfium) 20 minutes prior to the procedure. Dextromoramide may be given orally, sublingually or by suppository. Wilkes also believes that incontinence is not a major problem in domiciliary nursing, as sterile disposable self-retaining catheters can be used. If blockage threatens the system it can be washed out with 1 in 5000 solution of Hibitane (chlorhexidine).

Patients often hesitate to complain about smell, perhaps in the belief that the doctor can do little about it. Wilkes found that where there is a fungating lesion in, for example, the breast, it is often possible, by trying various hormones such as oestrogens, non-virilizing androgens, steroids or progestogens or local cytotoxic drug applications to find an appropriate way to reduce the smell. It is important to note that topically applied cytotoxic agents, e.g. 5-fluorouracil, may produce myelosuppression and a check must be made for this at weekly intervals. The odour is due generally to anaerobic organisms and may be greatly reduced by systemic metronidazole or Augmentin. Charcoal impregnated pads will absorb and cut down smell.

The worrying noises that may accompany the final hours of a comatose patient may be due to stertorous breathing or the accumulation of mucus in the trachea or large bronchi. The noise due to stertorous breathing may be reduced by placing the head in the lateral position or by using an airway to prevent obstruction of the fauces by the tongue. The frightening noise of accumulated mucus may be abolished by injecting hyoscine hydrobromide 0.4 mg intravenously. Hyoscine may also be infused subcutaneously as a continuous infusion or given as an individual subcutaneous injection.

Physicians

The doctor must remember the importance of reassurance. In terminal illness this is essential, and it is often stated that people do not fear death but the process of dying. Time must be allocated by the doctor and his manner must be such that he invites questions from his patient and he will become his patient's friend. The seriously ill consider death as a possible outcome, and welcome the chance to talk about their feelings. The fact of sharing this fear with the doctor is in itself therapeutic, and promotes more confident communication between patients and doctors. The discussion of this fear whether or not it is founded in reality should be carried out only when the relationship between the doctor and the patient is sufficiently close. Both should have reached the stage where they are at ease with one another. The doctor is not trained to help in matters of a spiritual or theological nature, and it may be that the physician should not hesitiate to turn to the priest or minister to help. There should, of course, be good communication between the doctor and the chaplain, so that the latter may be sensitive to and be aware of the clinical situation in his approach to the patient.

Kubler-Ross (1970) has stated that there are five stages which most dying patients pass through:
1   The first is that of denial and isolation.
2   The next anger.
3   The third bargaining.

4   Then depression.
5   Finally the stage of acceptance.

These different stages require to be looked for and the patient should be encouraged to talk if he so desires.

Staff members handling dying patients should receive simple training courses, so that they can comprehend what is going on; they must understand the concept of empathy. They should realize that talking to the patients helps them in talking to the relatives, and here they must comprehend that the relatives may feel anxious, depressed, angry or guilty themselves. Great tact, sympathy and compassion are required, and the aggressive relative must not be answered by aggression but by explanation that may require constant repetition. At the initial stage of communication when the attempt is being made to tell a near relative that the patient is dying, it seems as if the relatives were deaf, and it is necessary to go over the same ground repeatedly and with simple words; not with scientific jargon.

The decision to tell a patient the correct diagnosis and that he is dying is one which remains a problem for each doctor and each individual patient. This step should be taken when a close relationship has been established with the ill old person and only after careful thought.

If a decision is made that there should be a conspiracy of silence then this must be complete and no well-meaning friend or relative without consultation should take it upon himself or herself to tell the patient the whole truth with the patient unprepared, unexpecting and perhaps unwanting to receive such information. It is necessary to make sure that the lines of communication are clearly established between doctor, nurses, relatives and patient, and if the patient is admitted to hospital, between hospital consultant, nurses, family doctor, relatives and patient. If, for example, the hospital consultant writes to the family doctor telling him of some operative procedure or medical preparation being advised for the patient, giving in his letter the diagnosis, the next sentence should tell the general practitioner the state of communication. Has the patient, or the patient's nearest relative, been told the diagnosis, if so what has been told to these people, and perhaps more importantly, if they have not been told the diagnosis, what exactly has been said to them? This saves much embarrassment, loss of confidence and eventually perhaps ill-feeling between patient and general practitioner.

In our planning we must allow time for the senior doctor to interview the relatives of those who are ill and who need explanation and guidance, but he needs time also to communicate what he has said to other members of the team; both within the hospital and without. This is an unfair burden to inflict on the most junior members of the medical staff.

Family doctor

Many family doctors visit a dying patient regularly and if hospital admission has taken place, on discharge of the patient they must be informed regarding the correct diagnosis. The doctor must be sure he is aware of the facilities available to his patient, for example, how to obtain a commode, or a night nurse or attendant. In the United Kingdom patients dying at home with cancer can usually obtain a night nursing service through the Marie Curie Foundation and services like this are supplied by varying authorities throughout the country. Many voluntary and religious bodies are active in helping this group of people.

Padre

Many elderly people are immensely comforted by a visit from their minister. This is easier in hospital if the padre is already a familiar figure in the ward. The minister should be given any necessary information from the ward sister or doctor. His visit may give great spiritual assistance to the dying patient and he may add greatly to the comfort of such people by listening carefully to any wish or desire expressed. The minister may be an invaluable link with the relatives and act as a helper in time of misunderstanding or doubt.

Domiciliary care

Older people often live in older housing lacking good amenities and it must also be recalled that approximately one-quarter of all people over 65 in the United Kingdom have no relatives and about one-third of this group live alone. Older people, thus, tend to be admitted to hospital while it is the younger age groups with nearby children and reasonable housing who still tend to die at home. There is a serious financial problem in nursing a dying patient at home. This may involve higher food bills for special diet, increased money spent on heating to keep the bedroom warm and in obtaining domestic assistance in addition to any statutory help provided because of the difficulty in coping in unsuitable housing.

Cartwright *et al.* (1973) found on enquiry from doctors that there were not sufficient hospital beds for some groups of patients, especially older people who were needing long-term nursing. These authors also concluded that the resources of the community services were often inadequate; nearly two-thirds of district nurses interviewed felt they would like to give more time to patients with a terminal illness. Home help services also were deficient. Help at night was more often needed, as was help with incontinent patients. In this study, outside lavatories were a problem, while washing machines, spin driers or telephones would often have been helpful in relieving the heavy burden of care. Better co-ordination of services was required.

Where should an elderly person die? From the point of view of the family it means care at home or care away. In fact, most people do their best to keep their elderly relatives at home when they are dying, but because they become exhausted with caring for their elderly relations, it may become necessary to admit the elderly relation to hospital, often with deep regret from the caring relatives. For this reason, an effort should be made to involve the relatives in the patient's further care when they are in hospital. The relatives also require reassurance, after admission has become unavoidable, in telling them what a splendid job they have done and how they could not have managed any longer to look after the patient at home. In fact, most elderly people are admitted to hospital primarily for nursing care, because they live alone or because the home is unsuitable.

In recent surveys it has been shown that some co-ordinator must be found to organize the many services required to care for an old person dying at home: the daily district nurse, night visiting, home laundry, the provision of nursing aids, such as commodes, bandages, and bed linen, the ways in which financial help can be given, and the arrangements made for friendly visiting if the ill person is isolated. Otherwise, the dying left at home may undergo the same sort of rejection by the community as those nursed in hospital. It is suggested that this co-ordinator may be the doctor, the health visitor, or the social worker, but it is essential to make sure that all the services are involved, or relatives may fail to make contact with anyone, and are left to struggle alone.

Macmillan and Marie Curie Foundation nurses visit patients suffering from cancer and give advice and help. In many areas there are nurses specially trained in stoma care who provide a skilled service for these special cases. The Crossroads Scheme helps those who care for such ill patients by providing a care attendant who will come at a time suitable to the carer on a regular basis free of charge. This allows some relief and in effect means that the patient can be kept longer at home if that is what is desired.

The use of geriatric departments

Death in the elderly may occur suddenly or be characterized by a slow decline, and in this instance, relatives are often more upset by the terminal process than elderly people who may be confused in mind and lacking in insight. Relatives may also be suffering from a sense of guilt in that they feel they have failed their elderly relations by not keeping them at home in their last illness. If dying people require hospital admission, this should be made simple, and it should be prompt. There are some old people who do not desire to die at home, wish to spare their spouse, or their relations, the worry and the trouble of a last illness, and are quite happy to go to hospital at that time, just as on the other hand there are relatives who greatly desire to take an old person home for the last few days of his terminal care. This means that there must be two-way traffic and a promise of immediate re-admission must be given to anxious relatives who are doing their best. To ensure continuity of therapy, use can be made of 5-day wards and of day hospitals for this type of patient. The trend towards dying in hospital continues and geriatric departments must be ready for this. All new geriatric units should have a large proportion of single rooms sited near the nursing station with excellent observation. If the ward sister and her nursing staff are carefully briefed and orientated towards the use of non-trained voluntary staff, near relatives can be encouraged to help with the physical aspects of nursing if they so desire, and in this way they can feel they are playing their part. It should be possible for them to stay in hospital for some days.

Support for the bereaved

It is essential that prompt help be given, especially to elderly people who have been bereaved. The family doctor, clergy, health visitor, social worker or voluntary worker all have parts to play.

Wilson (1970) studying the effect of bereavement on elderly people as a health visitor has suggested that this is a time when a continuity contact with a skilled visitor is of the utmost importance. The older person tends to withdraw from friends and society in general following bereavement. Wilson thinks that a most effective method of preventing social isolation and loneliness in old people is through support given at the time of greatest grief, ensuring that the old people do not become completely cut off from their families, friends and neighbours encouraging the intake of an adequate diet, and that some interest is found for them. Numerous studies have shown the deleterious effects of bereavement in older people's mental health.

Rees & Lutkins (1967) showed a significant difference in the mortality among surviving spouses and near relatives according to whether death took place at home or in hospital, the risk of the nearest relative dying within a year of bereavement was twice as great if the first death occurred in hospital than if it occurred at home.

Education

In general, all caring personnel should have training in the care of the dying. More professorial departments of geriatric medicine are needed to teach the practice and principles of the care of old people to medical students, nurses, para-medical staff, social workers, divinity students, students of architecture and voluntary helpers. This instruction should include the special needs of those old people who are dying. Reassurance to young and old alike is required as to the calm and quiet death which so many elderly people have.

Specialized hospices or units for the dying are often centres of excellence where the methods of handling patients, relatives and voluntary workers are first rate. Such places can play an important part in the training of medical students, nurses and para-medical staff. The rapid growth in the number of such hospices throughout the United Kingdom indicates how successful the hospice movement has been. For cancer patients the Marie Curie Foundation Homes have also been of great help. Based on these homes a few day hospitals have been established which in co-operation with the home visiting by the nurses have ensured a continuing domiciliary service. It has been demonstrated that the provision of an advisory service to families who were nursing a patient with incurable cancer at home enabled the patient to stay at home longer than he otherwise would and helped the family and the primary care team to cope with the added burden which resulted (Parkes 1980). Many hospices and Marie Curie homes provide such an advisory service.

For medical students and doctors there is a need to make sure that our problems are not increased by prolonging a living death for elderly individuals. The physician must plan each step in treatment with care, humanity and understanding for his older patient.

In modern societies demands have been made for euthanasia in the sense of medical manslaughter. This is abhorrent to most physicians who do understand the fear of the older people that they may be kept alive as vegetables and the horror of relatives who have to endure such events.

Euthanasia in its proper meaning, namely, gentle and easy death is something which all medical men desire for their patients and for themselves. This demands clinical judgement, not legal authority, and means relieving the suffering of the patient and comforting the relatives. Information about what is happening must be available to relations and friends and the quality of life in the remaining days or weeks must be of first importance – age is in essence a secondary point.

REFERENCES

Alderson M.R. (1970) Terminal care in malignant disease. *British Journal of Preventive and Social Medicine* **24**, 120.

Cartwright Ann, Hockey Lisbeth & Anderson J.L. (1973) *Life Before Death.* London, Routledge & Kegan Paul.

Cherry D.A., Gourley G.K., Cousins M.J. & Gannon B.J. (1985) A technique for the insertion of an implantable portal system for the long-term epidural adminsitration of opioids in the treatment of cancer pain. *Anaesthesia and Intensive Care* **13**, 145.

Exton-Smith A.N. (1961) Terminal care in the aged. *Lancet* **2**, 305.

Kubler-Ross Elizabeth (1970) *On Death and Dying.* London, Tavistock Publications.

Lao D.B., Batina R.R. & Ray M. (1978) Multiple primary malignancy in the elderly. *Journal of the American Geriatric Society* **26**, 526.

Leader (1986) Terminal dehydration. *Lancet* **1**, 306.

Marie Curie Foundation (1952) *Report of a National Survey Concerning Patients with Cancer Nursed at Home.* London.

McKeown Florence (1965) *Pathology of the Aged.* London, Butterworth.

Oliver D.J. (1985) The use of the syringe driver in terminal care. *British Journal of Clinical Pharmacology* **20**, 515.

Parkes C.M. (1980) Terminal care: evaluation of an advisory domiciliary service at St. Christopher's Hospice. *Postgraduate Medical Journal* **56**, 685.

Rees W.D. (1972) The distress of dying. *British Medical Journal* **3**, 105.

Rees W.D. & Lutkins S.G. (1967) Mortality of bereavement. *British Medical Journal* **4**, 13.

Saunders Cicely (1960) Management of patients in the terminal stage. In *Cancer*, (Ed. Raven R.W.), Vol. 6. Philadelphia J.B. Lippincott.

Saunders Cicely (1972a) *Care of the Dying. Nursing Times.* London, Macmillan, Publishers.

Saunders Cicely (1972b) A death in the family: a professional view. In *Care of the Dying*. Department of Health and Social Security. Reports on Health and Social Security, No. 5, p. 16. London, HMSO.

Spratt J.S. (1977) Multiple primary cancers. *Cancer* **40**, 1006.

Tempest Susan M. & Clarke I.M.C. (1982) The control of pain, I: by drugs; II: by non-drug methods. In *The Dying Patient* (Ed. Wilkes E.) Lancaster, MTP.

Twycross R.G. (1986) Symptom control. *British Journal of Hospital Medicine* **36**, 244.

Wilkes E. (1965) Terminal cancer at home. *Lancet* **2**, 799.

Wilkes E. (1973) Terminal illness at home. *Modern Geriatrics* **3**, 133.

Wilson F.G. (1970) Social isolation and bereavement. *Lancet* **2**, 1356.

Wilson J.A., Lawson P.M. & Smith R.G. (1987) The treatment of terminally ill geriatric patients. *Palliative Medicine* **1**, 149.

Wright B.M. & Callan K. (1979) Slow infusion using a portable syringe driver. *British Medical Journal* **2**, 582.

22
Organization of a Geriatric Service

Older people require a wide spectrum of services varying from housing to continuing care hospital accommodation where constant nursing attention is required. The elderly are particularly vulnerable as with failing physical health comes insult to mental health in the form of bereavement, fear, retirement and loss of status in the community. Geriatric medicine is concerned with the clinical, social, preventive and remedial aspects of illness and the maintenance of health in the elderly and certain prinicples must be stated. Old people are happier and possibly healthier in their own homes. They cannot distinguish early symptoms of disease from those that they attribute to ageing. They fare better in smaller communities and when they become physically or mentally ill and require continuing hospital care this is best provided in small units in their own community. In view of the large numbers of elderly people it is essential to try and cut down the time spent by older people in long-stay hospitals or private nursing homes, and this is of course necessary for humanitarian reasons.

A comprehensive geriatric health service includes several components:

A general practitioner service backed by an efficient primary care team supported by community based nursing, social, housing, private and voluntary agencies.

The availability to the general practitioner of domiciliary consultation with consultant doctors in the various specialities, with physiotherapists, occupational therapists, opticians, dentists, clinical psychologists, speech therapists, stoma control nurses and orthotists who would also give where necessary appropriate therapy.

Co-ordination of statutory and voluntary organizations with information on all services provided for old people in the appropriate area.

Those caring for the elderly must have a full knowledge of the special features of illness in the elderly.

Older people must be kept informed of any recommendation made on their behalf and given a choice before decisions are made.

Methodology

A methodology has been developed to assist the elderly (Fig. 22.1). Ascertainment, i.e. a seeking out process, is necessary to discover early

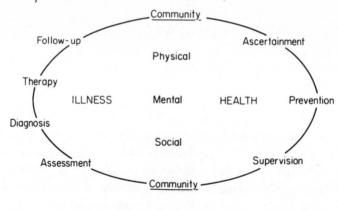

Fig. 22.1

illness and once this has been found preventive measures can be started to try and overcome or at least contain the illness detected and thus stop further deterioration. Such individuals at risk in the community must be supervised for life so that they can remain where they desire to be, in their own homes; the plan is to keep older people outwith institutions. Factors associated with illness in older people are physical disease, mental ill-health and social deprivation. Once illness has occured, accurate assessment, bearing in mind these factors mentioned above, and surveying the total disability is essential; a correct diagnosis or list of diagnoses must be made, appropriate therapy given and continued follow-up of the old person started. These are the broad lines of medical care for older people. In order to put these ways of caring for the health of the elderly into effect, it is necessary to plan a community service for old people. This can be organized from a general practitioner health centre, group practice or by a single-handed practitioner and the principles are detailed below.

Ascertainment

Self-reporting of disease by the elderly is not a satisfactory way of uncovering early pathological conditions. It is recognized that by 75 years a marked increase in morbidity has occurred and this is a possible time to commence preventive measures and all such people should be visited in their own homes. If the age of 75 and over is chosen then the person undertaking this work of ascertainment obtains job satisfacion in that morbidity to some considerable extent is uncovered. The person performing this home visit can be a nurse trained as a health educator and in the preventive aspects of illness, e.g. a health visitor. The physician commonly associated with disease who appears, uninvited, in the home of an elderly individual may not only cause apprehension but the suspicion that illness has occurred and someone has complained. The nurse who visits reports her findings to the old person's own doctor. On the other hand many general practitioners feel that they wish to do this work themselves and are well aware of all the pitfalls.

Prevention

Prevention of illness or of further disability includes measures such as attention to the patient's physical, mental or social health. For example, some adjustment in diet may be required, regular visiting by a voluntary worker may be advised, which may greatly improve the mental health, or assistance in housekeeping may be necessary. Ways may be found to entice older people out of their houses, i.e. to attend a lunch club, where they might receive remedial exercises, or join old-time dancing classes. Positive efforts should be made to encourage health. One of the main functions of the professional visitor, i.e. doctor or nurse, is to give advice on safety in the home and to encourage accident prevention. The patient's home may be quite unsuitable and a change of house may be required. If a nurse undertakes this work, in a small number of cases it may be essential for the old person to be referred to the general practitioner for examination to secure an accurate diagnosis, but many of the services required can be provided by the nurse after consultation with the general practitioner and the extra work load for the doctor is not great. Whatever is done, if the elderly person is discovered to be at risk it is necessary to arrange supervision from that time on.

Deafness is an important cause of disability in the elderly and the provision of a suitable hearing aid with correct counselling in its use is of great value (Beswick 1987).

Supervision

This supervision may be undertaken by a nurse, social worker or trained volunteer and watch is kept to try and prevent a recurrence of the factors which placed the old person at risk or caused the earlier breakdown. It is necessary also to make certain that any drugs prescribed by the physician are being taken as it is apparent from numerous studies that certain older people are not capable of taking drugs unsupervised. In such individuals, the trained visitor, in the absence of a relative, instructed specifically in administration of drugs, visits the patient's home each day and supervises the taking of the correct medicament. Repeat prescriptions in some cases result in drugs being given after they are no longer required and consultation with the general practitioner will overcome the problem. The regular visiting by a volunteer may completely transform the elderly person's life. There is no reason why elderly people cannot keep in touch with one another by telephone or why street wardens should not supervise a group of older people.

Community

Such measures give an outline of the attempt to keep older people happy and healthy in their own homes in the community. For the success of such a scheme a wide spectrum of domiciliary and community services are necessary. The domiciliary services include home helps (domestic assistants), home nursing service, friendly visitors (volunteers), chiropody (podiatry) at home, home physiotherapy or occupational therapy and meals-on-wheels. Night sitters-in are home helps who, in the absence of relatives, remain overnight in cases of acute short-term illnesses.

The work of the district nurse in the patient's own home is now mainly with the elderly and when it is possible to spread this over 24 hours it is of immense value. An important development has been the community psychiatric nurse specializing in work with older people and their familities in close collaboration with a psychogeriatric unit. Reference has already been made to the valuable use of nurses in cases of terminal illness.

For patients requiring more supervision, day hospitals are most useful for continuing therapy or observation. In many countries day centres are being constructed with a few beds to give respite care for relatives or other carers for 2–3 nights.

In many cases transport to enable old people to visit the doctor or to attend day centres or hospitals is a problem. Voluntary organizations may be able to help.

Continence of urine is of prime importance when an elderly person is being cared for at home and such an individual should have access to good advice on the prevention, treatment and management of incontinence. This can be attained by appointing a District Continence advisor who will help the professional domiciliary staff. Ideally each district should have a specialized hospital unit able to carry out urodynamic investigation to aid diagnosis in special cases. Advice regarding the management of incontinence is also needed in residential and nursing homes for elderly people (Horrocks 1986). An efficient domiciliary incontinence laundry service is essential if incontinent patients are to be cared for at home and the provision of equipment, e.g. commodes, or structural alteration to houses for individual disability should be available.

Services in the community also consist of lunch clubs or day centres (where physiotherapeutic exercises can be given), hobbies and crafts centres and counselling services. One of the great needs of the elderly is having someone to whom they can talk, and voluntary workers are now being trained to undertake this duty. Information must be given to older people on all the facilities available to them. Community services also include houses specially designed for the elderly and groups of sheltered houses with an intercommunication system connected to a caretaker. Pre-retirement training is of value (p. 13) and living in retirement courses can be arranged, and these encourage the development of a local community spirit which helps elderly people to form a group who desire to remain together when the period of instruction is over. These courses, in addition, inspire the fit elderly to help the frailer old person. In the future there will be an ever-increasing demand for continuing education for older people. Re-employment bureaux run by volunteers can supply work to those who have retired and wish a part-time post (p. 15). Many, especially in the 65–69 age group, want part-time paid employment but need help in finding it.

Ill old people

To undertake the methodology of the care of older people, a specialized geriatric service has been organized in many countries, and in the United Kingdom this arose primarily because of the pressure on hospital services for older people. It was soon discovered that when the old were standing in line for admission to hospital with the young the old tended to be pushed aside to wait. It was very understandable that if there was one acute hospital bed available and admission was requested for a patient of 25 years suffering from haematemesis and another of 75 with a cerebral infarction the choice of the doctor was usually in favour of the young patient. So beds were set aside in acute hospitals, teaching and district (the geriatric assessment unit), for the exclusive use of elderly people. This unit was founded in the belief that correct diagnosis was an essential component of the medical care of older people. It was also thought that in such special units increased knowledge about elderly ill people would be accumulated and doctors, nurses and all para-medical staff would become more skilled in dealing with elderly patients. A geriatric bed has been defined as one under the clinical control of a consultant physician in geriatric medicine and is intended for elderly patients of whom the majority are aged 75 and over who require the special skills of the department of geriatric medicine. In practice a comparison of the characteristics of elderly patients admitted to acute medical units and to geriatric units showed that those admitted to geriatric units were older, stayed longer and suffered mainly from chronic disorders. Those admitted to acute medical units had acute problems and were correctly placed. Very few elderly people were admitted for purely social reasons (Covell & Angus 1980). In some areas all patients with medical complaints 75 years and over are admitted to the geriatric units in district general hospitals.

Assessment

An old person who becomes ill and reports to the doctor is in the first instance best assessed at home, attention being paid not only to the possible diagnosis but also to the social conditions and the relationship that exists between the elderly individual and the relatives. There may of course be no relatives or there may be a deep misunderstanding and lack of affection between the old person and those who are present. This would influence the final decision as to placement when the patient is better. The home may be so unsuitable or so dirty that alternative accommodation may have to be found. If the old person requires admission to hospital these social conditions can be attended to, e.g. a dirty house cleaned, while the patient is being treated and discharge from the hospital is thus not delayed. It is the common practice for physicians in charge of the assessment wards to visit the old person at home prior to admission. The general practitioner who has requested hospital admission readily allows the physician to make this comprehensive assessment visit. This gives time, before admission, to make accurate plans about physical, social and mental rehabilitation. The relatives or neighbours are asked to build up the patient's mental health during the time the older person awaits hospital admission. Many elderly people still think they are being advised to enter hospital either because their relatives want rid of them or to die. The period before admission can be used to correct these impressions. This assessment visit gives the hospital physician a complete picture of the home circumstances and prevents discharge from hospital to totally unsuitable surroundings. It also is of great value in increasing empathy between the old person and the hospital doctor, e.g. the older patient after coming into hospital may recognize the physician who performed the home visit. Frequently following admission to a geriatric unit the older person, not surprisingly, wants to go home and tells the doctor a completely unrealistic story of home conditons. If the physician can reply with knowledge about the accurate state of the home the older individual accepts with amazing complacency the true situation. Caird & Judge (1979) have given excellent guidance on assessment of the elderly patient.

Diagnosis

The need for elderly patients is for accurate diagnosis or, more precisely, an accurate list of diagnoses. This is essential and fundamental to the working of any geriatric service. It is still not uncommon for quite serious illness to be missed as the symptoms are attributed to the ageing process. If the general practitioner has had previous knowledge of the elderly person or if this information has been supplied by the nurse who in routine preventive visits has previously seen this old person much time can be saved. The greatest problem in making an accurate diagnosis in older people is to find time for the doctor to take a detailed history and perform the necessary complete clinical examination.

Therapy

The patient is then given appropriate therapy. In many instances the elderly patient requires hospital admission as many conditions in the elderly, hemiplegia, mental confusion or incontinence, are extremely difficult to treat in the patient's own home. The special dangers of many drugs, e.g. digoxin, in older people must be kept in mind.

Follow-up

Once the therapy is completed and the patient has recovered at home or returned from hospital then follow-up visits should be organized and continuity of care ensured. These home visits can be paid by a nurse who makes sure that the old person has received, for example, any nursing or social services that have been requested and are required. The nurse also makes certain that the patient is taking only the medicines that have been ordered and reports back to the old person's own general practitioner (p. 344). The plan is to prevent recurrence of illness or re-admission and keep the old person in health in the community. There are indications, however, that the occasional visit by the general practitioner is of immense value.

The health centre

General practitioners working in groups of six to 12 in a health centre serving a population of 20–30 000 people are in an ideal position to help their elderly patients. In such a community there are approximately 3–4000 people over 65 (Fig. 22.2).

From the hospital, the consultant physician in geriatric medicine, the

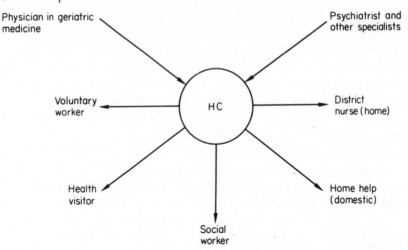

Physician in geriatric
medicine

Psychiatrist and
other specialists

Voluntary
worker

H C

District
nurse (home)

Health
visitor

Home help
(domestic)

Social
worker

Population served 20-30 000
containing 3-4000 elderly people (over 65)

Fig. 22.2 Health centre organization.

psychiatrist, and other specialists can come and meet the general practitioners at the centre. These specialists run an out-patient service, with a
session as often as is necessary, and the physician in geriatric medicine
also acts to guide the plan of regular visiting of elderly people in the community and encourage and stimulate his general practitioner colleagues in
the care of their elderly patients. The consultant physician in geriatric
medicine should make certain that the doctors at the health centre are kept
informed about any new developments in the provision of services for
elderly people and should advise on research projects especially for
obtaining accurate information of the local needs of the old people.

It is suggested that out of five or more general practitioners one might
have a special interest in diseases of and services for old people. He does
not see all the elderly people attending the centre, as each practitioner has
his own patients, but he is available for guidance in any special problem
should his advice be sought by his colleagues.

The district nurses and health visitors form the nursing team with the
district nurse performing her traditional role in the community, being
helped by nursing assistants, while the health visitor acts as the agent who
visits the 75 and over group. The nursing team works in close co-operation
with the doctors and with the chiropodist and is in a position to advise the
doctor when his patient requires the service of a chiropodist. The social
worker has an office in the health centre and is responsible for the co-
ordination of the social services and available for advice on problems of

housing and where social conditions are concerned. She acts as a psychosocial caseworker and as the guide to voluntary workers and is responsible in the main for provision of domiciliary services, such as meals-on-wheels, and is able to give advice on all services for the elderly including any necessary enquiries about financial aid. The home help service is organized from the health centre and the dietitian visits the centre from time to time giving advice to all those working in the patient's home about dietetic problems and making sure that the meals-on-wheels supplied are appropriate for the elderly. Representatives of voluntary organizations also attend the health centre and local ministers of religion look in and give them valuable support. A joint medical and social assessment of the older person's needs is essential. The physical and mental health of the individual must be estimated in association with the social circumstances. The social worker requires to correlate relevant medical and social information to make sure that the correct services are provided. The establishment of the health centre ensures a one-door service for all the old people in a local community so that they themselves or their relatives know where to ask for advice or help if need arises. Similar arrangements can be made in a group or a single-handed practice using the members of the health care team.

The area geriatric service

This is based on the teaching hospital or district hospital, and in the example discussed the population served is taken as 200 000. The geriatric services are under the control of four physicians in geriatric medicine with supporting medical staff who have a defined area with a definite population. The geriatric assessment unit is situated in the principal hospital where as well as acute beds there are also psychiatric beds; the out-patient department and the day hospital for the elderly are also situated there (Fig. 22.3).

The geriatric unit has in support of the assessment beds, beds in continuing treatment hospital units in two sites, one in the area served by the health centre and adjacent to the patient's own home and one as part of the teaching or district hospital. It is better in planning new services to avoid the use of the term long-stay and to call all such hospitals annexes, continuing treatment hospital units. The words 'long-stay' imply to the patient and his relatives that there is no active treatment when in fact skilled medical and nursing attention, occupational therapy and physio-therapy, chiropody and perhaps speech therapy may be taking place.

The components of the hospital service are:
1 Acute hospital beds for intensive care, reserved for patients of any age

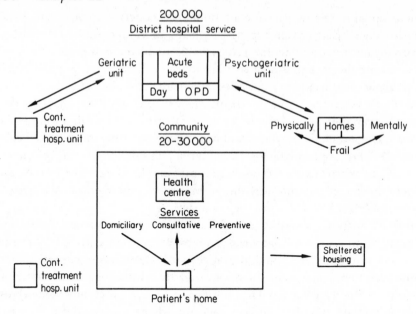

Fig. 22.3 Area geriatric service organization.

. who require urgent and specialized resuscitative measures.

2 A geriatric unit for illness requiring the special facilities for elderly people which it offers.

3 Psychiatric beds for those requiring the specialized treatment of the psychiatrist.

With a similar catchment area for the psychiatric beds, the acute beds and the geriatric unit, agreement between the general physicians, the physician practising geriatric medicine and the psychiatrist can be reached in the majority of ill old people. Those requiring intensive care should go to the intensive care unit; those with the sudden onset of illness who are elderly almost certainly go to the geriatric unit; while those with longstanding mental illness, requiring specialist psychiatrist advice continue to go to the separate psychiatric unit. Small psychogeriatric units have been used for these old people whom the psychiatrist considered unsuitable for his wards, the geriatric physician unacceptable for his unit, and for whom the social services director considered did not require admission to an old person's home. These ensure that no individuals are left uncared for in their own homes with the general practitioner being unable to obtain any help at all. In such units, jointly run by a psychiatrist interested in the elderly and a physician in geriatric medicine, around half of all people admitted directly can be sent home.

Over the years different ways of organizing geriatric assessment units in hospital have emerged. As mentioned above some are age-related and in others consultants in geriatric medicine in co-operation with general physicians run joint wards. The important element is that any ward admitting elderly patients needs full provision of staff with special training in the care of the elderly including the remedial professions and must offer facilities specifically suitable for the elderly. Of prime importance is that there should be an adequate number of beds with full investigational provision supported by continuing treatment beds. Admission of the elderly ill patient must be prompt; waiting lists are unacceptable.

Many hospitals have successful units under the supervision of the department of geriatric medicine and that of orthopaedics and consultation with other specialists is a consistent feature of geriatric medical practice. Stroke units have also been established with excellent results and a few hospitals have set aside beds for hospice-type care.

No elderly patient should be admitted directly from home or another hospital into a long-term hospital bed. Ideally no long-stay patient or resident should have anything but his or her own room and privacy is essential (Horrocks 1986).

The hospital service should also provide day hospital and out-patient facilities. Attached to each teaching and district hospital and essential for serving the geriatric assessment unit are continuing treatment hospital beds. These hospitals are best not to be too large and the unit used in the service in Glasgow is of 120 beds. Such units should be especially designed with such equipment as disposable bedpans and urinals, with many single rooms, with excellent observation for nursing staff, wide corridors and plenty of space for continuing rehabilitation, ample day space and physiotherapy and occupational therapy departments. Regular visiting of such beds by the consultant physician specializing in geriatric medicine is essential, and the morale of medical, nursing and para-medical staff must be maintained. This means good communication, the constant flow of new ideas and stimulation by teaching sessions.

Personalized clothing service including personal underwear makes a major contribution to rehabilitaton in continuing treatment and long-stay wards. Co-ordinators of voluntary services have also been of great help in spreading awareness of the contribution which voluntary workers can make working in wards for the elderly, e.g. in music classes or art therapy.

One suggested number of beds is that for each population sector of 200 000 the geriatric assessment unit in the district or teaching hospital should contain approximately 100 beds. Continuing treatment beds should be available to bring the total for the 200 000 inhabitants to about 400 beds. In our unit the ratio of assessment to continuing treatment beds has been estimated ideally to be 1:9 for females and 1:2.5 for males. An estimate of the number of geriatric beds required varies from 10 per 1000 elderly to 18 per 1000 over 65 years. This figure depends on many factors; the number of women available as nurses and for ancillary work in the area, the housing services available for old people, the extent of private beds outwith the health service and the wealth of the local population are some. Traditionally there have been a greater number of beds for the elderly in hospitals in Scotland; this may have been due to the smaller number of private nursing home beds. Figures have now been given for the minimum number of beds and staff (Table 22.1).

Table 22.1 (from Andrews & Brocklehurst 1987)

Minimum numbers per 1000 population 75 years and over	
Hospital beds	22.0
Consultant physicians in geriatric medicine (at least	
two geriatricians in each district)	0.21
Trained occupational therapists	0.45
Trained physiotherapists	0.47
Nurses (a maximum of beds per nurse)	
Morning and afternoon	4.8
Evening	6.9
At night	10.0

A major time of difficulty is in making safe arrangements for a smooth transition of the older patient from hospital to home. In many units after careful consultation with the carers and arrangements for appropriate domiciliary services, a district nurse attached to the geriatric unit visits the patient's home either the day of discharge or shortly after to ensure that any services arranged have actually been provided. The drug therapy can be re-checked with the patient and the carer and a general assessment can be made of the prospective success of the discharge.

Community services

The other constituents of the area geriatric services are homes for both the physically and mentally frail and sheltered housing. At present there is an outstanding demand for places in homes, purposely built for physically frail old people. Such homes should be specially designed and have no steps or stairs, wide doors on the lavatories, freestanding baths, ample lounge accommodation and wash-hand basins and WCs for every room. In Scotland, the numbers in such homes have been restricted to about 60 people; these are mainly single or widowed women.

It is likely in the future that homes for the mentally frail will also be essential for individuals who have passed through the diagnostic net of the geriatric physician and the psychiatrist and for whom no further hospitalization is necessary. It should be a rule that no one should enter these specialized homes without preliminary complete assessment and diagnosis by, preferably, both geriatric physician and psychiatrist interested in the elderly. By careful design a therapeutic environment can be created and elderly mentally confused people improve markedly. Trained nursing staff can be minimal and a grouping of around 30 old people is usual.

Regular visits by the physician specializing in geriatric medicine should be made to homes for the physically frail, and the psychiatrists interested in the elderly should also visit the homes for the mentally frail regularly. Where these latter homes have been constructed they have taken a tremendous load off the hospital service. It can be dogmatically stated, however, that shortage of beds in one part of the service produces overloading or breakdown in other sectors.

Adequate cover by consultants is essential for all hospital units to ensure that the consultant does not have overall care of too many beds. In psychiatry, as in geriatric medicine, it is essential that assessment beds are adequately equipped to make a correct and comprehensive diagnosis possible.

Over recent years there has been a rapid and massive increase in the numbers of private nursing home beds in the United Kingdom. Many of them are occupied by elderly patients not so severely disabled as those in long-term hospital units. Patients in nursing homes were far less dependent than those in long-term care wards (Capewell *et al.* 1986). Careful clinical assessment is essential before a patient is admitted to a nursing home.

Homes for the physically and mentally frail should not be regarded as final or an end point in a system. Older people admitted to these homes may, with care, attention and continued therapy improve so much that they can advance to protected or sheltered housing. This type of housing has, in the main, taken over from the traditional old person's home and with 24-hour supervision by a warden can give the old person both freedom of action and the opportunity to communicate in a friendly way with neighbours while still protected by someone on call all the time. This is best accomplished by an intercommunication system between each elderly person and the warden's flat, and if the design of the sheltered housing is good the warden's office is situated at the entry to the housing so that an eye can be kept open for unwanted visitors or vandals and thus the housing is protected by the presence of the warden and also by trying to ensure that unwanted visitors are kept out. There is great need for rapid expansion of this type of housing, and it is recommended that 50 sheltered houses be provided for every 1000 elderly people (p. 351).

Geriatric teamwork

In the geriatric unit there is a team consisting of physicians in geriatric medicine, supporting medical staff, specially trained nurses, physiotherapists, occupational therapists, chiropodists, speech therapists and secretarial assistance. The domiciliary team based on the health centre consists of district nurse, health visitor, physiotherapist, occupational therapist, chiropodist, social worker and voluntary worker. Co-ordination is accomplished by the physician in geriatric medicine coming from the hospital to the health centre and by the social worker in the hospital being in contact with the social worker in the health centre. The district nurse, health visitor and members of the preventive and therapeutic team are with the general practitioner and under his guidance members of the health care team.

At the geriatric unit in the hospital there is a weekly case conference when each member of the ward team, i.e. doctors, nurses, physiotherapists, occupational therapists and social workers, meet. The present condition of every patient in the ward is discussed in detail regarding progress, continuing therapy and prospects and planning for discharge. At this meeting the district nurses attached to the unit who have followed up the older patients who have been discharged to their own homes report on any problems encountered. Team work is an essential ingredient of an organized geriatric service.

Patients requiring the skills of the psychiatrist or of the geriatric physician and those in the intensive care unit and the acute beds, day hospital and out-patient department are all in the same hospital area.

In addition to the services mentioned above, there is ample scope for voluntary service in the form of sheltered housing in the locality of the health centre or as nursing homes for those suffering from cancer or those who are dying, again run by voluntary organizations.

The flow through geriatric units in the teaching or district hospital depends on the provision of the correct personnel, equipment and amenity and cannot be accomplished without adequate continuing treatment hospital accommodation, day hospital and day-centre facilities. Linked to this must be adequate follow-up services based on the health centre with appropriate accommodation for physically and mentally frail older people, adequate provision of sheltered housing and a wide range of domiciliary services.

In addition to the services mentioned above, night sitters-in during short-term illness, laundry for the incontinent, provision of specialized equipment on loan and adaption of houses where required to suit disabled people are all essential. The growing importance of training for retirement, of hobbies and crafts centres for those retired and retired employees' associations have been mentioned before, and while every attention must be given to the long-stay patient every effort must also be made to try and prevent disability and to improve the morale and mental health of the aged person.

Teaching in geriatric medicine has placed an additional but necessary duty on physicians practising geriatric medicine and instruction to professional and non-professional carers must be continued and expanded.

The growing realization of the need to help the carers means that post-discharge contact with relatives is important. There is a growing number of support groups, e.g. for suffers from Alzheimer disease and parkinsonism, and these can provide valuable guidance and help. Many geriatric day hospitals run stroke clubs while the Crossroads Care Attendant Scheme is of immense assistance (p. 353). In certain countries, e.g. New Zealand, the carer of a long-term invalid is entitled by law to 14 days holiday every year either by admission of the invalid to suitable accommodation or by building up services in the invalid's own home. Intermittent hospital admission while not without its problems (Rai *et al.* 1986) may be essential to protect the health of the carer. In the practice of geriatric medicine there is one fundamental rule when re-admission to hospital is promised if home care fails this re-admission must be immediate otherwise faith in the service will disappear and mutual trust vanish.

Brotherston (1969) writing on the National Health Service stated: 'Demographic change and the development from a comparatively young society produced by the large Victorian birth-rates, to a society with a more normal proportion of elderly, the so-called ageing society, still seems to take us by surprise. Although it has been emerging inevitably and has been publicized and discussed for many years, it is extraordinary that there should still be a prevailing atmosphere almost of grievance that this should have happened to us. . . . Perforce we must come to terms with the fact that the aged are here to stay and in increasing numbers; this is the kind of society we live in. Two things seem certain. Nothing will really flow smoothly in the Health Service until we reach an adequate stage of provision in our society for the elderly. This means many things apart from hospital beds. The other is that a major phenomenon of the elderly vis-à-vis the Health Service is under-demand not over-demand. Later generations of elderly may benefit in health from having been nurtured in earlier years in a better environment. But they will not be so stoic in the face of disability or so unwisely sparing of the medical services as are our contemporary veterans.'

REFERENCES

Andrews K. & Brocklehurst J. (1987) *British Geriatric Medicine in the 1980s.* London, King Edward's Hospital Fund.

Beswick K.B.J (1987) Today, there's none so deaf as cannot be helped. *Geriatric Medicine* **17**, 55.

Brotherston J.H.F. (1969) Change and the National Health Service. *Scottish Medical Journal* **14**, 130.

Caird F.I. & Judge T.G. (1979) *Assessment of the Elderly Patient.* Tunbridge Wells, Pitman Medical.

Capewell Ann E., Primrose W.R. & MacIntyre Celia (1986) Nursing dependency in registered nursing homes and long term care geriatric wards in Edinburgh. *British Medical Journal* **292**, 1719.

Covell B. & Angus Margaret M. (1980) A comparison of the characteristics of elderly people admitted to acute medical wards and general wards. *Health Bulletin (Edin)* **38**, 64.

Horrocks P. (1986) The components of a comprehensive district health service for elderly people – a personal view. *Age and Ageing* **15**, 321.

Rai G.S., Birlawska G., Murphy P.J. & Wright G. (1986) Hazards for elderly people admitted for respite (holiday admissions) and social care (social admissions). *British Medical Journal* **292**, 240.

Appendix I
Services Available for Old People

In the United Kingdom there is a wide variety of services available to old people which can help the general practitioner in the care of elderly patients (Horrocks 1986). Legislation in recent years has tended to divide these services into separate compartments rather than to unify them.

Any doctor entering general practice in a new area should contact the director of social service, the nearest geriatric unit, the director of housing and the secretaries of the local housing associations. He should also make himself known to the secretaries of voluntary organizations such as Age Concern (The Old People's Welfare Committee), Help the Aged, Crossroads Care Attendant Scheme, the British Red Cross Society and the Women's Royal Voluntary Service. An active liaison with the clergymen of the locality is also strongly recommended. The application of common sense to the problem of the elderly person and the seeking of assistance from the most appropriate organization is of immense help to the patient.

The general aim of the services organized by the health and social services is to keep old people in their own homes rather than in residential accommodation or in hospital. This is done by providing the form of service most appropriate to the need of the elderly individual. The organization of such services for old people include domiciliary, residential, housing, hospital and community facilities.

Domiciliary services

Home helps

The local authority social service department provides a home help service but the amount of time actually spent in the house by the home help varies greatly from district to district. In some areas no charge is made to all old people for this service but it is usual for an elderly individual living alone on supplementary benefit to pay nothing. In other places charges are graduated in line with the individual's personal income. The home help's main duties are to keep the house clean, to cook and shop for the household, and to do all washing where this is practicable.

The home help is not usually expected to attend on a Saturday

343

afternoon or a Sunday but many social service departments* have a Sunday morning service for old people living alone who require this attention. An evening service is also available in most areas. In some parts of the country a night service is provided where the home help sits in with the patient during the night and thus allows the family a good night's sleep. For a short-term illness this service can prevent the need for a hospital bed if the old person desires to remain at home and be treated by the family doctor provided he is willing to cope. The home help night-sitter is not a nurse and cannot be expected to do more than an interested and well-intentioned relative.

Home nursing

The home nursing service is provided by the area health authority and is of course well known to the general practitioner. This group of nurses is an invaluable aid to the doctor and the elderly benefit greatly from this help. In many districts a domiciliary night nursing service is available, and where this is not provided night nursing in the patient's home may be obtained in some areas for those suffering from cancer from the Marie Curie Foundation. The Foundation provides nurses as sitters-in during the night who will also undertake nursing duties. Both the Marie Curie Foundation and the Macmillan nurses provide an advisory service for patients with cancer. The initial introduction of this service, however, depends on a doctor's request.

After-care

Many general practitioners now have health visitors and district nurses attached to their own practices and these nurses are of great use in visiting initially all patients discharged from geriatric units.

In many geriatric assessment units district nurses are seconded in a part-time capacity from the area health authority. The nurses follow up the patients who have been discharged from the geriatric unit and ensure continuity of care. These same nurses also inform the general practitioner of what is happening to the patient and keep in regular touch. While the patient is in hospital, the district nurse joins the ward round and can visit if so desired, the old person's home, making sure that it is being prepared for the patient's return. These nurses can also keep the hospital physician responsible for the patient's treatment informed as to the present social conditions of his patient. On occasion the district nurse

*Social service department is called social work department in Scotland.

accompanies the patient when discharged from hospital, but more commonly she calls the next day to check that all the services requested are in operation. She can find out if the home help has come, if the fire is lit and if there is food in the house. The first 2 days following the patient's discharge from hospital are often the most difficult and certainly the most worrying from the hospital doctor's point of view.

This type of liaison is described only to show the great advantages of close co-operation, and there is ample scope for experiments of this kind to ensure that continuity of patient care occurs. The general practitioner is notified in the usual way when his patient is discharged from hospital by an immediate discharge note, but the district nurse can help him greatly by the routine visiting of those patients. The aim of such a service is to make sure that all concerned with the care of the old ill person are fully acquainted with the present medical and social circumstances.

Where the services of a specially trained nurse in the care of patients with a stoma are available this is most helpful.

Laundry services

In many areas a free or low-price laundry service is provided for the elderly, particularly the incontinent aged; this is a most valuable social service.

Chiropody service

Local health authorities are empowered to provide a chiropody service for the elderly and various schemes are in operation throughout the country. Visits by chiropodists to the elderly person's home can be arranged.

Physiotherapy and occupational therapy

Home treatment by physiotherapists is available and the services of an occupational therapist can also be arranged. As previously noted these experts are of great help in suggesting alterations to houses or equipment to make life much easier for the elderly person. Day hospitals for continuing supervision and therapy are attached to many geriatric and psychogeriatric units.

Meals-on-wheels

Meals-on-wheels, i.e. hot meals distributed to the homes of old people, is another service provided often by voluntary organizations but with social service department monetary grants. Social service departments have powers to provide directly domiciliary services such as meals-on-wheels for old people, or they can organize their supply with the assistance of such bodies as the Women's Royal Voluntary Service, or Age Concern (Old People's Welfare Committee). The people who receive this service are nominated by, for example, a health visitor, a social worker or a voluntary worker. Meals-on-wheels are seldom provided every day of the week; often only on 2 days per week, and are intended for housebound individuals. Besides meals-on-wheels, there are lunch clubs in most areas for those who can walk unaided, in old people's clubs or day centres run by voluntary organizations. Small charges are made for these meals; the service being subsidized by the local authority.

Home adaptations

It is on occasion desirable that adaptations be made to the homes of old people to help them to retain their independence. Handrails and fitments, e.g. around WCs and other adaptations considered essential can be provided as welfare services for the disabled under the Social Work Act to suit the needs of old people by the social service department. Consultation with the physician specializing in geriatric medicine may result in additional suggestions of help to the patient. These adaptations are usually arranged following a visit to the patient's house by an occupational therapist on the staff of the social service department whose advice is often invaluable.

Home medical and nursing equipment

The provision of home medical equipment is granted under the general principle that appliances which must be tailor made to individuals are the responsibility of the area health authority. On discharge from hospital special equipment required by a patient without which he would have to remain in hospital for treatment is the responsibility of the health authority. Items of home nursing equipment, e.g. a commode or bedpan, recommended by the general practitioner other than those prescribed on Form EC 10 should be provided by the social work department. In many areas the British Red Cross Society and other voluntary organizations also supply such items. If there is occasional incontinence in bed, incontinence pads should be provided. For the patient who is incontinent and ambulant it may be necessary to obtain plastic pants with an insert of an incontinence pad (Kanga Pants). There are many gadgets that are of use to older disabled people and some are described in *Home Made Aids for Handi-*

capped People (1974) and by Nichols (1981). *Modern British Geriatric Care* (1970) covers a wide variety of useful subjects such as co-ordination of services for the elderly and of help for old people with mental illness. Many helpful references and addresses are given by Muriel Skeet (1982), and the use of hoists for disabled people is comprehensively described by Christine Tarling (1980).

Invalid chairs supplied on a permanent basis are the responsibility of the area health authority, but voluntary bodies, such as the British Red Cross Society, usually lend a wheelchair for a temporary period if one is required. Health authorities also supply, on a temporary basis, such items as spinal carriages, hospital-type beds and self-lifting apparatus, where in the opinion of the hospital authorities such items are required for the continuation of treatment begun in hospital or if the patient would still have been in hospital if he had not obtained them. If an elderly person at home, however, requires a hydraulic-type hoist to make the nursing care possible and to get him in and out of bed then this apparatus can be provided by the local authority.

General practitioner service

The general practitioner provides the medical service for the elderly sick person and is the person who has the greatest power to help his elderly patient and his advice and experience can be of the utmost value. The preventive aspects of geriatric medicine have been discussed (p. 7), and some method of ensuring a regular medicosocial check on elderly people, especially those living alone, seems urgently necessary. Older people benefit greatly from a routine medical examination and some cases require investigation in hospital. It is important to try and define the different categories of old people so that a decision may be made as to which type of accommodation is most suitable to meet the needs of the older citizen. The best place for the great majority of older people is their own home and the best person to care for them when they are ill is their own general practitioner. The doctor should enlist help whenever it is required from people such as the district nurse, health visitor, social worker, home help or voluntary worker and should obtain any necessary apparatus for home nursing, e.g. a commode, through the district nursing service, the British Red Cross Society or appropriate authority. After the illness is over and if the elderly person has no relatives or has been left in a state of extreme frailty it may have to be decided whether an independent existence can be maintained, and the three factors of physical health, mental health and social conditions are assessed.

Residential accommodation

The social service department has referred to it, old people who are getting near the stage of requiring residential accommodation. The request may come from relatives, from friends, clergymen or doctors. Such old people are visited in their own homes by social workers who can discuss their problems and if necessary arrange welfare accommodation. If the old person does not wish to enter such residential accommodation the services at home can be built up.

Residential accommodation for persons, who by reason of age, infirmity or any other circumstances are in need of care and attention not otherwise available to them, is provided by the social service department which also has a duty to provide temporary accommodation for persons who are in need under such circumstances as the local authority may in any particular case determine. In relation to old people, temporary accommodation is valuable when its provision allows relatives caring for the elderly to have a holiday.

Many social service departments now provide purpose-built hostels which can care for elderly frail people: the frail ambulant home. Older people should not be advised to go into residential accommodation until they can no longer look after themselves in their own homes. The physical and mental health of the individual remains in a better state if he has to think and act for himself. There are, however, always exceptions to any principle and some older people do like the company of others. The frail ambulant home is of the greatest help to the physician practising geriatric medicine as it provides an outlet from hospital for the very old and less robust people.

The decision as to whether an older person should be admitted to hospital or to frail ambulant accommodation is sometimes difficult. It must be recalled that if there is a possible doubt about diagnosis or any chance of improving the patient's physical or mental health a preliminary period in hospital is worthwhile. This applies particularly to those being considered for admission to a nursing home. Some of the other guiding principles in common use are simply these; the acutely ill or those needing continuous nursing care or supervision are the responsibility of the hospital. The hospital service must also retain those of the elderly sick who have completed active treatment but still require further rehabilitation in hospital. These old people who are confused or disturbed to a degree making it impossible to care for them in a residential home are also a hospital responsibility. Lastly, older people who remain incontinent of urine or faeces must be treated in hospital; those with occasional urinary incontinence can be cared for in frail ambulant homes.

It is always worth keeping in mind that the cause of the incontinence must be sought and that doctors attending patients in frail ambulant accommodation should seek the help of the hospital consultant in order to make a firm diagnosis before assuming that the incontinence is irremediable.

Local authority residential accommodation should undertake the care of residents during minor illnesses that may involve a period of bed rest and that are of the type normally treated by the general practitioner and district nurse in a patient's own home.

The care of the infirm old person who may need help in dressing, assistance to the lavatory, and who may have to live on one level because he cannot climb stairs, should be the responsibility of the local authority.

In recent years the social service departments have taken responsibility for the mildly mentally confused old person who does not require continuous nursing care or supervision. These people should have been examined by a psychiatrist or a physician in geriatric medicine and a diagnosis made and all appropriate treatment given. If, in spite of this, the patient remains in the same condition, permanent accommodation may have to be found for him. Some social service departments have constructed purpose-built hostels for these slightly mentally disordered people. In other areas these individuals are accepted into frail ambulant homes and cared for there. The homes for mentally disordered old people appear very satisfactory provided a complete assessment of the patient's physical and mental condition is performed before the old person is admitted to such a hostel (de Zoysa & Blessed 1984). Many physicians in geriatric medicine advise a short period of admission to a geriatric unit for assessment or alternatively assessment in a mental hospital by a psychiatrist before a final decision is made about the old person's proper destination.

It has been repeatedly recommended that if the resident in a residential home develops an illness that is likely in the doctor's opinion to be rapidly fatal and for which he feels that no active surgical or specialized hospital treatment is necessary, the patient should be left where he is. In other words, the patient if he had had a home of his own would have remained there when it was considered that no further treatment or nursing care was going to be of value. The domiciliary services can be employed to help the staff of the old person's home when this added support is required. However, there are occasions when several old people are seriously ill and the sheer weight of nursing responsibility makes it impossible for the elderly patients to be kept in the home. A commonsense attitude must therefore be adopted and hospitals should be prepared to accept old people gravely ill with terminal diseases from old people's homes when the official in charge is no longer able to carry what may be a very heavy burden. In many areas there are voluntary homes run by the Marie Curie Foundation or various religious organizations who have a valuable and highly important function in caring for patients irremediably ill with carcinoma. In many areas there are excellent hospices for those requiring admission and most of them run an advisory service. Some consultant physicians have developed terminal care as a speciality and their advice is most helpful in the patient's own home while the specialist oncologist is also available to assist in many districts. The care of the dying is a most essential service in a community where so many elderly people have no relatives and when in skilled hands and with modern therapy ease of mind and relief of pain can be given when the patient's need is greatest.

Residential homes should not, however, accept responsibility for prolonged nursing care for the bedfast or those who are persistently incontinent. They are best used in caring for the frail elderly person. When discussing accommodation in a residential home with the elderly, mention must be made that the residents in such places pay for their maintenance according to their means. Assistance is given when necessary from the Department of Health and Social Security. In every case the resident is left with a small weekly income as pocket money.

In summary, residential homes are suitable for old people who are feeble and weak but who would be able to live in their own homes assisted by an unskilled relative if they possessed such advantages.

Special housing for the elderly

A housing authority must provide special housing and flats for the elderly. Some authorities have small houses or flatlets grouped together in a community with a warden who keeps a general watch over the residents. Crookston Home in Glasgow was a pioneer centre for such a scheme; the people there have their own small houses and are issued with rations to cook their own morning and evening meals and odd cups of tea but are served with a mid-day meal in small pleasant communal dining rooms. Visits are paid regularly by nursing sisters to make sure all is well.

In some areas voluntary agencies have bought houses and given each old person a room with cooking apparatus, which they furnish themselves, and varying degrees of domestic help are supplied; one resident housekeeper supervises six to eight people. In this respect much accommodation is provided through the agency of voluntary organizations. The social service department has a duty to co-operate with and co-ordinate these invaluable voluntary services which have such a large part to play in services for the elderly, such as home visiting. It must be kept in mind that arrangements do vary considerably from district to district. The idea of grouped flatlets that are warden supervized has much to commend it and many housing authorities have built sheltered houses for the elderly and have also co-operated with voluntary housing associations to provide additional similar protected housing (p. 339). These associations have expanded greatly and some have constructed extracare sheltered housing with additional supportive staff for those very elderly people with increasing frailty.

Hospital service (p. 335)

An elderly person may require to be admitted to hospital as an emergency case because of obstruction of the bowels, a fractured femur, myocardial infarct or a pneumonia, and in most cases he should be sent to the intensive care or the appropriate surgical or medical unit. The acute medical and surgical wards should not be closed to old ill people and the physician in geriatric medicine should try to play his part in ensuring that these acute beds are not occupied by elderly patients no longer in need of these facilities. A geriatric unit would be indicated if the elderly patient required investigation or assessment and rehabilitation. The practice of hospital medicine is changing and while the present trend of the establishment of intensive care units persists it would indeed be inadvisable to have separate units of such high quality for young and old. Thus the acutely ill old person, if necessary, should be admitted to an intensive care area. Other ill old people not requiring the expert attention of the surgical team or other specialist care, e.g. gynaecologist, ophthalmologist, orthopaedic surgeon or dermatologist, tend more and more to be referred to the geriatric service.

Local custom and the preference of individual general practitioners frequently decides the destination of the patient, but the physician in geriatric medicine should be regarded as particularly qualified in the complete investigation and assessment of elderly ill people and their rehabilitation and restorative therapy. In some districts all people over 75 years except those requiring acute surgical attention are admitted to the geriatric unit. Patients with long-term illness or terminal illnesses requiring medical or nursing care should be admitted to the geriatric service. Various systems of combining medical and geriatric wards are in operation with the expert knowledge of the physician in geriatric medicine being available.

If, in the opinion of the general practitioner, relatives need relief from the continuous care of an elderly invalid the geriatric unit should be prepared to help so that a holiday or at least a rest can be obtained by the family. In like manner the frail old person should be admitted to accommodation provided by the social service department in order to give the relatives a holiday if this is desired or becomes essential.

The special skill in rehabilitation of the physician in geriatric medicine should be kept in mind by physicians and surgeons when an elderly person has shown a limited response to treatment and where mobility has not been restored. This is particularly relevant in the care of patients with strokes and the therapeutic environment of the geriatric unit is of great help to such individuals. Watch must be kept that the opportunity for rehabilitation is not missed and chronic disability allowed to develop. Persistent incontinence of urine or faeces or both should be regarded as an urgent indication for early admission to a geriatric unit and it should only be exceptional for the continuously incontinent patient to be discharged home unless services, including laundry, can be provided for the patient. The advice of the physician in geriatric medicine should be sought promptly.

Hospitals are of prime importance in the early diagnosis of difficult medical problems of the elderly. The insidious onset of disease, the slow appearance of almost unnoticable symptoms and the happy results that follow correct diagnosis should lead to a full use of the diagnosis and treatment facilities of the hospital. Early admission, full and correct diagnosis, discharge home: these are the aims of a hospital service. The geriatric day hospital is an extension of in-patient care and forms a bridge between hospital and community. Elderly patients are referred to a day hospital for rehabilitation, maintenance treatment, medical or nursing investigation or if requiring too much care, e.g. nursing, for the day centre, for social companionship. The attendance at the day hospital by the old person provides a time of relief for many overworked relatives. The transport of the elderly disabled person is the main problem in organization. The future of day hospitals and evaluation of costs have been reviewed by Hildick-Smith (1981; 1984).

Community services

It has already been recommended that the practising doctor in any area should consult his local director of social service. He should also contact the secretary of the local Age Concern (Old People's Welfare Committee) who should be able to tell him of the work done for older people by the local branch of the Women's Royal Voluntary Service, the British Red Cross Society, the local churches, in many areas the Rotary Club, and the Council of Social Service. Reference has been made to the Scottish Retirement Council and the Retired Employees' Associations, and inquiry from the personnel officers of the larger industrial firms in the area may often reveal schemes for helping older people which are not generally known. On a national level Age Concern, formerly the National Old People's Welfare Council, the Centre for Policy on Ageing and the Pre-Retirement Association in London provide useful and most relevant information. Help the Aged now play a most important part in funding new services for old people and in publishing useful booklets.

Voluntary organizations provide such services as old people's homes, old people's clubs, some of which are all-day, lunch clubs, and, in co-operation with the local authority, meals-on-wheels. Many such organizations arrange routine home visits to housebound people and some, e.g. Crossroads, provide care attendants to relieve overburdened relatives. Help with repairs in the home, holidays at reduced rates and home entertainment are some of the activities of these bodies. Retired Employees' Associations are playing an important part in the welfare of the retired worker. Many people feel that the local authorities in the larger areas should appoint a doctor with special knowledge and interest in the elderly to co-operate with the local physician specializing in geriatric medicine.

Day centres and clubs for older people are provided by statutory bodies like the social service departments and also by many voluntary organizations. Some are open all day and supply morning coffee, lunch and afternoon tea with facilities for social activities of many kinds. Chiropody, hairdressing and laundry services are available in some. These day centres and clubs encourage local community spirit and improve the nutrition of those attending. By providing keep-fit classes and lectures on health education the physical and mental health of the elderly are improved. Until some form of notification of old people living alone is introduced, clubs and day centres provide a most valuable way of finding out about the elderly in a local community. Once a person has joined a club his name appears on the club register, and if he is not attending then a member of the club on the home visiting committee can pay a call at his home and find out what is happening. By this means many an ill and isolated old person can be brought to the notice of the relevant authorities and appropriate action taken.

In many districts older people especially those living alone are supplied with communicators, e.g. pendants with a red button. When the button is pressed a central receiving unit presents on a screen the elderly person's name and address and other relevant information, e.g. the name of the individual's own doctor and nearest relative. Depending on the system a mobile warden in a specially equipped car may proceed to the house or one of three named relatives or friends may be informed of the need for assistance.

Department of health and social security

A pension can be provided from this service for old people who have not paid the necessary contributions to enable them to draw a retirement pension. Other grants previously awarded have been withdrawn under new legislation and explanatory documents are expected soon. Advice should be obtained from the social service department in any case where there is the slightest suggestion of hardship due to insufficient income.

Many and varied are the services available for old people and as our welfare and hospital services mature more flexibility, more freedom of choice and more co-ordination will be achieved.

Some helpful booklets include the *Supplementary Benefits Handbook* obtainable from HM Stationery Office or booksellers, while Age Concern publish a pamphlet *Your Rights* which gives clear guidance. *Caring with Confidence* (1979), a booklet published by the Scottish Health Education Unit is a most useful guide for those caring for the elderly and more recently for the elderly in co-operation with Help the Aged a manual entitled *Take Care of Yourself* (1988) has been produced.

REFERENCES

Caring with Confidence (1979) Edinburgh, The Scottish Health Education Unit.

Hildick-Smith Marion (1981) The future of day hospitals. In *Advanced Geriatric Medicine*, (Eds. Caird F.I. & Evans J.), Vol. 1. London, Pitman Books.

Hildick-Smith Marion (1984) Geriatric day hospitals – changing emphasis in costs. *Age and Ageing* **13,** 95.

Home Made Aids for Handicapped People (1974) London, The British Red Cross Society.

Horrocks P. (1986) The components of a comprehensive district health service for elderly people – a personal view. *Age and Ageing* **15,** 321.

Modern British Geriatric Care (1970) Supplement to *Hospital Management*, September/October. London, Whitehall Press.

Nichols P. (1981) *Disabled*. Newton Abbot, David & Charles.

Skeet Muriel (1982) *The Third Age*. London, Darton, Longman & Todd Ltd.

Take Care of Yourself (1988) London, Help the Aged.

Tarling Christine (1980) *Hoists and their Use*. London, Disabled Living Foundation by William Heinemann Medical.

Your Rights (1983) Mitcham, Age Concern England.

de Zoysa A.S. R. & Blessed G. (1984) The place of the specialist home for the elderly mentally infirm in the care of mentally disturbed old people. *Age and Ageing* **13,** 218.

Appendix II
Training of Physicians in Geriatric Medicine

The specialty

Geriatric medicine has been regarded as that branch of medicine which deals with the clinical, psychological, rehabilitative and social problems of the elderly. In 1881 Charcot had written his lectures on diseases of old age and chronic sickness and he stated 'The importance of a special study of the diseases of old age would not be contested at the present day' and that 'This very interesting part of medicine has been long neglected and hardly in our own days has it succeeded in gaining its independence'. Geriatric medicine was not established as a specialty in the United Kingdom until the 1940s. An early pioneer in the field, Marjory Warren stated that 'There is much to recommend geriatrics as a specialty, comparable to paediatrics. The creation of such a specialty would stimulate those with a leaning to this type of work and raise the standard of the work done.' (Warren 1946). Throughout the 1960s and 70s the specialty developed as an academic subject and by 1986, 16 of the 27 British clinical medical schools had university departments of geriatric medicine and there were 650 consultants practising the specialty in the United Kingdom.

The geriatrician

The specialist geriatrician in addition to having the qualities of the general physician should have a certain facility in weighing up physical, mental and domestic factors relating to elderly patients and should assess from these when an attempt to restore activity is on and when it is not (Adams 1964). The doctor in geriatric medical practice encounters most of the diseases met by the general internal physician but he has to use rehabilitative techniques and co-ordinate health and social services for the elderly in the community and in continuing care institutions. The most frequent reasons given by newly appointed consultants for a career choice of geriatric medicine include a preference for working with a wide range of medical problems, good career prospects and an opportunity for involvement in multidisciplinary teamwork (Barker & Williamson 1986).

355

Training requirements

The medical student should have some training in geriatric medicine during his undergraduate course and he should have a grasp of the core knowledge of the specialty (Table II.1).

Table II.1 Educational objectives for medical undergraduates.

Ageing
Demographic changes
Attitudes to old age
Presentation of disease in old age
Management of illness in the elderly

In the United Kingdom the newly qualified doctor must be employed in approved pre-registration posts for a period of 1 year. The aspiring specialist will then undergo periods of general professional training followed by higher specialist training (Joint Committee on Higher Medical Training 1987).

General professional training will normally be the same as for general internal medicine and will include 3 years of post-registration experience in the hospital service. This period should be used to obtain wide experience in general internal medicine and associated specialties. The trainee might spend a period of time in an active geriatric medical service to find out if he or she likes caring for elderly sick people. The training requirements for a consultant in geriatric medicine or a specialist general physician with an interest in geriatric medicine include the need to obtain the Membership of the Royal Colleges of Physicians of the United Kingdom, MRCP (UK), or its equivalent.

Higher specialist training usually covers a 4-year period in approved training posts. The trainee is usually a senior registrar and should gain experience, in departments of geriatric medicine, of the clinical care of elderly patients in a variety of settings. Training in the administrative aspects of geriatric medicine is required and experience in the psychiatry of old age is especially desirable (Table II.2).

The trainee may aspire to one of two types of career posts:
Consultant physician in geriatric medicine (for those who wish to practise in the specialty; 85% of consultant posts in geriatric medicine in the United Kingdom). Within the 4-year approved geriatric medical training programme, periods totalling not more than 2 years may be spent gaining experience in other medical specialties, for example general internal medicine, community medicine, rheumatology, rehabilitation medicine or in relevant medical research.

Consultant general physician with special responsibility for the elderly (15% of consultant posts in the United Kingdom). Within the 4-year period of higher specialist training, normally 2 years will be spent in posts approved for training in geriatric medicine and 2 years in posts approved for training in general internal medicine. This training may include rotation to other specialties, for example cardiology, neurology or rheumatology. Trainees are normally accredited in both specialties.

Table II.2 Elements of specialist training in geriatric medicine.

Acute assessment
Rehabilitation
Continuing care
Day hospital care
Home visits
Administration of a geriatric service
Hospital consultations – other services
Research methods
Teaching others
Psychiatry of old age

REFERENCES

Adams G.F. (1964) Clinical undertaking. *Lancet* **1**, 1055.
Barker W.H. & Williamson J. (1986) Survey of recently appointed consultants in geriatric medicine. *British Medical Journal* **293**, 896.
Charcot J.M. (1881) *Clinical Lectures on Senile and Chronic Diseases*. London, The New Sydenham Society.
Joint Committee on Higher Medical Training (1987) *Training Handbook*. Royal College of Physicians of London.
Warren M.W. (1946) Care of the chronic aged sick. *Lancet* **1**, 841.

Appendix III
Useful Addresses

Abbeyfield Society
186–192 Darkes Lane,
Potter's Bar,
Hertfordshire EN6 1AB.

Age Concern, England
Bernard Sunley House,
60 Pitcairn Road, Mitcham,
Surrey CR4 3LL.

Age Concern, Northern Ireland
128 Great Victoria Street,
Belfast BT2 7BG.

Age Concern, Scotland
33 Castle Street,
Edinburgh EH2 3DN.

Age Concern, Wales
1 Park Grove, Cardiff CF1 3BJ.

Age Research
49 Queen Victoria Street,
London EC4N 4SA.

Alzheimer's Disease Society
Bank Building,
Fulham Broadway,
London SW6 1EP.

Alzheimer's Disease Society
40 Shandwick Place,
Edinburgh EH2 4RT.

Arthritis Care
6 Grosvenor Crescent,
London SW1 7ER.

Association of Carers
21–23 New Road,
Chatham, Kent ME4 4QJ.

BASE
(British Association for Service
    to the Elderly)
Lloyd Girling,
19 Hillpark Drive,
Birkhill, Dundee DD2 5QZ.

British Association for the Hard
    of Hearing
16 Park Street, Windsor,
Berks SL4 1LU.

British Deaf Association
36 Victoria Place, Carlisle,
Cumbria CA1 1EX.

British Diabetic Association
10 Queen Anne Street,
London W1M OBD.

British Geriatrics Society,
1 St Andrew's Place,
Regent's Park,
London NW1 4LB.

British Red Cross
9 Grosvenor Crescent,
London SW1X 7EJ.

British Red Cross
204 Bath Street,
Glasgow G2 4HL.

British Telephones for the Blind
Fund
Mynhurst Leigh, Near Reigate,
Surrey.

British Wireless for the Blind
Fund
226 Great Portland Street,
London W1N 6AA.

Cancer Aftercare and
Rehabilitation Society
Lodge Cottage, Church Lane,
Timsbury, Bath, Avon.

Carter's (J and A) Ltd
Alfred Street, Westbury,
Wilts BA13 3DZ.

Central Register of Charities
(Charity Commission)
St Albans House,
57 Haymarket,
London SW27 4PZ.

Centre for Policy on Ageing
Nuffield Lodge, Regent's Park,
London NW1 4RS.

Chest, Heart and Stroke
Association
Tavistock House North,
Tavistock Square,
London WC1L 9LE.

Clos-o-mat (GB) Ltd
2 Brooklands Road,
Sale, Cheshire.

Counsel and Care for the
Elderly
131 Middlesex Street,
London E1 7JF.

Crossroads Care Attendant
Scheme Trust
94 Cotton Road, Rugby,
Warwickshire CV21 4LN.

Crossroads Care Attendant
Scheme
Scottish Headquarters
24 George Street
Glasgow G2 1EG.

Cruse
126 Sheen Road, Richmond,
Surrey.

Department of Health and
Social Security
Disablement Services Branch,
3 Government Buildings
Warbreck Hill Road, Blackpool,
Lancs.

The Disabled Living Foundation
380–384 Harrow Road,
London W9 2HU.

Downs Surgical Ltd
Church Path, Mitcham,
Surrey.

Extend
(Exercise and Training for the
  Elderly and Disabled)
Mrs Penny Copple
The Boulevard, Sheringham,
Norfolk NR26 8LJ.

Health Education Authority
PO Box 413,
London SE99 67E.

Health Education Council
78 New Oxford Street,
London WC1A 1AH.

Hearing Aid Council
40a Ludgate Hill,
London EC4 7DE.

Help the Aged
16–18 St James' Walk,
London EC1R OBE.

International Glaucoma
  Association
King's College Hospital,
Denmark Hill,
London SE5 9RS.

John Bell and Croyden
50 Wigmore Street, London W1.

Kanga Hospital Products
PO Box 39, Bentinck Street,
Bolton.

Kylie Advisory Service
  (absorbent bed sheets)
Nicholas Laboratories,
225 Bath Road,
Slough SL1 4AV.

Loxley Medical Supplies Ltd
Bessingby Industrial Estate,
Bridlington, North Humberside.

Marie Curie Memorial
  Foundation,
28 Belgrave Square,
London SW1X 8QG.

Mecanaids Ltd
St Catherine Street, Gloucester.

Mental After Care Association
Eagle House, 110 Jermyn Street,
London SW1Y 6HB.

Mental Health Foundation
8 Hallam Street,
London W1N 6BH.

MIND (The National
  Association for Mental Health)
22 Harley Street,
London W1N 2ED.

National Benevolent Fund for
  the Aged
New Broad Street House,
35 New Broad Street,
London EC2M 1NH.

National Council for Carers and
  their Elderly Dependants
(exists to help those who have
  or have had the care of elderly
  or infirm relatives)
29 Chilworth Mews,
London W2 3RG.

National Council for Voluntary
  Organizations
26 Bedford Square,
London WC1B 3HU.

National Federation of Housing
  Associations
30–32 Southampton Street,
London WC2E 7HE.

National Society for Cancer
  Relief
Room 128 Anchor House,
15–19 Britten Street,
London SW3 3TZ.

Nuffield Nursing Homes Trust
71–91 Aldwych,
London NW1 4RS.

Parkinson's Disease Society
36 Portland Place,
London W1N 3DG.

Pre-Retirement Association
19 Undine Street,
London SW17 8PP.

Royal Association for Disability
  and Rehabilitation
25 Mortimer Street,
London W1N 8AB.

Royal Medical Benevolent Fund
24 King's Road, Wimbledon,
London SW19.

Royal National Institute for
  the Blind
224 Great Portland Street,
London W1N 6AA.

Royal National Institute for
  the Deaf
105 Gower Street,
London WC1E 6AH.

Royal Society for the Prevention
  of Accidents
Cannon House, The Priory,
Queensway,
Birmingham B4 6BS.

Scottish Council on Disability
Princes House,
5 Shandwick Place,
Edinburgh EH2 4RG.

Scottish Health Education
  Group
Health Education Centre,
Woodburn House,
Canaan Lane,
Edinburgh EH10 4SG.

Scottish Retirement Council
212 Bath Street,
Glasgow G2 4HW.

Scottish Trust for the Physically
  Disabled
Pritchard House,
32 Inglis Green Road,
Edinburgh EH14 2ER.

Smith and Nephews
  (Southalls) Ltd
Alum Rock Road, Birmingham.

Charles F. Thackray Ltd
Viaduct Road, Leeds.

Ulverscroft Large Print Books
The Green, Bradgate Road,
Anstey, Leics. LE7 7FU.

Vernon Carus Ltd
Penwortham Mills, Preston,
Lancashire.

Wireless for the Bedridden
20 Wimpole Street,
London W1M 8BQ.

Women's Royal Voluntary
   Service
234–244 Stockwell Road,
London SW9 9ST.

Workers Education Association
Temple House, 8 Berkley Street,
London W1 8BY.

Appendix IV
American Drugs Equivalent to those Mentioned in Text

| Approved name | Proprietary names | |
	UK	USA
Acetazolamide	Diamox	Diamox
Acyclovir	Zovirax	Zovirax
Allopurinol	Xyloric	Zyloprim
Amantadine	Symmetrel	Symmetrel
Amiloride	Midamor	Colectril
Aminophylline	Theodrox	Lixaminol
Amitriptyline	Tryptizol	Elavil
Amoxycillin	Amoxil	Amoxil
(USA: Amoxicillin)		
Amphotericin	Fungilin, Fungizone	Fungizone
Ampicillin	Penbritin	Penbritin
Atenolol	Tenormin	Tenormin
Azathioprine	Imuran	Imuran
Bendrofluazide	Aprinox	Benuron
(USA: Bendroflumethazide)		
Benzhexol	Artane	Artane
(USA: Trihexyphenidyl)		
Bethanidine	Esbatal	Esbatal
Bisacodyl	Dulcolax	Dulcolax
Bromocriptine	Parlodel	Parlodel
Bumetanide	Burinex	Bumex
Busulphan	Myeleran	Myeleran
Calcitonin	Calcitare,Calsynar	Calcimar
Captopril	Capoten	Capoten
Carbachol	–	Carcholin
Carbamazepine	Tegretol	Tegretol
Carbimazole	Neomercazole	Neomercazole
Cephalexin	Ceporex	Keflex
Chenodeoxycholic acid	Chendol, Chenofalk	Chenix
Chlorambucil	Leukeran	Leukeran
Chloramphenicol	Chloromycetin	Chloromycetin
Chlordiazepoxide	Librium	Librium
Chlormethiazole	Heminevrin	Heminevrin
Chloroquine	Aralis, Nivaquine	Aralen
Chlorpromazine	Largactil	Thorazine
Chlorpropamide	Diabinase	Diabinase
Cimetidine	Tagamet	Tagamet
Clofibrate	Atromid-S	Atromid-S
Clonazepam	Rivotril	Clonopin
Cloxacillin	Orbenin	Cloxapen
Co-trimoxazole	Septrin, Bactrim	Septra, Bactrim

Approved name	Proprietary names UK	USA
Cyclophosphamide	Endoxana	Cytoxan
Deglycyrrhizinised Liquorice	Caved-S	Ulcedal
Dexamethasone	Decadron	Decadron
Diazepam	Valium	Valium
Diflunisal	Dolobid	Dolobid
Digoxin	Lanoxin	Lanoxin
Dihydroergotamine Mesylate	Hydergine	Hydergine
Disopyramide	Norpace, Rhythmodan	Norpace
Doxapram	Dopram	Dopram
Droperidol	Droleptan	Inapsine
Enalapril	Innovace	Vasotec
Erythromycin	Erythrocin	Emycin
Ethambutol	Myambutol	Myambutol
Ferrous Gluconate	Fergon	Fergon
Ferrous Sulphate	Feospan	Feosol
Fludrocortisone	Florinef	Florinef
Flurbiprofen	Froben	Froben
Fluphenazine Decanoate	Modecate	Prolixin Decanoate
Fosfesterol	Honvan	Stilphostrol
Frusemide (USA: Furosemide)	Lasix	Lasix
Gentamicin	Genticin	Garamycin
Glyceryl Trinitrate (USA: Nitroglycerin)	Trinitrin	Nitrol
Haloperidol	Serenace	Haldol
Heparin	Pularin	Hepathrom
Hydrallazine (USA: Hydralazine)	Apresoline	Apresoline
Hydroxocobalamin	Neocytamen	Alpharedisol
Hydroxychloroquine	Plaquenil	Plaquenil
Hydroxyurea	Hydrea	Hydrea
Ibuprofen	Brufen, Fenbid	Motrin, Rufen
Imipramine	Tofranil	Tofranil
Indomethacin	Indocid	Indocid
Iron-Dextran	Imferon	Imferon
Iron-Sorbitol-Citric Acid	Jectofer	Astrafer
Isoniazid	Rimifon	Nydrazid
Isoprenaline (USA: Isoproterenol)	Saventrine	Isuprel
Isosorbide Dinitrate	Isordil	Isordil
Ketoconazole	Nizoral	Nizoral
Levodopa	Brocadopa, Larodopa	Dopar, Larodopa
Lignocaine (USA: Lidocaine)	Xylocaine	Xylocaine
Melphalan	Alkeran	Alkeran
Methadone	Physeptone	Dolophine
Methicillin	Celbenin	Celbenin
Methotrexate	Maxtrex	Folex, Mexate
Methyldopa	Aldomet	Aldomet
Methylphenidate	Ritalin	Ritalin
Methyltestosterone	Perandren	Metandren

Approved name	Proprietary names	
	UK	USA
Metoclopramide	Maxolon	Regulan
Metoprolol	Betaloc, Lopresor	Lopressor
Miconazole	Daktarin	Micatin
Minoxidil	Loniten	Loniten
Nalidixic Acid	Negram	Negram
Naproxen	Naprosyn	Naprosyn
Neomycin	Neomin	Mycifradin
Nifedipine	Adalat	Procardia
Nitrofurantoin	Furadantin	Furadantin
Norethandrolone	Nilevar	Nilevar
Nystatin	Nystan	Mycostatin
Orciprenaline	Alupent	Alupent
Orphenadrine	Disipal	Disipal
Oxymetholone	Anapolon	Adroyd
Paracetamol	Panadol	Tempra
(USA: Acetaminophen)		
Penicillamine	Distamine, Pendramine	Cuprimine, Depen
Pethidine	–	Dolantin
(USA: Meperidine)		
Phenoxybenzamine	Dibenyline	Dibenzyline
Phenylbutazone	Butazolidin	Butazolidin
Phenytoin	Epanutin	Dilantin
Pholcodine Linctus	Ethnine	Ethnine
Piroxicam	Feldene	Feldene
Prazosin	Hypovase	Minipress
Prednisolone	Deltacortril	Deltasone
Primidone	Mysoline	Mysoline
Probenecid	Benemid	Benemid
Promethazine	Phenergan	Phenergan
Propantheline	Pro-Banthine	Probanthine
Propranolol	Inderal	Inderal
Quinestradol	Pentovis	Estrovis
Ranitidine	Zantac	Zantac
Rifampicin	Rimactane, Rifadin	Rimactane, Rifadin
(USA: Rifampin)		
Salbutamol	Ventolin	Ventolin
Sodium Cromoglycate	Intal	Intal
Sodium Etidronate	Didronel	Didronel
Spironolactone	Aldactone	Aldactone
Streptokinase	Kabikinase, Streptase	Kabikinase, Streptase
Sulindac	Clinoril	Clinoril
Sulphasalazine	Salazopyrin	Azulfidine
(USA: Sulfasalazine)		
Temazepam	Normison, Euhypnos	Cerepax
Terbutaline	Bricanyl	Bricanyl
Thioridazine	Melleril	Mellaril
Thyroxine	Eltroxin	Synthyroid
Tolbutamide	Rastinon	Orinase
Triamterene	Dytac	Dyrenium
Warfarin	Marevan	Coumadin

Index